REGENERATIVE PHARMACOLOGY

Regenerative medicine is broadly defined as the repair or replacement of damaged cells, tissues, and organs. It is a multidisciplinary effort in which technologies derive from the fields of cell, developmental, and molecular biology; chemical and material sciences (i.e., nanotechnology); engineering; surgery; transplantation; immunology; molecular genetics; physiology; and pharmacology. As regenerative medicine technologies continue to evolve and expand across the boundaries of numerous scientific disciplines, they remain at the forefront of the translational research frontier with the potential to radically alter the treatment of a wide variety of disease and dysfunction. The goal of this book is to draw attention to the critical role that the pharmacological sciences will undeniably play in the advancement of these treatments. This book is invaluable for advanced students, postdoctoral Fellows, researchers new to the field of regenerative medicine and its companion field, tissue engineering, as well as experienced investigators looking for new research avenues. This is the first state-of-the-art book in this rapidly evolving field of research.

GEORGE J. CHRIST is Professor of Regenerative Medicine and Translational Science and head of the Program in Cell, Tissue and Organ Physiology at the Wake Forest Institute for Regenerative Medicine. He is an affiliate faculty in the Molecular Medicine and Molecular Genetics Programs, as well as the Virginia Tech–Wake Forest University School for Biomedical Engineering and Sciences. He also holds appointments in the Departments of Urology and Physiology and Pharmacology and the Sticht Center for Aging. He is the former director and founder of the Institute for Smooth Muscle Biology at the Albert Einstein College of Medicine. Dr. Christ is an internationally recognized expert in muscle physiology. He is the past chairman of the Division of Systems and Integrative Pharmacology of the American Society of Pharmacology and Experimental Therapeutics (ASPET) and past president of the North Carolina Tissue Engineering and Regenerative Medicine Society. He currently serves on the Executive Committee of the Division for Integrative Systems, Translational and Clinical Pharmacology of ASPET. He is on the editorial board of five journals and has authored more than 200 scientific publications. Dr. Christ has served on both national and international committees related to his expertise and has also served on NIH study sections in the NIDDK, NICHD, NCRR, and NHLBI. He has chaired working groups for both the NIH and the World Health Organization. Dr. Christ is a co-inventor on more than 24 patents (national and international), which are either issued or pending, related to gene therapy for the treatment of human smooth muscle disorders and tissue engineering technologies. He is a co-founder and directing member of Ion Channel Innovations, LLC, a development-stage biotechnology company pioneering the use of gene therapy for the treatment of human smooth muscle disorders. In addition, he is a co-founder and board member of Creative Bioreactor Design, Inc., another early-stage biotechnology company in the expanding field of regenerative medicine and tissue engineering.

KARL-ERIK ANDERSSON, MD, PhD, is Professor of Regenerative Medicine and Urology at Wake Forest Institute for Regenerative Medicine. He also holds appointments in the Departments of Physiology and Pharmacology and Molecular Medicine at Wake Forest University School of Medicine. He has Swedish Specialist Degrees in internal medicine and clinical pharmacology and a PhD in pharmacology from the University of Lund, Sweden. From 1978 to 2006, he was Professor and Chairman of the Department of Experimental and Clinical Pharmacology, University of Lund, and from 1993 to 2000, he was Vice Dean of the Medical Faculty at the University of Lund. Dr. Andersson has received several awards, including a Lifetime Achievement Award from the Society for Urodynamics and Female Urology. Dr. Andersson is a member of many international societies, including the American Urological Association, the European Association of Urology, and the International Society for Sexual Medicine. He has served on both national and international committees related to his expertise in basic and clinical physiology and pharmacology and has also served on NIH study sections in the NIDDK. He has chaired working groups for the International Consultation of Urogenital Diseases, supported by the World Health Organization. He also serves on the editorial boards of several journals, including the *Journal of Urology* (section editor), *Neurourology and Urodynamics* (associate editor), *and European Urology*, and is editor-in-chief of the *Urotoday International Journal*. Dr. Andersson has authored more than 800 articles in peer-reviewed international journals. His current research interests include clinical and basic physiology and pharmacology of the urogenital tract and regenerative medicine.

This book is dedicated to our parents, families, mentors, students, and colleagues.

Contents

Color plates appear after page 234

Contributors

Karl-Erik Andersson, MD, PhD
Professor
Wake Forest Institute for Regenerative Medicine
Wake Forest School of Medicine
Winston-Salem, NC

Anthony Atala, MD
Chair, Department of Urology
Director, Wake Forest Institute for Regenerative Medicine
Wake Forest School of Medicine
Winston-Salem, NC

Atta Behfar, MD, PhD
Assistant Professor
Marriott Heart Disease Research Program
Division of Cardiovascular Diseases
Mayo Clinic
Rochester, MN

Timothy A. Bertram, DVM, PhD
President, Research & Development
Chief Science Officer
Tengion, Inc.
Winston-Salem, NC

Stefanie Biechler, PhD
Biomedical Engineering Program
University of South Carolina School of Medicine
Columbia, SC

Peter R. Brink, PhD
Professor and Chair, Department of Physiology and Biophysics
Institute for Molecular Cardiology
Stony Brook University
Stony Brook, NY

David Burmeister, PhD
Postdoctoral Fellow
Wake Forest Institute for Regenerative Medicine
Wake Forest School of Medicine
Winston-Salem, NC

Martin K. Childers, DO, PhD
Professor
Department of Rehabilitation Medicine
Institute for Stem Cell and Regenerative Medicine
University of Washington
Seattle, WA

George J. Christ, PhD
Professor
Wake Forest Institute for Regenerative Medicine
Wake Forest School of Medicine
Winston-Salem, NC

Ira S. Cohen, MD, PhD
Professor, Department of Physiology and Biophysics
Director, Institute for Molecular Cardiology
Stony Brook University
Stony Brook, NY

Stephen A. Fann, MD
Associate Professor
Department of Surgery
Medical University of South Carolina
Charleston, SC

Harold I. Friedman, MD
Professor and Chief
Department of Surgery, Division of Plastic Surgery
University of South Carolina School of Medicine
Columbia, SC

Mark E. Furth, PhD
Chief Technology Officer
Comprehensive Cancer Center
Wake Forest School of Medicine
Winston-Salem, NC

Peter A. Galie
Graduate Research Assistant
Department of Biomedical Engineering
University of Michigan
Ann Arbor, MI

Gautam S. Ghatnekar, DVM, PhD
CEO and President
FirstString Research Inc.
Charleston, SC

Richard L. Goodwin, PhD
Associate Professor
Department of Cell Biology and Anatomy
University of South Carolina School of Medicine
Columbia, SC

Robert G. Gourdie, PhD, FAHA
Professor and Center Director
Virginia Tech Carilion Research Institute and
Virginia Tech–Wake Forest University School of Biomedical Engineering
   and Sciences
Roanoke, VA

Roche de Guzman, PhD
Postdoctoral Fellow
Virginia Tech–Wake Forest University School of Biomedical Engineering
   and Sciences
Virginia Polytechnic Institute and State University
Blacksburg, VA

Benjamin S. Harrison, PhD
Associate Professor
Wake Forest Institute for Regenerative Medicine
Wake Forest University Health Sciences
Winston-Salem, NC

Johnny Huard, PhD
Stem Cell Research Center
Department of Orthopedic Surgery
Department of Bioengineering
McGowan Institute of Regenerative Medicine
University of Pittsburgh
Pittsburgh, PA

Emily Ongstad, MS
Graduate Student
Clemson University–Medical University of South Carolina
    Bioengineering Program
Virginia Tech Carilion Research Institute
Charleston, SC

Jay D. Potts, PhD
Associate Professor
Department of Cell Biology and Anatomy
University of South Carolina School of Medicine
Columbia, SC

Lola M. Reid, PhD
Professor
Department of Cell and Molecular Physiology
    and Program in Molecular Biology and Biotechnology
University of North Carolina at Chapel Hill
Chapel Hill, NC

Justin M. Saul, PhD
Associate Professor
Department of Chemical and Paper Engineering
School of Applied Engineering and Science
Miami University
Oxford, OH

G. Sitta Sittampalam, PhD
National Center for Advancing Translational Sciences
National Institutes of Health
Therapeutics for Rare and Neglected Diseases
Rockville, MD

Bert Spilker, PhD, MD
Pharmaceutical Consultant
Bethesda, MD

Jan P. Stegemann, PhD
Associate Professor
Department of Biomedical Engineering
University of Michigan
Ann Arbor, MI

Andre Terzic, MD, PhD
Professor
Marriott Heart Disease Research Program
Division of Cardiovascular Diseases
Mayo Clinic
Rochester, MN

Panagiotis A. Tsonis, PhD
Professor, Department of Biology
Director, Center for Tissue Regeneration and Engineering at Dayton
University of Dayton
Dayton, OH

Virginijus Valiunas, PhD
Research Associate Professor
Department of Physiology and Biophysics
Institute for Molecular Cardiology
Stony Brook University
Stony Brook, NY

Mark Van Dyke, PhD
Associate Professor
Virginia Tech–Wake Forest University School of Biomedical Engineering
  and Sciences
Virginia Polytechnic Institute and State University
Blacksburg, VA

J. B. Vella, MD, PhD
Stem Cell Research Center
Department of Orthopedic Surgery
Department of Bioengineering
University of Pittsburgh
Pittsburgh, PA

M. Natalia Vergara, PhD
Postdoctoral Fellow
Wilmer Eye Institute
Department of Ophthalmology
Johns Hopkins University, School of Medicine
Baltimore, MD

Belinda J. Wagner, PhD
President
Biographic Design Consulting
Winston-Salem, NC

J. Koudy Williams, DVM
Professor
Wake Forest Institute for Regenerative Medicine
Wake Forest School of Medicine
Winston-Salem, NC

James Yoo, MD, PhD
Professor and Chief Scientific Officer
Wake Forest Institute for Regenerative Medicine
Wake Forest School of Medicine
Winston-Salem, NC

Michael J. Yost, PhD
Associate Professor
Department of Surgery
Medical University of South Carolina
Charleston, SC

Foreword

Regenerative pharmacology is poised to revolutionize human treatment options in medicine and define a new medical frontier. Prepared minds have recognized the convergence of discoveries in pharmacology, molecular biology, and genetics with those of nanotechnology, advanced analytical techniques, and biomaterials resulting in the ability to initiate differentiation and regeneration of cells, tissues, and organs.

Dating back thousands of years, ancient civilizations documented how they imagined being able to regenerate limbs lost in battle or trauma. For centuries, the regenerative characteristics of salamanders, chicks, and other animals were known but it was only within the past four decades that scientists began to mobilize the integrative thinkers, resources, and enabling technologies to identify and address the reality of cellular differentiation. Understanding of hematopoietic stem cell differentiation led to the first life-saving regenerative intervention for bone-marrow transplantation in the mid 1970s and, over the next 15 years, scientists refined genetic engineering to succeed at more complicated hematopoietic cell interventions resulting in FDA-approved recombinant therapies to enhance regeneration of red blood cells and granulocytes. Yet, to take regenerative therapies to the next level, where pluripotent cells could be differentiated, de-differentiated, and reprogrammed, it meant that the nature of the regenerative biomedical research community itself needed to be remodeled.

Centers of Excellence in stem-cell and regenerative research were established and now serve as welcoming institutions where creative "new alloy" scientists, who possess a wide range of interdisciplinary expertise and skills in enabling technologies, can work toward a similar goal. These multidisciplinary scientists are funded to focus on teamwork and characterizing regenerative interventions that unite specific biology, physics, genetics, chemistry, and enabling technologies in a way that was only imagined in the past. Following his discoveries of alpha and beta adrenergic receptors in 1948, and therapeutic use of beta-blockers for the treatment of blood pressure and heart disease, Dr. Raymond P. Ahlquist remarked "... at this time being a pharmacologist is akin to being a physiologist with a screwdriver." Today, a regenerative pharmacologist must surely be equipped with a hardware store of tools.

The impending impact of regenerative therapeutic intervention cannot be overstated in considering improvements to quality of life and reductions in healthcare costs. In the near term, the pharmaceutical industry will seek the talent and technology to develop research and interventions requiring partnerships with the NIH and with the FDA for approvals. The negative long-term physical, emotional and financial impact of birth deformities, traumatic injury, and dismemberment will be mitigated with future regenerative therapies and definitive treatments for life-long illnesses like diabetes and cardiovascular disease will be part of our history. With the complexity of the human organism itself, interdisciplinary teams of biomedical scientists are now identifying and replicating the sequence and symphony of essential factors that initiate, modulate, differentiate, de-differentiate, and remodel cells and tissues for organ regeneration. Today, scientists are pharmacologically able to guide pluripotent cells to differentiate along predictable paths of development, producing various heart cells and valves, cardiac tissues, urinary bladders, and other tissues with histologically appropriate layers, differentiation, innervations, and functionally appropriate contractions.

Dr. George J. Christ and Dr. Karl-Erik Andersson are congratulated for an outstanding book, *Regenerative Pharmacology*, which should be required reading for all biomedical scientists, medical students, integrative pharmacologists/physiologists, and indeed contemporary healthcare practitioners, regardless of specialty. *Regenerative Pharmacology* is a premier foundational treatise that introduces the topic and complexities of regenerative medicine and specifically describes new major developments in regenerative therapies. The book captures the evolution of many proposed regenerative interventions and, in an unassuming manner, the authors communicate in conversational style, to deliver details of their work in extensively referenced chapters.

Regenerative Pharmacology is a milestone publication and a definitive reference work for truly state-of-the-art discussions on stem and progenitor cells, bioreactor technology, and wound healing. This reference provides for in-depth understandings of regeneration of cardiac, kidney, bladder, and muscle cells and tissues, as well as micro/nano technology for delivery of therapeutic agents, active factors embedded in biomaterials, enabling technologies, implanted materials, and tissue-engineered constructs.

Congratulations to the editors for compiling this work. Congratulations to the editors and chapter authors for sharing their world-level expertise and for the manner in which the fundamentals of their work are introduced in understandable terms and then built upon to state-of-the-art discussions and future directions. The authors are among the top experts in this new frontier of biomedical research and truly represent the "new alloy" scientists and pioneers who will shape our lives with their regenerative research and therapies of the future.

Dennis C. Marshall, RN, MS, PhD
Immediate Past Chairperson, Executive Member,
Division for Integrative System, Translational and
Clinical Pharmacology, American Society
for Pharmacology and Experimental Therapeutics and
Subcommittee for Clinical and Translational Research,
Federation of American Societies for
Experimental Biology and
Executive Director,
Medical Affairs Ferring Pharmaceuticals Inc.

Preface

The concept for this book, although based on years of prior research and learning, was definitively established several years ago when we coined the phrase "regenerative pharmacology," and moreover, wrote our first article introducing the topic and the potential implications for pharmacologists (Andersson & Christ, Mol. Int., 2007). Since that time, the field has truly exploded, although the underlying purpose for this first edited volume on the subject remains the same: namely, to get pharmacologists more involved in this field of research by exposing them to the tools, opportunities, challenges, and expertise that will be required to ensure awareness and galvanize involvement. In addition, we hope that the excellent material provided by the diversity of experts in this volume will spark new multidisciplinary conversations among all of the stakeholders. In our opinion, the field of regenerative medicine and its companion field, tissue engineering, would benefit significantly from the more rigorous application of pharmacological sciences. Specifically, despite enormous progress and promise, regenerative medicine and tissue engineering would still profit from a greater focus on the evaluation of functional outcomes and endpoints. In particular, a more extensive characterization of basic pharmacodynamics (excitation-contraction coupling mechanisms, rigorous analysis of concentration-response curve (CRC) data using standard pharmacological analyses/methods, estimation of receptor affinity, receptor subtypes, intrinsic activity, efficacy, potency, etc.) is required. In addition, we posit that greater emphasis on the pharmacology and physiology of various regenerative medicine and tissue engineering approaches is critical to increase understanding of tissue/organ regeneration and repair processes, as well as to enhance the rate of technology development and eventual clinical translation. In this volume we have brought together diverse fields of research, ranging from materials chemistry and functionalized biomaterials to stem cells, high-throughput drug screening and bioreactors for in vitro tissue engineering, as well as in vivo studies of wound healing and tissue and organ regeneration and repair. Again, we hope that the outcome will be recognition by all parties of the importance of the cross-fertilization of ideas and tighter integration of the pharmacological sciences into the regenerative medicine and tissue engineering translational research enterprise. In fact, the image on the cover of this book, a 3D torus, is a simile for the ultimate complexity (and beauty) of tissue and organ regeneration and repair, as well as their eventual manipulation by pharmacology. That is, once we understand the properties of the knot, we can use pharmacology to drive regenerative medicine and tissue engineering technologies toward the creation of very precisely regulated tissue and organ structures with the requisite functional characteristics. We envision this book as the first volume of a series that will grow in parallel with this exciting field of research, and moreover, describe the journey at various points along the path. We look forward to the enormous possibilities for improved human health that can result from further development of regenerative pharmacology, and remind the reader that this is only the beginning of a long voyage.

George J. Christ, PhD
Karl-Erik Andersson, MD, PhD
Winston-Salem, NC, USA

Acknowledgments

So many people have provided the inspiration and guidance required to complete this edited volume, which reflects many years of thought and preparation. We appreciate the understanding and encouragement of all our friends and family over the years. Above all, we would especially like to thank our most immediate families: Gina, Brandon, Jamie, Bryan, and Jake (George Christ); and Dagmar, Kristian, Mikael, and Karl (Karl-Erik Andersson), who paid the greatest price, but were always supportive and saw the greater good in this effort, while sharing love and laughs and many important moments throughout the years that led to the creation of this book. In addition, we would like to thank the folks at Cambridge University Press, especially Amanda O'Connor. Peggy Rote and her team at Aptara, Inc., also did an amazing job with the production of the book. Finally, we are grateful to Donna Tucker who helped organize and coordinate the final phase of copyediting and production among all of the authors and editors.

Section I

Basic Principles of Regenerative Pharmacology

Introduction to Regenerative Pharmacology: A Short Primer on the Role of Pharmacological Sciences in Regenerative Medicine

GEORGE J. CHRIST AND KARL-ERIK ANDERSSON

Regenerative medicine technologies continue to evolve and expand across the boundaries of numerous scientific disciplines, remaining at the forefront of the translational research frontier with the potential to radically alter the treatment of disease and dysfunction from a variety of causes. For the purposes of this book, regenerative medicine is broadly defined as the repair or replacement of damaged cells, tissues, and organs. This interdisciplinary effort includes, but is not necessarily limited to, the fields of cell, developmental, and molecular biology; chemical and material sciences (e.g., nanotechnology); engineering; surgery; transplantation; immunology; molecular genetics; physiology; and pharmacology. The goal of this book is to draw attention to the critical role that the pharmacological sciences will undeniably play in this process. In this regard, in 2007 [1], we defined "regenerative pharmacology" as "the application of the pharmacological sciences to accelerate, optimize and characterize (either in vitro or in vivo), the development, maturation and function of bioengineered and regenerating tissues" and posited that it would be of widespread utility to the sustained growth, expansion, and translation of regenerative medicine technologies. Since that publication, there has been a robust expansion of pharmacological approaches and applications to regenerative medicine. Many aspects of that growth are captured in the chapters included in this volume.

When viewed from a broader context, the timing of the regenerative pharmacology effort is auspicious and could leverage ongoing national efforts. One example is the creation of the Armed Forces Institute of Regenerative Medicine (AFIRM; http://www.afirm.mil). The AFIRM consists of two civilian research consortia working with the U.S. Army Institute of Surgical Research (USAISR) in Fort Sam Houston, Texas. Each consortium is a multi-institutional network, together comprising more than 30 academic and 15 for-profit members. Moreover, a national strategy for regenerative medicine has been outlined by the recently established Alliance for Regenerative Medicine (http://www.alliancerm.org/), a Washington, DC–based nonprofit organization. The mission of this organization is to educate key policy makers about the potential of regenerative medicine and furthermore to advocate for public policies that will create the favorable environments for funding, regulatory approval, and reimbursement strategies, among others, that will be required to move the field forward. In addition, the National Institutes of Health (NIH) has recently published a fact sheet on the past, present, and future of regenerative medicine research and clinical translation (http://report.nih.gov/NIHfactsheets/Pdfs/RegenerativeMedicine(NIBIB).pdf). More recently, the Regenerative Medicine Promotion Act of 2011 (HR 1862) was introduced in the House of Representatives in May. Finally, the NIH recently established a Center for Regenerative Medicine: crm.nih.gov. Clearly, these are very exciting times for expanding the role of pharmacologists and the science of pharmacology into the realm of regenerative medicine and tissue engineering.

Therefore, the explicit aim of this chapter is to provide a conceptual framework from which to view the potential impact of regenerative pharmacology on the wider fields of regenerative medicine and tissue engineering. When viewed in this context, there is an important distinction between regenerative pharmacology and the more traditional applications of the pharmacological sciences to the development of small molecules (<500 Da), delivered systemically, for the palliation and symptomatic treatment of human disease (see Chapter 9 for additional details). More specifically, regenerative pharmacology seeks not only to create a new generation of therapies for improved symptomatic treatment of disease (i.e., fewer side or off-target effects caused by improved mechanisms of action [MOAs], enhanced localization, and cellular and subcellular specificity), but rather to maximally leverage existing multidisciplinary expertise for the development of transformational curative therapies through implementation of the science of pharmacology in the domains of regenerative medicine and tissue engineering. The focus on curative pharmacological therapies represents a paradigm shift for this longstanding field of medical research that has already had an enormous worldwide impact on healthcare delivery.

Importantly, organ and tissue engineering and the application of regenerative medicine technologies to patients also have a long and distinguished history. The necessity for these technologies grows logically out of the shortage of donor organs for replacement and transplantation, as well as the need for reconstructive procedures in patients experiencing tissue loss as a result of trauma, disease, or other congenital or acquired conditions [2,3]. The historical details of the field are well beyond the scope of this chapter; therefore, interested readers are referred to several other excellent expert opinions, reports, and textbooks [4–8], as well as other chapters in this volume that review some of the key developments. Without question, though, regenerative medicine represents a continuously evolving interdisciplinary biotechnology enterprise with global roots. However, as recently pointed out by Ingber and Levin [9], interdisciplinary distinctions can become quite blurred when dealing with a subject as complex as tissue and organ regeneration and engineering. Nonetheless, this field of translational research offers tremendous potential to positively impact and

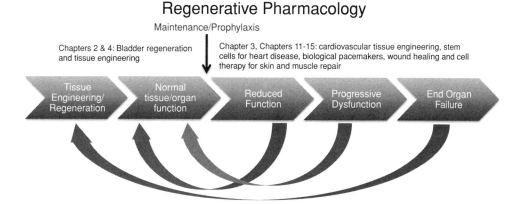

Figure 1-1. Schematic depiction of the utility of regenerative pharmacology to tissue engineering and regenerative medicine for the treatment of end-organ disease or failure. As illustrated, because of a variety of circumstances or causes, normal tissue or organ function can be compromised and transit through a series of stages starting with reduced function, eventually leading toward increasingly progressive dysfunction and finally end-organ failure. At each point along this path, demarcating the initiation and progression of tissue or organ dysfunction, regenerative strategies using or incorporating pharmacological strategies can be envisioned for restoration of function. However, at the point of end-organ failure, there is, by definition, not enough viable tissue remaining that any conventional gene- or drug-based strategy will be useful, and therefore, tissue engineering strategies would be required for whole organ replacement or alternatively, strategies for promoting endogenous organ regeneration. However, irrespective of the precise cause and degree of dysfunction, regenerative pharmacology provides an opportunity for restoration of normal organ and tissue function. Certainly, the exact strategies and technologies applied will depend on the magnitude and duration of dysfunction, as well as the organ or tissue of interest. The *arrow* denoting maintenance or prophylaxis indicates the possibility that after the process is sufficiently well understood, it might be possible to develop strategies for the maintenance of normal tissue or organ homeostasis or to slow the initiation and progression of tissue or organ dysfunction. Guidance concerning the relevance of each chapter to this overall scheme is provided. However, it is important to emphasize that the chapter denotations are the editors' (not the authors') and, moreover, are merely meant to reflect more general aspects of their relationship to the process being depicted. DDS = drug delivery system; HTS = high-throughput screening.

extend the useful lifespan of a seemingly ever-aging U.S. and world population, and the goal of this chapter (and book) is to begin to outline the numerous ways in which pharmacology can assume a primary role in this process.

The potential scope of regenerative pharmacology ranges from enhancing cellular therapy to optimizing bioengineered tissue and organ replacements to promoting endogenous tissue and organ repair. Figure 1-1 presents a conceptual framework for thinking about the application(s) of regenerative pharmacology during the initiation,

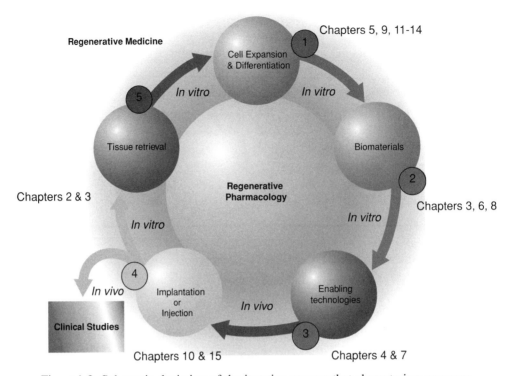

Figure 1-2. Schematic depiction of the iterative process that characterizes regenerative pharmacology. As illustrated, at all five steps along the path to clinical translation, regenerative pharmacology may be used to promote or direct the regenerative process as well as to report or dissect the impact of that process on established tissue or organ function(s). In this scenario, regenerative pharmacology is relevant to augmentation of cell expansion and differentiation (step 1) and furthermore can be combined with various nanotechnologies to create functionalized biomaterials or drug delivery systems (steps 2 and 3) as well as bioreactor technologies (step 3; note that a host of other enabling technologies, including but not limited to organ or tissue printing, vascularization, and innervation strategies might also be required) to further facilitate the tissue engineering or regenerative process before implantation (step 4) and tissue retrieval (step 5; preclinical analysis). Although one cannot rule out the possibility that at some point in the future technologies might exist to recapitulate embryonic development in adults in vivo (e.g., blastema formation, as described in Chapter 15), at the present level of technological development, this seems a reasonable research strategy for improved treatment of a variety of human diseases and dysfunctions. Regardless of the particular strategy used, regenerative pharmacology would play an important role in further augmenting or accelerating organ or tissue development at all five steps in the process. Again, an attempt has been made by the editors to position the main purpose of the various chapters in the context of the overall iterative regenerative pharmacology process. (Modified from Andersson and Christ [1].)

development, and progression of tissue or organ disease and dysfunction. Figure 1-2 provides a more comprehensive breakdown of the potential contribution of regenerative pharmacology to the each step in the iterative process that leads to advancement or creation of new regenerative medicine or tissue engineering technologies for the treatment of organ or tissue disease and dysfunction. For the convenience of readers, the editors have noted where the individual chapters in this volume primarily impact these overarching themes. The numerous excellent contributions in this volume cover virtually the entire spectrum of regenerative pharmacology as originally described [1], with a few notable exceptions, which are described briefly in this chapter.

As illustrated, regenerative pharmacology can be used to both dissect and direct the regenerative process, and examples of this are provided in the chapters in this volume. In the former role (i.e., dissect) regenerative pharmacology is clearly more akin to "classical" pharmacology (see Chapters 2 and 3), but the latter role, that is, using pharmacological technologies to direct the development and regeneration of engineered and endogenous organs in vitro and in vivo, is clearly a more novel area of investigation, and thus, the vast majority of chapters in this volume are devoted to further exploration of this concept (see Chapters 4 to 15). Recent work from our group provides examples of how regenerative pharmacology can be used to dissect pertinent characteristics of regenerating and engineered organ and tissues in vitro and in vivo. For example, these studies have shown the utility of this approach in investigating de novo bladder regeneration, which is discussed in detail in Chapter 2. In this chapter, we briefly describe other examples of regenerative pharmacology to the in vitro investigation of bioreactor-derived tissue-engineered blood vessels (TEBVs; [10]) as well as after retrieval of implanted bioengineered vessels [11] or tissue-engineered skeletal muscle repair [TEMR] constructs [12,13]. Both TEBV and TEMR constructs were created using in vitro bioreactor technologies. TEBVs are being developed for the repair and replacement of damaged and diseased blood vessels (e.g., coronary artery bypass, peripheral artery disease, and dialysis access grafts) and were used as an interposition graft in the carotid artery of a sheep model. The TEMR constructs are being developed for the treatment of volumetric muscle loss (VML) and the associated irrecoverable functional deficits produced by these injuries. VML injuries may be caused by trauma as well as a variety of congenital and acquired conditions. To assess the utility of tissue engineering approaches to the treatment of VML injuries, we have examined the ability of implanted TEMR constructs to repair surgically created VML injuries of the latissimus dorsi (LD) muscle in a murine model (see Figs. 1-3 and 1-4 for details).

Briefly, our experience with the TEBV and TEMR constructs reveals the importance of bioreactor preconditioning in vitro to tissue formation and function in vivo and points to the current limitations of in vitro tissue engineering. More specifically, in these two instances, currently available bioreactor technology and methods produce relatively immature bioengineered tissues in vitro, with respect to both their physiological characteristics and pharmacological responsiveness [10–13]. The most salient features of these published studies with respect to their implications for regenerative pharmacology are summarized in Figures 1-3 and 1-4. A key feature of regenerative pharmacology that is emphasized in Figure 1-2 is the importance of bioengineered

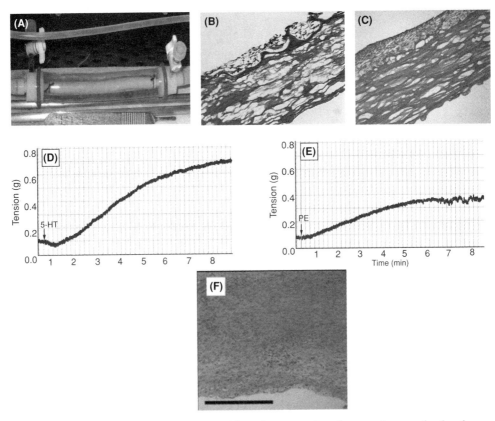

Figure 1-3. Illustration of the applicability of regenerative pharmacology to the development of tissue-engineered blood vessels (TEBVs). (**A**) Bioreactor flow system containing the scaffold seeded with endothelial cells (ECs) on the luminal side and with smooth muscle cells (SMCs) on the abluminal side. The bioreactor provides an external media bath, optical access, a bypass system, control over flow and pressure conditions, and the ability to maintain sterility. (**B**) Hematoxylin and eosin (H&E) stain of representative example of statically seeded SMCs on a decellularized construct after 48 hours and (**C**) after longer-term (3–4 weeks) bioreactor preconditioning. As shown, this period of bioreactor conditioning is sufficient to cause formation a substantive medial SMC layer. As noted by Yazdani et al. [10], Fura-2–based digital imaging microscopy experiments revealed no receptor mediated increases intracellular calcium levels. However, as indicated by the representative tracings shown in (**D**) and (**E**), retrieval of TEBV 4 months after implantation as a carotid artery interposition graft in sheep (Neff et al. [11]), revealed pharmacologically mediated contractile responses to 10 μM 5-Hydroxytryptamine (**D**) and 10 μM phenylephrine (**E**). *Arrows* indicate the application of agonists. (**F**) Representative H&E staining of a retrieved TEBV 4 months after implantation. Scale bar = 400 μM (Modified from Yazdani et al., 2009; Neff et al., 2011). (See color plate 1.)

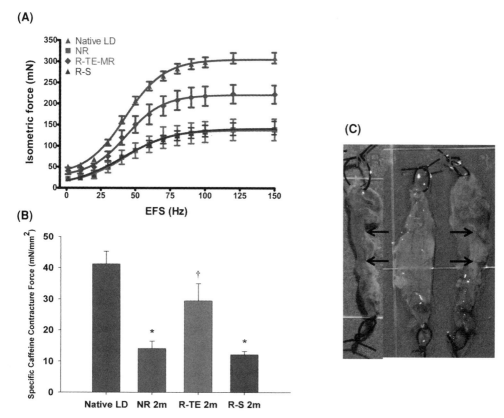

Figure 1-4. Morphologic assessment and functional recovery of retrieved tissues from the mouse volumetric muscle loss (VML) injury model. For these studies, bioengineered skeletal muscle implants were sutured into a surgically created VML injury by removal of approximately 50 percent of the murine latissimus dorsi (LD) muscle (see Machingal et al. [12] for details). (**A**) The mean values for the electrical field stimulation (EFS)–induced contractions observed on all retrieved tissues 2 months after injury or implantation. The sample sizes are native LD = 20, no repair (NR) (see C) = 5, repair with tissue-engineered muscle repair implantation (R-TE-MR) = 5, and R-S (repaired with a scaffold alone – no cells) = 5. The isometric absolute force (mN) is displayed as a function of stimulation frequency. Additionally, in (**B**) after force-frequency testing contralateral native LD muscles ($n = 6$), NR ($n = 4$), R-TE-MR ($n = 3$), or R-S ($n = 4$) at the 2-month time point were subjected to twitch contractions at 0.2 Hz in the presence of a maximally stimulating concentration of caffeine (50 mM). The *asterisk* denotes that group means are significantly different from that of control ($p < .05$). Values are means ± standard error of the mean. *Dagger* indicates that the group mean is significantly different from that of all other groups ($P < .05$). (**C**) shows representative examples of the gross morphology of retrieved LD tissues for an NR, native LD, and TEMR animal. *Arrows* indicate the original site of the surgical defect. Morphologic examination of tissue demonstrates robust tissue formation and remodeling of the TEMR construct but little or no tissue formation in the NR group. (Modified from Machingal et al. [12]). (See color plate 2.)

tissue characterization after implantation and retrieval (step 5 in the iterative process). As illustrated in Figures 1-3 and 1-4, after implantation in vivo, both TEBV and TEMR constructs produce new tissue formation and integration with host tissue, resulting in a dramatic increase in tissue physiology and pharmacological responsiveness to relevant stimuli. Nonetheless, and quite interestingly, despite quite remarkable functional recovery after implantation, both technologies reveal suboptimal physiological characteristics with respect to comparison with their native tissue counterparts. For example, the TEBVs in this study produce only approximately 20 to 30 percent of the contractile force of a native carotid artery to the same level of pharmacological stimulation. Although an improvement over prior work, which documented less than 10 percent functional recovery [14], there is clearly still room for improvement. In addition, although the TEMR-repaired LD muscles recover approximately 60 to 70 percent of native LD contractility to electrical field stimulation in the murine model, they still revealed evidence for altered excitation–contraction coupling; therefore, it appears that a component of the regenerating muscle may still be experiencing disruption in the EC coupling process, which would contribute to voltage-induced force deficits [15,16] (Fig. 1-4).

In short, with respect to both the TEBV and TEMR technologies, pharmacological studies have shed important mechanistic insight on the characteristics of the engineered and regenerating tissues (both in vitro and in vivo) that provide critical guidance for future technology developments. More data and additional pharmacological probes (with improved selectivity profiles) and bioactive agents would certainly aid in the continued development of regenerative pharmacology for vessel and muscle engineering. Of course, these represent just two examples, but they are further reinforced by the information contained in Chapters 2 and 3, which focus on the urinary bladder.

The applications of regenerative pharmacology continue with Chapter 4, which begins to examine the importance of matrix biology and mechanical forces on the differentiation of mesenchymal stem cells with specific emphasis on cardiovascular applications. Whereas Chapters 2 and 3 largely emphasize the utility of pharmacology to dissect aspects of the regeneration, this work highlights the ability of pharmacology to both dissect and direct regeneration. It is difficult to overestimate the value of this type of pharmacological data or information (to the nature of the regenerative process) and its importance to the improved understanding and clinical application of tissue engineering and regenerative medicine technologies.

Another major focus of this volume, and one to which the majority of chapters are devoted, is on the utilization of regenerative pharmacology to direct organ or tissue regeneration and engineering. Chapters 5 and 9, for example, deal with stem cells. The ability of pharmacology to modulate the behavior of stem and progenitor cells will be a key to the explicit goal of promoting the development, maturation, and function of bioengineered and regenerating organs and tissues. In this regard, stem cell source(s), characterization, and differentiation are the subject of Chapter 5, and the development of the high-throughput screening methods for stem cell expansion and differentiation that would be required for efficient clinical translation and implementation are described in Chapter 9.

As noted in two recent articles, the field of biodegradable materials (i.e., biomaterials) represents a natural interface for pharmacology and regenerative medicine, yet there remains a paucity of successful clinical or commercial applications [17,18]. Consistent with their continuously evolving role [19], biomaterials, nanotechnologies, and their applications to the development of next generation gene and drug delivery systems (i.e., functionalized biomaterials) represent some of the most important and exciting new areas of applied pharmacology and are covered in Chapters 6 and 8. In fact, a variety of extant biomaterial-based technologies are available for tuning spatial and temporal delivery of bioactive agents. The applications of such technologies to regenerative medicine and tissue engineering are virtually endless and will undoubtedly open up new vistas of scientific enquiry.

Regenerative medicine technologies will likely need to be both organ specific as well as patient specific. For example, patients with diminished regenerative capacity may require more advanced technologies; therefore, one might suspect that more organ or tissue development will be required in vitro for successful regeneration after implantation in vivo. In this regard, significant tissue or organ maturation in vitro will require the use of bioreactors (i.e., the laboratory instruments or devices that are used to seed or precondition engineered tissues or organs by providing a biomechanical environment and milieu that mimics key aspects of the in vivo characteristics of the tissue or organ of interest) [20]. The complexity and sophistication of bioreactors may need to be enhanced to accommodate these more demanding requirements. Chapter 7 provides some examples of how this might transpire, and one can easily imagine how these devices could assume a pivotal role in regenerative medicine and the applications of regenerative pharmacology, perhaps especially with respect to the eventual transportation of the clinical product.

Another key aspect of regenerative pharmacology is the selection of animal models for studying the time course and characteristics of endogenous regeneration as well as the regenerative response that occurs after implantation of bioengineered organs and tissues. In this regard, efficient clinical translation requires the use of the most appropriate animal model for a given organ or tissue. Matching the pharmacology of the organ or tissue of interest to the corresponding human condition is therefore of paramount importance. There are many considerations and possibilities, and Chapter 10 provides an excellent summary of current knowledge and opportunities for selection of the most translational animal models.

Chapters 11 to 14 provide examples of ongoing applications of regenerative pharmacology to the treatment of a variety of diseases and disorders. More specifically, these range from the development of biologic pacemakers for cardiac disease (see

Chapter 11), stem cell therapy for cardiac repair (see Chapter 12), and pharmacology and cell therapy for wound healing and repair of damaged muscle (see Chapter 13) to regenerative pharmacotherapy for skin and heart. Not only do these chapters highlight the obstacles and promise of regenerative medicine and the impact of pharmacology from leading experts in the field, but importantly, they also identify numerous molecular targets for future consideration and development. In short, these "state-of-the-art" approaches point to the many exciting potential applications of pharmacology to regenerative medicine and tissue engineering.

Finally, Chapter 15 describes the current status of research in the amphibian kings of regeneration. Undoubtedly, there is much we can learn from the awesome regenerative capacity of the urodeles (newts and salamanders), which is characterized by complete wound healing and functional regeneration of a wide variety of tissues and organs. The molecular fingerprint and pharmacological blueprints uncovered by these investigations may one day provide important clues and novel approaches for enhanced clinical treatment of numerous age- and disease-related degenerative conditions of cells, tissues, and organs in patients.

There are clearly aspects and applications of regenerative pharmacology that are not covered in this initial volume on the subject. The most notable among these are potential applications to central nervous system (CNS) disorders. Thus, although important aspects of peripheral nerve regeneration are covered in Chapter 8, applications of regenerative pharmacology to a wide variety of CNS disorders (e.g., Parkinson's disease, Alzheimer's disease), including spinal cord injuries, is well beyond the intended scope of this book. However, the potential applications of nanotechnology, particularly to assist with transiting drugs and pharmaceuticals across the blood–brain barrier, have been well codified elsewhere [21,22]. In addition, we do not consider potential applications of regenerative pharmacology to genetic diseases, although clearly, regenerative pharmacology may provide an immediate therapeutic opportunity to slow down the decline of muscle function or loss in patients with, for example, muscular dystrophy [23]. The rationale for this particular application is that targeting key events downstream of the genetic defect can compensate, at least partially, for the pathological consequences of the disease. Finally, the use of drug-eluting stents for the treatment of vascular disease is not covered in this book, although we do recognize that there is obvious overlap between stent use and other aspects of the regenerative pharmacology applications that are covered herein. In short, these omissions are consistent with the main intent of this first volume on the subject, which is to provide readers with a reasonably comprehensive introduction and familiarity with the possibility of regenerative pharmacology but not an exhaustive recitation of all potential and current applications. We anticipate that this will be a very fast-moving field of research; therefore, application coverage can be even further expanded in subsequent updates as the field matures.

In summary, there exists an extraordinary opportunity for pharmacologists to get involved in this quickly developing research and development effort. As outlined throughout this volume, regenerative pharmacology is a relatively recent field of endeavor, but it is one with enormous potential to move regenerative medicine and tissue engineering technologies more rapidly forward toward clinical translation. One particularly striking feature of the application of pharmacology to regenerative medicine is that it has the intrinsic potential to be curative rather than palliative, although improved treatment of symptoms would also be welcome. As noted earlier, this type of thinking represents a paradigm shift from the more traditional view of small molecule-based systemic therapeutics, which are designed to provide symptomatic relief. Regenerative pharmacology is equally applicable whether the loss of viable tissue occurs as a result of congenital anomalies, traumatic injury, inflammation, infection, or surgery or as a complication of another chronic disease. In each instance, regenerative pharmacology holds the promise of providing a curative therapeutic solution for end–organ and tissue failure, whether it is through augmentation of endogenous regeneration or enhancement of engineered replacement tissues and organs.

When considered in its entirety then, regenerative pharmacology is an enormous field of endeavor, and undoubtedly, this volume can provide only a glimpse into the huge scope and virtually endless possibilities of this burgeoning field of research. As such, we have necessarily focused on only a few examples to demonstrate the point, recognizing that, of course, there is still much below the "tip of the iceberg." This chapter, as well as prior reports [1,24], have provided some specific examples of regenerative pharmacology that begin to address the important role of the pharmacological sciences in tissue engineering and regeneration. In this book, we build on that conceptual base but expand our consideration to include a broader and more detailed discussion of the spectrum of pharmacological approaches currently being used or contemplated for regenerative medicine. In this scenario, the use of not only biomaterials but also cells as drug delivery vehicles for enhancing regenerative capacity and extending the applications of tissue engineering and regenerative medicine will also be explored.

References

1. Andersson KE and Christ GJ. Regenerative pharmacology: the future is now. *Mol Interv* 7: 79–86, 2007.
2. Orlando G, Baptista P, Birchall M, De Coppi P, Farney A, Guimaraes-Souza NK, Opara E, Rogers J, Seliktar D, Shapira-Schweitzer K, Stratta RJ, Atala A, Wood KJ, and Soker S. Regenerative medicine as applied to solid organ transplantation: current status and future challenges. *Transplant Int* 24: 223–232, 2011.
3. Vacanti J. Tissue engineering and regenerative medicine: from first principles to state of the art. *J Pediatr Surg* 45: 291–294, 2010.
4. Atala A. Engineering organs. *Curr Opin Biotechnol* 20: 575–592, 2009.
5. Atala A. Recent applications of regenerative medicine to urologic structures and related tissues. *Curr Opin Urol* 16: 305–309, 2006.
6. Mikos AG, Herring SW, Ochareon P, Elisseeff J, Lu HH, Kandel R, Schoen FJ, Toner M, Mooney D, Atala A, Van Dyke ME, Kaplan D, and Vunjak-Novakovic G. Engineering complex tissues. *Tissue Eng* 12: 3307–3339, 2006.

7. Vacanti CA. The history of tissue engineering. *J Cell Mol Med* 10: 569–576, 2006.
8. Vacanti JP. Editorial: tissue engineering: a 20-year personal perspective. *Tissue Eng* 13: 231–232, 2007.
9. Ingber DE and Levin M. What lies at the interface of regenerative medicine and developmental biology? *Development* 134: 2541–2547, 2007.
10. Yazdani SK, Watts B, Machingal M, Jarajapu YP, Van Dyke ME, and Christ GJ. Smooth muscle cell seeding of decellularized scaffolds: the importance of bioreactor preconditioning to development of a more native architecture for tissue-engineered blood vessels. *Tissue Eng Part A* 15: 827–840, 2009.
11. Neff LP, Tillman BW, Yazdani SK, Machingal MA, Yoo JJ, Soker S, Bernish BW, Geary RL, and Christ GJ. Vascular smooth muscle enhances functionality of tissue-engineered blood vessels in vivo. *J Vasc Surg* 53: 426–434, 2011.
12. Machingal MA, Corona BT, Walters TJ, Kesireddy V, Koval CN, Dannahower A, Zhao W, Yoo JJ, and Christ GJ. A tissue-engineered muscle repair construct for functional restoration of an irrecoverable muscle injury in a murine model. *Tissue Eng Part A* 17: 2291–2303, 2011.
13. Corona BT, Machingal MA, Criswell T, Vadhavkar M, Dannahower A, Bergman C, Zhao W, Christ GJ. Further development of a tissue engineered muscle repair (TEMR) construct in vitro for enhanced functional recovery following implantation in vivo in a murine model of volumetric muscle loss (VML) injury. *Tissue Eng Part A*. 18: 1213-1228, 2012.
13. Moon du G, Christ G, Stitzel JD, Atala A, and Yoo JJ. Cyclic mechanical preconditioning improves engineered muscle contraction. *Tissue Eng Part A* 14: 473–482, 2008.
14. Niklason LE, Gao J, Abbott WM, Hirschi KK, Houser S, Marini R, and Langer R. Functional arteries grown in vitro. *Science* 284: 489–493, 1999.
15. Corona BT, Balog EM, Doyle JA, Rupp JC, Luke RC, and Ingalls CP. Junctophilin damage contributes to early strength deficits and EC coupling failure after eccentric contractions. *Am J Physiol Cell Physiol* 298: C365–376, 2010.
16. Ingalls CP, Warren GL, Williams JH, Ward CW, and Armstrong RB. E-C coupling failure in mouse EDL muscle after in vivo eccentric contractions. *J Appl Physiol* 85: 58–67, 1998.
17. Vert M. Degradable and bioresorbable polymers in surgery and in pharmacology: beliefs and facts. *J Mater Sci Mater Med* 20: 437–446, 2009.
18. Vert M. Degradable polymers in medicine: updating strategies and terminology. *The Int J Artif Organs* 34: 76–83, 2011.
19. Williams DF. On the nature of biomaterials. *Biomaterials* 30: 5897–5909, 2009.
20. Goldstein AS and Christ G. Functional tissue engineering requires bioreactor strategies. *Tissue Eng Part A* 15: 739–740, 2009.
21. Boulaiz H, Alvarez PJ, Ramirez A, Marchal JA, Prados J, Rodriguez-Serrano F, Peran M, Melguizo C, and Aranega A. Nanomedicine: application areas and development prospects. *Int J Mol Sci* 12: 3303–3321, 2011.
22. Ellis-Behnke RG, Teather LA, Schneider GE, and So KF. Using nanotechnology to design potential therapies for CNS regeneration. *Curr Pharm Des* 13: 2519–2528, 2007.
23. Mozzetta C, Minetti G, and Puri PL. Regenerative pharmacology in the treatment of genetic diseases: the paradigm of muscular dystrophy. *Int J Biochem Cell Biol* 41: 701–710, 2009.
24. Furth ME and Christ GJ. Regenerative pharmacology for diabetes mellitus. *Mol Interv* 9: 171–174, 2009.

2

Regenerative Pharmacology of the Bladder

DAVID BURMEISTER, KARL-ERIK ANDERSSON, AND GEORGE J. CHRIST

Regenerative pharmacology can be defined as "the application of pharmacological sciences to accelerate, optimize and characterize (either in vitro or in vivo) the development, maturation and function of bioengineered and regenerating tissues" (Andersson & Christ, 2007). Generally, two approaches may be used: (a) the "active" (i.e., directing) approach, exemplified by the use of growth factors and different pharmacological agents or bioactive molecules to alter cell proliferation, differentiation, and function in a desired fashion, and (b) the "passive" (i.e., dissecting) approach, as illustrated through the use of established pharmacological methods to evaluate and compare salient characteristics of endogenously regenerated or bioengineered cells and tissues (e.g., how closely do the requisite signal transduction mechanisms of an engineered or regenerating tissue or organ compare with the native tissue or organ?). Both of these approaches are currently used in regenerative medicine, and the goal of this chapter as well as Chapter 3 is to illustrate these basic principles in detail using organ regeneration as observed in the bladder.

Why the bladder? Somewhat surprisingly perhaps, the bladder has actually been at the leading edge of clinical translation in tissue engineering and regenerative medicine. This is partly attributable to the rather extensive intrinsic regenerative capacity of this organ (Table 2-1). Regenerative pharmacology has been used as a tool to understand not only the phenomenon of endogenous bladder regeneration (with and without the use of scaffolds or cells) but also to optimize bioengineered bladder constructs for implantation (see Chapter 3 for more details). Because of the bladder's natural regenerative capacity, regenerative pharmacology not only can be used to characterize "normal" bladder regeneration (e.g., functionally, structurally, molecularly) but can also be used to identify mechanisms to improve regeneration in scenarios in which it is compromised.

In this regard, the distinction between "accelerating" or "augmenting" organ or tissue regeneration on the one hand and "characterizing" functional restoration in the regenerating organ or tissue is not trivial and indeed is at the heart of "directing"

Table 2-1. *A summary of clinical experiences with De Novo bladder regeneration*

Reference	Major clinical finding
Sisk et al. 1939	A 58-year-old man underwent extensive STC (leaving 3 × 3 cm of posterior bladder wall) and voided through his urethra 8 weeks later
Folsom et al. 1940	Eight women with interstitial cystitis underwent STC, resulting in bladder capacities up to 600 mL (one failure caused by pyelonephritis)
Richardson 1952	A 66-year-old man had removal of necrotic bladder tissue above trigone with normal cystogram and urination and a 350-mL capacity 1 year later
Bohne et al. 1957	Seven patients with carcinoma underwent STC, and bladder regeneration did occur; however, infections prevented success in some
Portilla Sanchez et al. 1958	A 65-year-old patient with bladder cancer underwent STC with a plastic mold; 3 months later, a bladder with a transitional epithelium grew larger than the mold
Baker et al. 1959	70 patients with bladder cancer underwent STC, with most resulting in sufficient bladder regeneration (∼20% incidence of asymptomatic ureteral reflux)
Liang 1962	11 patients underwent ∼75% STC without molds, suggesting a mechanical stretch stimulus for bladder regeneration
Tucci et al. 1963	A 45-year-old man underwent 80%–90% STC for bladder cancer, leaving only the ureterovesical junction and bladder neck; normal urination and 400-mL bladder capacity were observed 6 months later
Baker et al. 1965	Several patients presenting with recurring multiple transitional cell carcinomas underwent total mucosal excision; complete epithelial regeneration occurred without the incidence of cancer
McCallum 1965	A 36-year-old man had necrotic tissue (entire bladder except for part of the trigone) removed; bladder capacity increased from ∼45 mL to ∼300 mL in 6 weeks with normal bladder function

STC = subtotal cystectomy.

versus "dissecting" regenerative pharmacology, respectively. As mentioned earlier, the directing approach involves using pharmacological agents to actively modify different aspects of bladder physiology and function during regeneration and repair and could include treatments such as stem cell therapy or the delivery of growth factors as well as a host of other bioactive molecules. Although regenerative pharmacology can also be used to control, for example, stem cell growth or differentiation in vitro for eventual use in bladder repair, that topic is the subject of other chapters (see Chapters 5 and 9).

In contrast to the "directed" or "active" approach, the "dissecting" approach simply uses pharmacological methods to evaluate the characteristics of functional restoration during regeneration. As illustrated in Figure 2-1 and further discussed in Chapter 3, the regenerative process is evaluated using multidisciplinary investigations ranging from studies of bladder function in vivo (via cystometry) to cell and tissue function

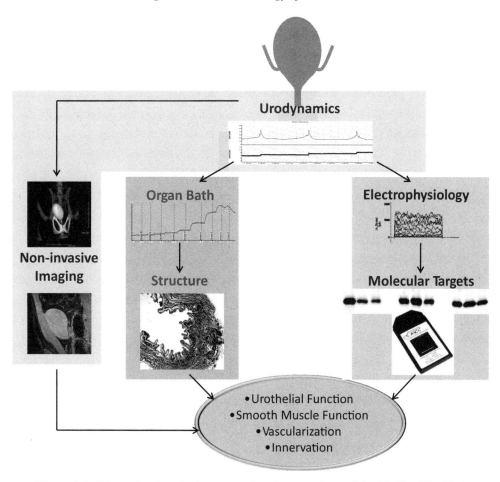

Figure 2-1. Dissecting (passive) regenerative pharmacology of the bladder. The bladder can be used as a model system that integrates multidisciplinary studies to evaluate organ regeneration (i.e., function and structure) on the whole organ (*green text*), tissue (*red text*), and cellular (*blue text*) levels. In vivo urodynamic studies can be used to examine overall bladder function. After euthanasia, bladder tissue can be cut into strips and stimulated to contract in an organ bath system (pharmacological studies), or sliced into sections for structural analysis (histological studies). Additionally, both gene and protein levels can be evaluated (molecular studies) and patch clamp methods can be used (electrophysiological studies) to study regenerated tissue. Noninvasive CT and MR imaging can be used longitudinally to examine organ morphology during regeneration, and possibly provide information on aspects of tissue phenotype gained via other methods. The information obtained from these studies can be used to design therapeutic interventions (see Fig. 2-2). (See color plate 3.)

in vitro via a variety of standard as well as state-of-the-art assays. In the remainder of this chapter, we will focus on discussion of the strategies outlined earlier with specific emphasis on animal models of intrinsic bladder regeneration. Additionally, the unique regenerative properties of the bladder will be addressed, not only in terms of the current clinical need and available technologies but also with respect to how bladder derivatives per se can be used in regenerative pharmacology.

Regenerative Pharmacology and Bladder Disease

The aim of regenerative pharmacology is, ideally, to facilitate the restoration of normal organ function. This can be accomplished in conjunction with tissue engineering strategies to replace a nonfunctioning organ (end-stage disease). Alternatively, regenerative pharmacology can enhance endogenous regenerative capacity when sufficient viable bladder tissue remains in the face of functional impairments. From a physiological perspective, normal bladder function involves storage of urine at increasing volumes (without increasing intravesical pressure or spontaneous bladder contractions) until complete voluntary emptying is required. Diverse disease etiologies (e.g., neurogenic, congenital, trauma, infections) that compromise the low-pressure, high-volume function (decreased compliance) of the bladder lead to a number of lower urinary tract symptoms such as urgency, urgency incontinence, frequency, and nocturia. Without a doubt, there is enormous room for improved therapeutics, and regenerative pharmacology may be applicable to a number of these scenarios.

In this regard, antimuscarinic drugs (e.g., oxybutynin, solifenacin, darifenacin) are now the first-line therapy for treatment of detrusor overactivity and the overactive bladder syndrome. Lower urinary tract symptoms can also be treated with α-adrenoreceptor (AR) blockers (e.g., doxazosin) alone or in combination with antimuscarinics (Kaplan et al. 2006; Chapple et al. 2009). However, in cases of neurogenic bladder overactivity, in which one of the main aims of treatment is to prevent damage to the upper urinary tract, bladder contractility can be reduced with these treatments, necessitating the use of clean intermittent catheterization in some cases. With such diverse etiologies for bladder dysfunction and such a large demand (more than 50 million people are estimated to have some type of urgency incontinence), many different classes of drugs have been investigated (Andersson et al. 2009). These include, for example, β-3 AR agonists (e.g., mirabegron) and botulinum toxin-A, but a more detailed discussion of all current pharmacological interventions is well beyond the scope of this chapter, and moreover, these interventions are discussed in detail elsewhere (Andersson et al. 2009).

Most importantly, severe cases of bladder dysfunction are largely refractory to conventional pharmacological treatments. In this scenario, high bladder pressures may develop and lead to upper urinary tract deterioration (i.e., end-stage renal disease [ESRD]), particularly if the intravesical pressure exceeds 40 cm H_2O. Patients who display poorly compliant bladders caused by structural or neurogenic causes are at risk for ESRD and are thus candidates for surgical intervention (Reyblat et al. 2008). Currently, the gold standard treatment in these situations has been bladder augmentation. This procedure has been performed in patients with bladder diseases arising from many different etiologies, including spinal cord injury, myelomeningocele, interstitial cystitis, idiopathic detrusor overactivity, radiation cystitis, multiple sclerosis, and schistosomiasis. Thus, the potential applications of regenerative pharmacology to the treatment of bladder dysfunction and end-organ bladder disease are truly enormous.

The purpose of bladder augmentation is to maintain low intravesical pressures while increasing bladder capacity (Gurocak et al. 2007). Attempts to increase bladder capacity can be traced back to the late 1800s and throughout the twentieth century with many different materials both natural (fascia, dura mater, intestinal segments) and synthetic (Teflon, polyvinyl) (Schwartz 1891; Kudish 1957; Bono et al. 1966; Kelami et al. 1970; Gleeson et al. 1992; Cheng et al. 1994). By the middle of the twentieth century, the use of intestinal (usually ileal) segments became commonplace, but this procedure was still associated with side effects such as urinary stones, pyelonephritis, metabolic imbalances, infections, and mucus production (Flood et al. 1995). This, along with the lack of tissue available for donor bladder transplantation, pointed to the need for regenerative medicine or tissue engineering technologies for the bladder (Aboushwareb et al. 2008). Although this approach is also covered in Chapter 3, we discuss some relevant background herein to provide important context to an improved understanding of endogenous bladder regeneration, which is the focus of this chapter.

In one of the first successful neo-organ transplants, bladders were constructed by seeding dome-shaped synthetic scaffolds (collagen or collagen–polyglycolic acid composites) with urothelial cells on the inside and smooth muscle cells on the outside that were subsequently implanted into patients with myelomeningocele (Atala et al. 2006). The regenerative pharmacology aspects of this work (which were crucial for the success of these neo-bladders) are covered in detail in Chapter 3. Although these studies indicate that an autologous, engineered tissue can be safely implanted and may have clinical utility for the treatment of neurogenic bladder, the clinical experience is still limited, and the technology is not yet ready for wide dissemination (Atala 2011). In this regard, it is clear that greater mechanistic insight of the endogenous regenerative process would be beneficial to further improve this technology for broader clinical applications. Such is the focus of this chapter.

The successful application of tissue engineering approaches to bladder augmentation in patients may not be surprising given the long known regenerative capacity of the bladder in both animal models and humans. There are numerous indications that the human bladder possesses significant regenerative capacity (e.g., after subtotal cystectomy [STC]) as outlined in Table 2-1. Sisk and Neu reported one of the first clinical experiences in 1939, describing a patient who voided through the urethra 8 weeks after STC leaving only a 3-by-3 cm patch of the posterior bladder wall (Sisk et al. 1939). Later studies described presumptive regeneration in bladder cancer patients. For example, one study reported that only 6 months after removal of the entire bladder, except for the ureterovesical junction and bladder neck, bladder capacity reached 400 mL (Tucci et al. 1963). Even though unsuccessful accounts of bladder regeneration also exist (Bohne et al. 1957; Ross et al. 1969; Goldstein et al. 1970; Taguchi et al. 1977; Barros et al. 2006) citing complications such as infections, taken together, the extant literature clearly indicates that under certain circumstances, the human bladder can regenerate in situ. However, a more precise identification of the requirements for human bladder regeneration has not been codified, and the continued use of bladder augmentation techniques ensures that this avenue will not be pursued until further understanding of the natural process is obtained. To this end, the use of animal models allows researchers to study bladder regeneration under tightly controlled conditions. Indeed, Daniel Liang in the 1960s attempted to leverage this idea and reported similar findings of STC-induced bladder growth both in humans and rats (Liang 1962; Liang et al. 1963).

The utility of the bladder as a model organ system to study the characteristics of endogenous regenerative capacity and the role of regenerative pharmacology in characterizing this process is highlighted in Figure 2-1. As described in Chapter 1, the use of regenerative pharmacology to modulate the regenerative process (see Fig. 2-2) is iterative. Through this approach, one can identify, for example, biologically active molecules (e.g., small molecules and growth factors) that can be utilized to further optimize functional bladder regeneration.

Passive Regenerative Pharmacology of the Bladder

As noted earlier, the underlying premise for this line of research is that strategies aimed at harnessing the body's natural capacity for regeneration will undoubtedly benefit from a basic understanding of de novo bladder regeneration. Given that there is a lack of knowledge on endogenous organ regeneration per se in well-characterized and easily studied systems, it is not entirely surprising that so few strategies to enhance this process have been discovered. As a first step in this direction, we have recently published the first studies we are aware of that used a multidisciplinary approach to characterize bladder regeneration (Burmeister et al. 2010; Peyton et al., 2012). In the initial report (Burmeister et al., 2010), trigone-sparing cystectomy (STC) was performed in 12-week-old female rats. Computed tomography revealed a time-dependent increase in bladder volume at 2, 4, and 8 weeks after STC that positively correlated with restoration of bladder function. Bladders emptied completely at all time points studied, that is, we observed functional regeneration, albeit in the presence of significantly diminished contractility (see later discussion for details). Moreover, the bladder displayed urothelial, lamina propria, and detrusor muscle layers and regained normal thickness upon histologic evaluation. Immunohistochemical staining also showed expression of proliferating cell nuclear antigen and a population of CD117 (c-kit)–positive cells after STC that was not seen in control bladders.

More recently (Peyton et al., 2012), fluorescent bromodeoxyuridine (BrdU) labeling was used to quantify the spatiotemporal characteristics of the proliferative response

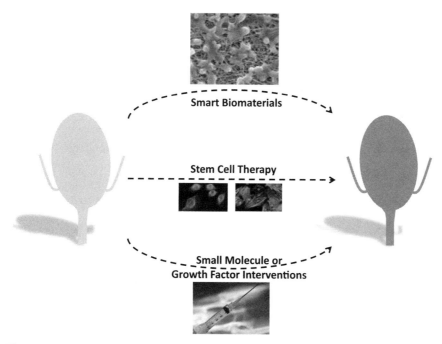

Figure 2-2. Directing (active) regenerative pharmacology of the bladder. Dissecting the process of bladder regeneration (Fig. 2-1) can identify specific processes (e.g., cell proliferation, differentiation, angiogenesis, innervation, and stem cell migration) that can be manipulated pharmacologically to direct tissue engineering and regenerative medicine strategies for the bladder. (*Top*) Tissue-engineered constructs currently used for bladder augmentation techniques can be altered to include, for example, different cell types and/or controlled oxygen delivery to enhance regeneration. (*Middle*) Supplementation of stem cells may modulate different aspects of bladder regeneration in a paracrine fashion. (*Bottom*) Pharmacological manipulation with small molecules or growth factors may be used to target specific signaling cascades involved in bladder regeneration. The ultimate goal with any of these interventions is to maximize bladder regeneration to restore normal bladder function. (See color plate 4.)

that mediates this robust functional regeneration during the first week post-STC. Less than 1 percent of cells in the bladder wall were labeled with BrdU in control bladders, but this percentage significantly increased by 5–8-fold at all time points post-STC. Specifically, the spatiotemporal characteristics of the proliferative response were defined by a significantly higher percentage of BrdU-labeled cells within the urothelium at 1 day than in the muscularis propria (MP) and lamina propria (LP). A time-dependent shift at 3 and 5 days post-STC revealed significantly fewer BrdU-labeled cells in the MP than LP or urothelium. By 7 days, the percentage of BrdU-labeled cells was similar among urothelium, LP, and MP. STC also caused an apparent increase in immunostaining for Shh, Gli-1, and BMP-4. In summary, the early stages of functional bladder regeneration are characterized by time-dependent changes in the location of the proliferating cell population in bladder wall layers, and expression of several evolutionarily conserved developmental signaling proteins. This report extends previous observations and further establishes the rodent bladder as an excellent model for studying novel aspects of mammalian organ regeneration.

Interestingly, although we have indeed observed functional regeneration (as reflected by the fact that animals are continent, with low-pressure, high-volume reservoirs), the regeneration process still does not result in full restoration of a bladder with identical properties as native bladders. More specifically, we observed a decrease in bladder smooth muscle contractility to both muscarinic and electrical field stimulation (EFS). Cholinergic activation resulted in contractile responses that were approximately 20 percent of that observed in normal bladder tissue of age-matched control participants. Although we observed a time-dependent increase in detrusor contractility, when bladder volume was completely restored (i.e., 8 weeks after STC), maximal steady-state contractions were still only about 37 percent of normal values. This diminished contractility occurs despite the apparent recovery of bladder wall innervation as judged by the presence of contraction to EFS (and staining to protein gene product 9.5). These observations are in agreement with an earlier study by Frederiksen et al. (2004) in which whole-mount staining of acetylcholinesterase was performed to visualize the pattern of "normal" innervation after regeneration. They found that regenerating bladder tissue contained nerves on the anterior aspect of the bladder that were more slanted against the longitudinally running muscle bundles compared with control participants. This pattern of innervation was more reminiscent of the trigonal region of the bladder (i.e., the tissue that was still present after cystectomy) than in native bladder wall from control animals.

In fact, this same group had already posited that the newly forming bladder tissue after STC most closely resembles the remaining supratrigonal tissue. In 2004, Frederiksen et al. (2004) provided the first and most complete description of the pharmacology of newly forming bladder tissue (after STC) at that time. In those studies, transverse strips were excised from the bladder body 15 weeks after STC in female rats and were evaluated by investigating the possibility of regional differences in contractility. The authors used agonists and antagonists of muscarinic receptors and α_1-AR, as well as an agonist and desensitizing agent of P2X1 receptors (α,β-methylene adenosine triphosphate [ATP]). Their findings showed that contractility in response to EFS was not affected by α1-AR blockade, and strips from just above the trigone contracted similarly (in terms of percent maximal response) when muscarinic receptors were blocked. However, in more distal (i.e., equatorial) preparations, muscarinic blockade produced a greater inhibition of contractility in control bladders than that from animals that had undergone STC. The result of this investigation was consistent with prior work and supported the supposition that although the newly formed bladder smooth muscle is well innervated, the pharmacological properties are most reminiscent of the trigonal tissue from which it had developed.

The process of bladder regeneration also shows species variations in the extent of restoration of bladder capacity. For example, Lin et al. (1989) performed cystometric and pharmacological experiments examining the rabbit bladder 8 weeks after STC. They evaluated in vitro contractile responses of five transverse detrusor muscle strips (upper body, lower body, mid bladder, upper base, and lower base) in response to bethanechol, ATP, isoproterenol, and epinephrine. They showed that the absolute contractile responses of bladder strips taken from the bladder dome (but not the bladder base) were lower in animals subjected to STC when stimulated with EFS, bethanechol, or ATP. Although this reduction in contractility is similar to that seen in other species, morphologic and cystometric studies led the authors to the conclusion that small increases in capacity were due to an increased size of the bladder base.

This impaired ability to restore normal bladder capacity is similar to what was seen by Zhang et al. in a canine model (Zhang et al. 2006). In this severe, 90 percent cystectomy model in dogs, STC alone was used as a control group for augmentation cystoplasty. They found that even 9 months after cystectomy, there was still a 72 percent reduction in bladder capacity. These types of species differences in the response of the bladder after STC dictates that appropriate animal models must be chosen. Clearly, in certain circumstances, steps may need to be taken to assist with the restoration of bladder volume, especially when 90 percent of the bladder is removed.

Because endogenous regeneration is not sufficient to restore bladder function in all animal species, additional studies have focused on provisions of biomaterials (i.e., scaffolds) or cells to enhance regenerative capacity. Such studies are described in detail in Chapter 3 by Bertram and colleagues. Scaffolds with and without seeded cells have been used in augmentation surgeries to enhance bladder regeneration. Examining the pharmacological performance of regenerated bladders after incorporation of a scaffold is certainly important to ensure normal bladder performance. Bertram et al. reported on the contractility of bladder smooth muscle 9 months after bladder scaffold implantation (Bertram et al. 2008). Upon examination of bladder strips, there were no differences in contractile responses to cholinergic, AR, or EFS when compared with control participants.

The importance of seeding cells on scaffolds used for bladder augmentation was highlighted in a study by Oberpenning et al. (1999). In this study, dogs underwent STC, and their bladders were augmented with a polyglycolic acid scaffold alone or a scaffold seeded with urothelial and smooth muscle cells. Augmentation with the polymer alone resulted in small, poorly compliant bladders, but bladders that were augmented with cell-seeded scaffolds displayed normal bladder capacity and compliance up to 11 months after STC. Additionally, bladders from this group showed normal histologic architecture, with minimal evidence of the fibrosis that was seen in the scaffold-only group. Expression of cytokeratin markers, smooth muscle actin, and S-100 demonstrated the presence of nerves in the dog bladders that received cell-seeded scaffolds.

More studies are required to elucidate why the provision of these exogenous cells and biomaterials components appear to compensate for diminished regenerative capacity. Although a fair amount of data has already been generated in this model system, more work needs to be done to fully characterize the many different aspects of bladder pharmacology during and after regeneration. Nonetheless, improved understanding of normal bladder regeneration in vivo would assist in further optimization of the tissue engineering process by providing guidance with respect to improvements in both the preferred cell type and the most advantageous biomaterials or scaffolds. Moreover, improved understanding of the mechanistic basis for diminished bladder contractility observed even in the presence of functional regeneration in vivo would likewise have huge implications for further improving endogenous regeneration. For example, alterations in receptor populations, ion channel properties, or second messengers may cause diminished contractility. Identifying such mechanisms or any other differences in transmembrane or transcellular signal transduction would logically point toward improved therapeutic strategies for regeneration, including the application of bioactive molecules (see later discussion).

Active Regenerative Pharmacology of the Bladder

Application of tissue engineering approaches via scaffold incorporation opens the door for the local administration of many different pharmacologically active agents in order to improve the regeneration of the urinary bladder (i.e., active regenerative pharmacology). As a proof of concept study, Kanematsu et al. analyzed the ability of bladder acellular matrix (BAM) to carry a loaded growth factor (basic fibroblast growth factor [bFGF]) (Kanematsu et al. 2003). They demonstrated sustained release of bFGF from the acellular scaffold both in vivo and in vitro. Moreover, 4 weeks after use in an augmentation cystectomy model in rats, bFGF-rich scaffolds were able to promote angiogenesis and inhibit shrinkage of the implant in a dose-dependent manner. This study not only supports the potential use of growth factors for bladder regeneration but also suggests the possibility to "load" scaffolds used for augmentation with growth factors.

Another logical growth factor candidate is vascular endothelial growth factor (VEGF), a widely used bioactive molecule with known angiogenic potential. Youssif et al. (2005) demonstrated that incubation of BAM scaffolds with VEGF164 and subsequent injection of VEGF164 into the bladder wall during augmentation surgery increased bladder capacity and decreased residual volume 4 weeks after surgery compared with control participants. Evidence for enhanced angiogenesis was seen at this time point, and higher smooth muscle content was observed at all time points studied. Moreover, VEGF supplementation led to an increased amount of nerve growth factor (NGF)–positive cells up to 8 weeks after surgery, suggesting a chemotactic effect of VEGF that can upregulate other growth factors.

A synergistic effect of VEGF and NGF has also been postulated by Kikuno et al. (2009), in a study examining augmentation techniques in spinal cord injured rats. Eight weeks after initial spinal cord injury, female Sprague-Dawley rats underwent augmentation cystoplasty using BAM alone or BAM loaded with NGF, VEGF, or NGF and VEGF. Eight weeks after augmentation surgery, animals that received both growth factors displayed much higher bladder capacity and compliance and increased smooth muscle and nerve content than in any other group. Taken together, these studies indicate that both NGF and VEGF provide examples of how growth factors or other bioactive molecules may be extremely beneficial in restoring bladder function and architecture during the regenerative process.

The complexity and potential biologic redundancy of bladder regeneration was illustrated by DiSandro et al (1997). They implanted excised bladders from wild-type and epidermal growth factor receptor (EGFR) knockout mice into the bladders of athymic rats and subsequently performed bladder augmentation with BAM scaffolds in these same rats. They found that although mouse urothelial and smooth muscle cells invaded the regenerated matrix, there was no difference in the contributions of normal and knockout (KO) mouse bladders histologically, and both seemed to promote bladder regeneration after augmentation. However, the authors pointed out that EGFR signaling may still play a synergistic role in bladder regeneration even though compensatory pathways exist.

In another study (in yet another species), Loai et al. implicated the VEGF pathway described earlier but also demonstrated an importance of hyaluronic acid in a porcine model of augmentation cystoplasty (Loai et al. 2010). This study showed that using this glycosaminoglycan and a growth factor in combination produced the best epithelialization, neovascularization, and smooth muscle regeneration 10 weeks after surgery compared with BAM scaffolds with hyaluronic acid alone. Although few studies have examined the incorporation of multiple growth factors, it is conceivable that delivery of many different growth factors, small molecules, or other compounds may aid in regeneration of the urinary bladder. In short, the extant literature suggests that a completely functional regenerative response might require a "cocktail" of small molecules, growth factors, and perhaps even cells. This seems a reasonable supposition, keeping in mind that even "normal" bladder regeneration, when it is found to occur (in rodents; see Burmeister et al. 2010) is associated with diminished detrusor contractility. It follows logically that the greater the impairment in regenerative capacity, the more ingredients that will be required in the "cocktail."

In addition to well-defined conditions incorporating known amounts of pharmacological agents such as those described earlier, reports have studied the effects of stem and progenitor cell populations on bladder regeneration (Chung et al. 2005; Zhang et al. 2005; Drewa et al. 2009; Jack et al. 2009; Sharma et al. 2010a, 2010b; Zhu et al. 2010). Nonetheless, the rationale for including stem cells relies, at least in part, on their ability to create a favorable cytokine environment for tissue repair

Table 2-2. *Summary of approaches used for tissue-engineered augmentation in animal models*

Reference	Cells used	Scaffold used	Finding
Chung et al. 2005	BM MSCs	SIS	Increased MHC, decreased collagen expression with cell-seeded scaffolds
Zhang et al. 2005	BM stromal cells	SIS	Canine augmentation resulted in good smooth muscle formation if scaffolds were cell seeded
Drewa et al. 2006	3T3 fibroblasts	PGA	Urothelial proliferation was aided with fibroblast seeding of scaffolds used for rat bladder augmentations
Drewa et al. 2009	Hair follicle stem cells	BAM	Thicker muscle layers were seen in rat bladders augmented with stem cell–seeded scaffolds
Jack et al. 2009	ADSCs	PLGA	12 weeks after augmentation in nude rats, cell-seeded scaffolds produced superior muscle contraction in vitro
Sharma et al. 2010a	BM MSCs	Poly(1,8-octanediol-co-citrate)	Cell-seeded scaffolds used for augmentation in nude rats led to increased muscle-to-collagen ratios
Sharma et al. 2010b	SMCs, UCs	SIS	Augmentation cystoplasty in baboons showed greater fibrosis in unseeded scaffolds
Zhu et al. 2010	ADSCs	BAM	Cell seeding for implantation into rabbits led to better muscle and nerve regeneration

ADSC = adipose-derived stem cells; BAM = bladder acellular matrix; BM MSC = bone marrow–derived mesenchymal stem cells; PGA = polyglycolic acid; PLGA = poly (lactic-co-glycolic) acid; SIS = small intestinal submucosa; SMC = smooth muscle cell; UC = urothelial cell.

and regeneration. In this instance then, the cell can even be the drug, or at least the therapeutic delivery vehicle (see Chapter 12). Most often, an acellular scaffold is used in a cystectomy model and compared with a scaffold that has been seeded with bone marrow mesenchymal stem cells, adipose-derived stem cells, or even hair follicle stem cells. The variety of animal models, cell types, and methodologies used thus far prevents straightforward comparisons among the strategies used; therefore, it is difficult as yet to identify a "gold standard" approach. Nonetheless, it is evident that stem and progenitor cells seem to promote a faster and more complete regenerative response in terms of smooth muscle regeneration and nerve regeneration with several studies demonstrating an increased bladder capacity as well. These findings are summarized in Table 2-2. Mechanistic insight into the scientific rationale for these strategies will prove to be of utmost value for regenerative pharmacology. Although the biomaterial alone can provide structure and a template for tissue growth and repair, the inclusion of a cellular component has been found to assist with the following:

- immune responses
- fibrosis
- smooth muscle formation and maturation
- urothelial migration and maturation
- contractility
- innervation
- bladder capacity and compliance

However, to date, no definite cocktail has been identified, which is further complicated by the need to explore a seemingly ever-expanding list of different components and ingredients.

In this regard, another question that undoubtedly has clinical implications involves the inflammatory response that occurs after injury or scaffold implantation. As a first step in this direction, Ashley and colleagues have begun to characterize the immune response after bladder reconstruction with small intestinal submucosa (SIS) scaffolds (Ashley et al. 2009, 2010). They found that although most inflammatory cells were present in similar levels in graft and native bladder regions, neutrophils were more abundant in scaffold sections. Moreover, their finding that regional differences in where the intestinal segment was taken from (i.e., proximal vs. distal small intestine) led to different inflammatory profiles indicates yet one more variable that may play a pivotal role in whether approaches using SIS are successful. Clearly, there is a need to understand what cytokines, monocytes, and other inflammatory processes are implicated in successful regeneration. However, after this information is in hand, intuitively it seems that one would want to develop regenerative pharmacology strategies that do not require a cellular component.

Bladder Acellular Matrix as a Vehicle for Growth Factors

As indicated by many of these studies, the bladder is rapidly repaired after injury and is therefore a logical organ to study in terms of the contribution of the extracellular matrix (ECM) to this process as a potential guide for development of novel regenerative pharmacology strategies (Hodde 2002). BAM was first studied in 1975 and is derived from the lamina propria layer of the bladder (Meezan et al. 1975). This ECM supports growth and differentiation of different cell types, including the urothelium, which can rapidly proliferate in response to injury, and involves both de- and redifferentiation (Sutherland et al. 1996; Lai et al. 2005; Staack et al. 2005).

Upon analysis, BAM contains many different growth factors, including VEGF, platelet-derived growth factor (PDGF), keratinocyte growth factor (KGF), transforming growth factor β (TGF-β), epidermal growth factor (EGF), and bFGF, among others

(Badylak 2002). Additional studies have begun to more rigorously characterize the types and amounts of bioactive molecules. One study quantified these growth factors via enzyme-linked immunosorbent assays and showed their presence via Western blotting. In these studies, PDGF, KGF, and VEGF were the most predominant bioactive molecules identified (Chun et al. 2007). These investigators also showed that the protein extraction buffer used produced different yields of growth factors, and moreover, BAM protein extract was also shown to induce a dose-dependent increase in proliferation of fibroblasts in vitro. Taken together, these studies show that acellular bladder matrix alone has a large variety of molecules that may be of value to regenerative pharmacology.

Many different decellularization techniques have also been employed, leading to variability in removing cellular debris, which makes comparison between studies difficult (Farhat et al. 2008). Yang et al. (2010) compared several different decellularization protocols using either detergent or distension techniques. They found that using methods to optimize wash times, wash buffer temperatures, and pH values, as well as the use of proteinase inhibitors, preserved bioactive factors. This resulted in a decellularized porcine bladder with no cellular materials but well-preserved extracellular collagen, sulfated glycosaminoglycans, and levels of VEGF and PDGF. Moreover, a positive correlation was observed between the growth factor content and sulfated glycosaminoglycan content, suggesting that preservation of one may be indicative of the other. Further studies are required to determine which process is best for preserving the intrinsic regenerative template of BAM and what may be altered to produce the most beneficial BAM, which may vary from application to application. To date, BAM has been used not only for reconstruction of the urinary bladder as mentioned earlier but also for many other applications such as reconstruction of esophageal, myocardial, skeletal muscle, urethral, and penile applications (Badylak et al. 2005, 2006; Eberli et al. 2007; el-Kassaby et al. 2008; Moon du et al. 2008; Machingal et al. 2011; Corona et al. 2012).

Summary and Conclusions

The field of urologic tissue engineering has made great strides in the understanding and clinical application of regenerative medicine and pharmacology. Pharmacological principles have been applied to the evaluation of regenerating and engineered bladders as well as improving the tissue engineering and regeneration process. However, a more systematic and rigorous approach must be taken to optimize the many steps in the daunting process of applying regenerative pharmacology to improved therapy of bladder disease. Herein we have discussed a few of those steps (e.g., scaffold preparation, cell sources, growth factor selection) which are far from completely understood and moreover have not fully incorporated the use of pharmacological sciences to actively direct or dissect all aspects of the tissue engineering and regeneration processes. As this callow field of research continues to expand, we will begin to better define the boundary conditions for successful application of regenerative pharmacology to the improved treatment of diverse bladder diseases and disorders. Additionally, to permit more meaningful comparison of distinct regenerative strategies, the investigators in this field of research must codify a standardized experimental paradigm or methodology. Nonetheless, even at this early stage of development, the future looks bright for the utility of regenerative pharmacology to both hasten and broaden the clinical utility of regenerative medicine technologies to the bladder and beyond.

References

Aboushwareb, T. and A. Atala (2008). "Stem cells in urology." *Nat Clin Pract Urol* 5(11): 621–631.

Andersson, K. E., C. R. Chapple, L. Cardozo, F. Cruz, H. Hashim, M. C. Michel, C. Tannenbaum, and A. J. Wein (2009). "Pharmacological treatment of overactive bladder: report from the International Consultation on Incontinence." *Curr Opin Urol* 19(4): 380–394.

Andersson, K. E. and G. J. Christ (2007). "Regenerative pharmacology: the future is now." *Mol Interv* 7(2): 79–86.

Ashley, R. A., B. W. Palmer, A. D. Schultz, B. W. Woodson, C. C. Roth, J. C. Routh, K. M. Fung, D. Frimberger, H. K. Lin, and B. P. Kropp (2009). "Leukocyte inflammatory response in a rat urinary bladder regeneration model using porcine small intestinal submucosa scaffold." *Tissue Eng Part A* 15(11): 3241–3246.

Ashley, R. A., C. C. Roth, B. W. Palmer, Y. Kibar, J. C. Routh, K. M. Fung, D. Frimberger, H. K. Lin, and B. P. Kropp (2010). "Regional variations in small intestinal submucosa evoke differences in inflammation with subsequent impact on tissue regeneration in the rat bladder augmentation model." *BJU Int* 105(10): 1462–1468.

Atala, A. (2011). "Tissue engineering of human bladder." *Br Med Bull* 97: 81–104.

Atala, A., S. B. Bauer, S. Soker, J. J. Yoo, and A. B. Retik (2006). "Tissue-engineered autologous bladders for patients needing cystoplasty." *Lancet* 367(9518): 1241–1246.

Badylak, S. F. (2002). "The extracellular matrix as a scaffold for tissue reconstruction." *Semin Cell Dev Biol* 13(5): 377–383.

Badylak, S. F., P. V. Kochupura, I. S. Cohen, S. V. Doronin, A. E. Saltman, T. W. Gilbert, D. J. Kelly, R. A. Ignotz, and G. R. Gaudette (2006). "The use of extracellular matrix as an inductive scaffold for the partial replacement of functional myocardium." *Cell Transplant* 15 Suppl 1: S29–40.

Badylak, S. F., D. A. Vorp, A. R. Spievack, A. Simmons-Byrd, J. Hanke, D. O. Freytes, A. Thapa, T. W. Gilbert, and A. Nieponice (2005). "Esophageal reconstruction with ECM and muscle tissue in a dog model." *J Surg Res* 128(1): 87–97.

Baker, R., W. C. Maxted, and N. Dipasquale (1965). "Regeneration of transitional epithelium of the human bladder after total surgical excision for recurrent, multiple bladder cancer: apparent tumor inhibition." *J Urol* 93: 593–597.

Baker, R., T. Tehan, and T. Kelly (1959). "Regeneration of urinary bladder after subtotal resection for carcinoma." *Am Surg* 25(5): 348–352.

Barros, M., R. Martinelli, and H. Rocha (2006). "Experimental supratrigonal cystectomy. Evaluation of long-term complications." *Int Braz J Urol* 32(3): 350–354.

Bertram, T., G. J. Christ, K.-E. Andersson, T. Aboushwareb, C. Fuellhase, R. Soler, B. J. Wagner, D. Jain, J. W. Ludlow, R. Payne, and M. J. Jayo (2009). "Pharmacologic response of regenerated bladders in a preclinical model." *FASEB J* 23: 291.

Bohne, A. W. and K. L. Urwiller (1957). "Experience with urinary bladder regeneration." *J Urol* 77(5): 725–732.

Bono, A. V. and A. De Gresti (1966). "[Partial substitution of the bladder wall with teflon tissue. (Preliminary and experimental note on the impermeability and tolerance of the prosthesis)]." *Minerva Urol* 18(2): 43–47.

Burmeister, D., T. Aboushwareb, J. Tan, K. Link, K. E. Andersson, and G. Christ (2010). "Early stages of in situ bladder regeneration in a rodent model." *Tissue Eng Part A* 16(8): 2541–2551.

Chapple, C., S. Herschorn, P. Abrams, F. Sun, M. Brodsky, and Z. Guan (2009). "Tolterodine treatment improves storage symptoms suggestive of overactive bladder in men treated with alpha-blockers." *Eur Urol* 56(3): 534–541.

Cheng, E., R. Rento, J. T. Grayhack, R. Oyasu, and K. T. McVary (1994). "Reversed seromuscular flaps in the urinary tract in dogs." *J Urol* 152(6 Pt 2): 2252–2257.

Chun, S. Y., G. J. Lim, T. G. Kwon, E. K. Kwak, B. W. Kim, A. Atala, and J. J. Yoo (2007). "Identification and characterization of bioactive factors in bladder submucosa matrix." *Biomaterials* 28(29): 4251–4256.

Chung, S. Y., N. P. Krivorov, V. Rausei, L. Thomas, M. Frantzen, D. Landsittel, Y. M. Kang, C. H. Chon, C. S. Ng, and G. J. Fuchs (2005). "Bladder reconstitution with bone marrow derived stem cells seeded on small intestinal submucosa improves morphological and molecular composition." *J Urol* 174(1): 353–359.

Corona, B. T., M. A. Machingal, T. Criswell, M. Vadhavkar, A. Dannahower, C. Bergman, W. Zhao, and G. J. Christ (2012). "Further development of a tissue engineered muscle repair (TEMR) construct in vitro for enhanced functional recovery following implantation in vivo in a murine model of volumetric muscle loss (VML) injury." *Tissue Eng Part A* 18:1213–1228.

DiSandro, M. J., L. S. Baskin, Y. W. Li, Z. Werb, and G. R. Cunha (1997). "Development and regenerative ability of bladder in the transgenic epidermal growth factor receptor gene knockout mouse." *J Urol* 158(3 Pt 2): 1058–1065.

Drewa, T., R. Joachimiak, A. Kaznica, V. Sarafian, and M. Pokrywczynska (2009). "Hair stem cells for bladder regeneration in rats: preliminary results." *Transplant Proc* 41(10): 4345–4351.

Drewa, T., J. Sir, R. Czajkowski, and A. Wozniak (2006). "Scaffold seeded with cells is essential in urothelium regeneration and tissue remodeling in vivo after bladder augmentation using in vitro engineered graft." *Transplant Proc* 38(1): 133–135.

Eberli, D., R. Susaeta, J. J. Yoo, and A. Atala (2007). "Tunica repair with acellular bladder matrix maintains corporal tissue function." *Int J Impot Res* 19(6): 602–609.

el-Kassaby, A., T. AbouShwareb, and A. Atala (2008). "Randomized comparative study between buccal mucosal and acellular bladder matrix grafts in complex anterior urethral strictures." *J Urol* 179(4): 1432–1436.

Farhat, W. A., J. Chen, J. Haig, R. Antoon, J. Litman, C. Sherman, K. Derwin, and H. Yeger (2008). "Porcine bladder acellular matrix (ACM): protein expression, mechanical properties." *Biomed Mater* 3(2): 025015.

Flood, H. D., S. J. Malhotra, H. E. O'Connell, M. J. Ritchey, D. A. Bloom, and E. J. McGuire (1995). "Long-term results and complications using augmentation cystoplasty in reconstructive urology." *Neurourol Urodyn* 14(4): 297–309.

Folsom, A. I., H. A. O'Brien, and G. T. Caldwell (1940). "Subtotal Cystectomy in the treatment of Hunner Ulcer." *J Urol* 44: 650.

Frederiksen H., A. Arner, U. Malmquist, R.S. Scott, and B. Uvelius (2004). "Nerve induced responses and force-velocity relations of regenerated detrusor muscle after subtotal cystectomy in the rat." *Neurourol Urodyn* 23: 159–165.

Gleeson, M. J. and D. P. Griffith (1992). "The use of alloplastic biomaterials in bladder substitution." *J Urol* 148(5): 1377–1382.

Goldstein, A. M., V. Gualtieri, and P. L. Getzoff (1970). "Expansion mechanisms of the partially cystectomized bladder: an experimental study in rabbits." *J Urol* 104(3): 413–417.

Gurocak, S., R. P. De Gier, and W. Feitz (2007). "Bladder augmentation without integration of intact bowel segments: critical review and future perspectives." *J Urol* 177(3): 839–844.

Hodde, J. (2002). "Naturally occurring scaffolds for soft tissue repair and regeneration." *Tissue Eng* 8(2): 295–308.

Jack, G. S., R. Zhang, M. Lee, Y. Xu, B. M. Wu, and L. V. Rodriguez (2009). "Urinary bladder smooth muscle engineered from adipose stem cells and a three dimensional synthetic composite." *Biomaterials* 30(19): 3259–3270.

Kanematsu, A., S. Yamamoto, T. Noguchi, M. Ozeki, Y. Tabata, and O. Ogawa (2003). "Bladder regeneration by bladder acellular matrix combined with sustained release of exogenous growth factor." *J Urol* 170(4 Pt 2): 1633–1638.

Kaplan, S. A., C. G. Roehrborn, E. S. Rovner, M. Carlsson, T. Bavendam, and Z. Guan (2006). "Tolterodine and tamsulosin for treatment of men with lower urinary tract symptoms and overactive bladder: a randomized controlled trial." *JAMA* 296(19): 2319–2328.

Kelami, A., A. Ludtke-Handjery, G. Korb, J. Rolle, J. Schnell, and K. H. Danigel (1970). "Alloplastic replacement of the urinary bladder wall with lyophilized human dura." *Eur Surg Res* 2(3): 195–202.

Kikuno, N., K. Kawamoto, H. Hirata, K. Vejdani, K. Kawakami, T. Fandel, L. Nunes, S. Urakami, H. Shiina, M. Igawa, E. Tanagho, and R. Dahiya (2009). "Nerve growth factor combined with vascular endothelial growth factor enhances regeneration of bladder acellular matrix graft in spinal cord injury-induced neurogenic rat bladder." *BJU Int* 103(10): 1424–1428.

Kudish, H. G. (1957). "The use of polyvinyl sponge for experimental cystoplasty." *J Urol* 78(3): 232–235.

Lai, J. Y., P. Y. Chang, and J. N. Lin (2005). "Bladder autoaugmentation using various biodegradable scaffolds seeded with autologous smooth muscle cells in a rabbit model." *J Pediatr Surg* 40(12): 1869–1873.

Liang, D. S. (1962). "Bladder regeneration following subtotal cystectomy." *J Urol* 88: 503–505.

Liang, D. S. and R. J. Goss (1963). "Regeneration of the bladder after subtotal cystectomy in rats." *J Urol* 89: 427–430.

Lin, A. T., K. Kato, F. Monson, A. J. Wein, and R. M. Levin (1989). "Pharmacological responses of rabbit urinary bladder after subtotal cystectomy." *J Urol* 142(2 Pt 1): 409–412.

Loai, Y., H. Yeger, C. Coz, R. Antoon, S. S. Islam, K. Moore, and W. A. Farhat (2010). "Bladder tissue engineering: tissue regeneration and neovascularization of HA-VEGF-incorporated bladder acellular constructs in mouse and porcine animal models." *J Biomed Mater Res A* 94(4): 1205–1215.

Machingal, M. A., B. T. Corona, T. J. Walters, V. Kesireddy, C. N. Koval, A. Dannahower, W. Zhao, J. J. Yoo, and G. J. Christ (2011). "A tissue-engineered muscle repair construct for functional restoration of an irrecoverable muscle injury in a murine model." *Tissue Eng Part A* 17(17–18): 2291–2303.

McCallum, D. C. (1965). "Gangrene of the bladder with subsequent regrowth." *J Urol* 94(6): 669–670.

Meezan, E., J. T. Hjelle, K. Brendel, and E. C. Carlson (1975). "A simple, versatile, nondisruptive method for the isolation of morphologically and chemically pure basement membranes from several tissues." *Life Sci* 17(11): 1721–1732.

Moon du, G., G. Christ, J. D. Stitzel, A. Atala, and J. J. Yoo (2008). "Cyclic mechanical preconditioning improves engineered muscle contraction." *Tissue Eng Part A* 14(4): 473–482.

Oberpenning, F., J. Meng, J. J. Yoo, and A. Atala (1999). "De novo reconstitution of a functional mammalian urinary bladder by tissue engineering." *Nat Biotechnol* 17(2): 149–155.

Peyton, C. C., D. Burmeister, B. Petersen, K. E. Andersson, G. J. Christ (2012). "Characterization of the early proliferative response of the rodent bladder to subtotal cystectomy: a unique model of Mammalian organ regeneration." *PLoS One* (10):e47414. doi: 0.1371/journal.pone.0047414. Epub 2012 Oct 12.

Portilla Sanchez, R., F. L. Blanco, A. Santamarina, J. Casals Roa, J. Mata, and A. Kaufman (1958). "Vesical regeneration in the human after total cystectomy and implantation of a plastic mould." *Br J Urol* 30(2): 180–188.

Reyblat, P. and D. A. Ginsberg (2008). "Augmentation cystoplasty: what are the indications?" *Curr Urol Rep* 9(6): 452–458.

Richardson, E. J. (1952). "Bladder regeneration case report and review of the literature." *Minn Med* 35(6): 547–549.

Ross, G., Jr., I. M. Thompson, K. K. Keown, Jr., B. B. Judy, and G. E. Gammel (1969). "Further observations on the role of smooth muscle regeneration." *J Urol* 102(1): 49–52.

Schwartz, R. (1891). "Ricerche in proposito della rigenerazione della vescica urinaria." *Sperimentale* 45: 484.

Sharma, A. K., M. I. Bury, A. J. Marks, N. J. Fuller, J. W. Meisner, N. Tapaskar, L. C. Halliday, D. J. Matoka, and E. Y. Cheng (2010a). "A Non-Human Primate Model for Urinary Bladder Regeneration Utilizing Autologous Sources of Bone Marrow Derived Mesenchymal Stem Cells." *Stem Cells*.

Sharma, A. K., P. V. Hota, D. J. Matoka, N. J. Fuller, D. Jandali, H. Thaker, G. A. Ameer, and E. Y. Cheng (2010b). "Urinary bladder smooth muscle regeneration utilizing bone marrow derived mesenchymal stem cell seeded elastomeric poly-(1,8-octanediol-co-citrate) based thin films." *Biomaterials* 31(24): 6207–6217.

Sisk, I. R. and V. F. Neu (1939). "Regeneration of the Bladder." *Trans Am Assn G.U Surg* 32: 197.

Staack, A., S. W. Hayward, L. S. Baskin, and G. R. Cunha (2005). "Molecular, cellular and developmental biology of urothelium as a basis of bladder regeneration." *Differentiation* 73(4): 121–133.

Sutherland, R. S., L. S. Baskin, S. W. Hayward, and G. R. Cunha (1996). "Regeneration of bladder urothelium, smooth muscle, blood vessels and nerves into an acellular tissue matrix." *J Urol* 156(2 Pt 2): 571–577.

Taguchi, H., E. Ishizuka, and K. Saito (1977). "Cystoplasty by regeneration of the bladder." *J Urol* 118(5): 752–756.

Tucci, P. and G. Haralambidis (1963). "Regeneration of the Bladder: Review of Literature and Case Report." *J Urol* 90: 193–199.

Yang B, Y. Zhang Y, L. Zhou , Z. Sun, J. Zheng, Y. Chen, Y, Dai. (2010). "Development of a porcine bladder acellular matrix with well-preserved extracellular bioactive factors for tissue engineering." *Tissue Eng Part C Methods* 16: 1201–1211.

Youssif M., H. Shiina, S. Urakami, C. Gleason, L. Nunes, M. Igawa, H. Enokida, E. A. Tanagho, R. Dahiya. (2005). "Effect of vascular endothelial growth factor on regeneration of bladder acellular matrix graft: histologic and functional evaluation." *Urology* 66(1): 201–207.

Zhang, Y., D. Frimberger, E. Y. Cheng, H. K. Lin, and B. P. Kropp (2006). "Challenges in a larger bladder replacement with cell-seeded and unseeded small intestinal submucosa grafts in a subtotal cystectomy model." *BJU Int* 98(5): 1100–1105.

Zhang, Y., H. K. Lin, D. Frimberger, R. B. Epstein, and B. P. Kropp (2005). "Growth of bone marrow stromal cells on small intestinal submucosa: an alternative cell source for tissue engineered bladder." *BJU Int* 96(7): 1120–1125.

Zhu, W. D., Y. M. Xu, C. Feng, Q. Fu, L. J. Song, and L. Cui (2010). "Bladder reconstruction with adipose-derived stem cell-seeded bladder acellular matrix grafts improve morphology composition." *World J Urol* 28(4): 493–498.

3

Mechanical Control of Adult Mesenchymal Stem Cells in Cardiac Applications

PETER A. GALIE AND JAN P. STEGEMANN

Introduction: Mesenchymal Stem Cells and the Cardiac Microenvironment

Adult mesenchymal stem cells (MSCs) are multipotent progenitor cells that have shown promise in a wide range of regenerative treatments spanning fields as diverse as oncology, orthopedics, and cardiology. In recent years, MSCs have been implanted into patients with various myocardium-related pathologies, including dilated cardiomyopathy, concentric hypertrophy, and others related to heart failure. Although the mechanism by which these cells repair damaged tissue or restore function is currently a topic of debate, these cells have been shown to have beneficial effects in regenerating myocardial function upon injection [1,2,3–11]. It has been hypothesized that the implanted cells regenerate tissue through paracrine effects [12–14], cell fusion with damaged cells [15–18], as well as through differentiation into cardiomyocytes [19–22]. However, the extent to which damaged myocardium uses stem cell homing from the circulation as a repair mechanism is not clear, bringing into question the effectiveness of cell implantation [1]. Regardless of whether MSCs act by one of these mechanisms or a combination of them, controlling their phenotype is highly relevant to the repair of damaged myocardial tissue. This chapter focuses on the use of these cells for the regeneration of damaged myocardial tissue, particularly the effects of mechanical stimuli in controlling the phenotype and function of MSCs in cardiac applications.

The biochemical environment of the myocardium is characterized by a variety of messenger molecules that influence the contractility of the tissue. The cardiac action potential is governed by voltage-dependent channels that act as gates for sodium, potassium, and calcium, and the concentrations of these solutes are affected by β_1-adrenergic and muscarinic receptors, which in turn are acted on by soluble agents such as norepinephrine and acetylcholine. Because MSCs are implanted into damaged areas of the heart, there often are additional biochemical factors present as a consequence of local tissue fibrosis or ischemia. For example, hypertension

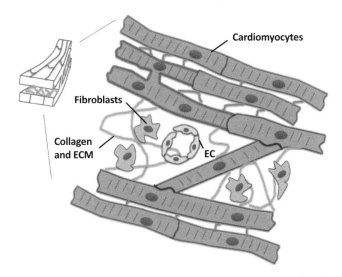

Figure 3-1. Microstructure of adjacent myocardium lamina. Branching is more preva-lent between myocytes on the same laminar sheet than between the sheets. The laminar sheets are connected by a network of extracellular proteins interspersed with cardiac fibroblasts and vascular-related cells. EC = endothelial cells; ECM = extracellular matrix.

can cause an imbalance of matrix metalloproteinases (MMPs) and tissue inhibitors of MMPs (TIMPs) [23]. In addition, ischemic conditions, as well as tissue necrosis factor (TNF), can cause MSC to release vascular endothelial growth factor (VEGF) through a signal transducer and activator of transcription 3 (STAT3) and p38 mitogen-activated protein kinase (MAPK)–dependent pathway [24,25]. It is postulated that VEGF may be an important factor in the mechanism by which MSCs repair damaged myocardium through paracrine action; further evidence indicates that VEGF may also be important in stimulating MSC differentiation to cardiomyocytes [21].

The structure of the extracellular matrix (ECM) is also specific to the myocardium. Cardiac tissue cells are surrounded by a matrix consisting mostly of type I colla-gen with lesser amounts of types III and V. The cardiac environment also is rich in fibronectin, elastin, and laminin. A schematic depiction of this environment is illus-trated in Figure 3-1. The majority of these components are synthesized by cardiac fibroblasts, which account for about two-thirds of the cells in the myocardium [26]. In an important study of MSC differentiation, it was shown that the compliance of adhesion substrates strongly affects MSC phenotype [27]. This finding has potential relevance to cardiac pathologies and therapies because the mechanical properties of the predominately collagen myocardium may influence cardiomyocyte phenotype. In particular, stiffer environments caused by cardiac fibrosis could disrupt MSC engraft-ment into host tissue and inhibit differentiation into cardiomyocytes. Hence, there has been increasing interest in designing tailored matrix microenvironments to direct differentiation of stem cells both before and after transplantation [28].

Cells in the heart walls experience a combination of compressive and tensile stresses, as well as fluid shear stress from the myocardium's interstitial fluid. The environment is also characterized by its dynamic nature because of the continual beating of the heart. Advances in finite element modeling have increased our understanding of myocardial mechanical loading, and computational fluid dynamics simulations have been used to simulate the flow of blood in the lumen of the ventricle and interstitial fluid through the tissue [29,30]. Recent studies have used this knowledge of cardiac mechanics to investigate how MSCs respond to the different components of the mechanical environment encountered when implanted into the myocardium. These studies have analyzed the effects of cyclic, uniaxial strain on the cells in both tension and compression [26,31–34], as well as how shear stress affects MSC phenotype [33,35,36]. As with biochemical and matrix factors, disease states can alter the mechanical environment of the myocardium and lead to changes in MSC behavior [37].

Current Status of Mesenchymal Stem Cell Implantation for Cardiac Repair

The ability to control MSC phenotype is of high importance in developing progenitor cell-based cardiac therapies. Clinical trials using MSC implantation to improve cardiac function already have been initiated, although our understanding of MSC phenotype control is primitive. Despite a number of excellent studies in the area, the specific mechanisms by which MSCs function in the heart remains unclear, especially in response to the mechanical microenvironment of the myocardium. It has been proposed that MSCs can differentiate into cardiomyocytes, produce cytokines or other paracrine factors, or fuse with existing tissue cells, but the control and relative contribution of these effects is not understood. There is even a question of how long these cells reside in the damaged myocardium after transplant. However, there is good evidence that implanting MSCs into failing hearts can improve function in both animal and human studies. This section gives examples of approaches used in applying MSCs to cardiac repair as naked cell injection, monolayer transplantation, and in scaffold-assisted approaches. Figure 3-2 is a schematic illustrating these different approaches.

Several animal injury models have been created to demonstrate the effect of injected MSCs on ischemic and fibrotic myocardial tissue. The two primary locations of MSC injection in the heart are directly into the myocardium (intramyocardial) and into the coronary artery (intracoronary). Both injection methods have demonstrated positive results despite the common obstacle of cell engraftment within the fibrotic myocardium. An advantage of injection into the vasculature is the resulting distribution of any paracrine factors released by the stem cells to perfused tissue [38,39]. However, fibrotic regions of the myocardium may suffer from reduced blood flow when the occluded artery remains blocked [40], and a recent study has

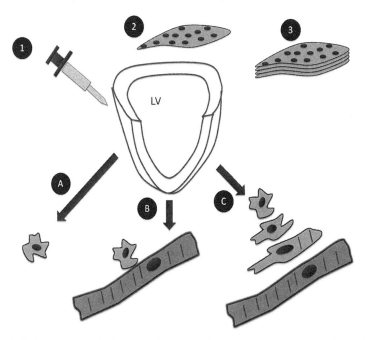

Figure 3-2. Delivery techniques and proposed mechanisms of mesenchymal stem cell implantation. LV = left ventricle.
 1) Naked cell delivery
 2) Monolayer transplantation
 3) Three-dimensional scaffold transplantation
    A) Paracrine effects
    B) Cell fusion
    C) Differentiation into a myocyte-related lineage

demonstrated that intracoronary injection is associated with reduced blood flow after the treatment [41]. The primary advantage of intramyocardial injection is the ability to localize the treatment directly to the fibrotic region. Cells injected in this manner often improve cardiac function through formation of new vasculature [5,6] and have even been associated with reduction of arrhythmias [9]. Using a rat model of idiopathic dilated cardiomyopathy (IDC), it was found that intramyocardially injected MSCs induced angiogenesis and myogenesis through direct differentiation into both vascular-associated cells and cardiomyocytes, as well as through the production of angiogenic, antiapoptotic, and mitogenic factors, including VEGF, hepatocyte growth factor, adrenomedullin, and insulin-like growth factor 1 (IGF-1) [2].

In addition to direct MSC injection, other methods of cell delivery to the heart have been investigated. For example, monolayers of cultured MSC without exogenous matrix support have been grafted onto the surface of scar tissue in the myocardium [42]. The cells produced significant amounts of ECM components while in culture, and the implanted cell sheet produced a substantial amount of new tissue that showed evidence of angiogenesis. The results suggested that the majority of MSC did not differentiate into cardiomyocytes but rather acted through paracrine action to stimulate formation new tissue and vasculature [42]. It was hypothesized that a major benefit of this extra tissue was to decrease overall wall stress on the damaged myocardium, but in other respects, the monolayer technique produced similar effects as an injection method used for a similar injury model [3]. Both studies suggested that paracrine effects of the implanted MSCs outweighed the benefit of direct differentiation into cardiomyocytes.

The idea of using a cardiac patch seeded with MSC applied directly to the epicardium also has shown promise. The concept behind this technique is to deliver cells while they are seeded into the type of matrix they will encounter in the native environment of the heart. For example, a study using a type I collagen patch populated with MSCs found a significant improvement in heart function in rat infarction models [43] without signs of rejection. However, the authors did not find any significant improvement in wall thinning. Another study used a polyethylene glycol–modified fibrin, a degradable material that allows the gradual release of MSCs into the affected area [44]. Using a murine postinfarct model, this patch was able to significantly improve the hemodynamic function of the heart, especially ejection fraction. A recent study used a portion of decellularized swine myocardium as a scaffold for a cellular patch seeded with bone marrow mononuclear cells [45]. Such patches attempt to reconstitute certain key aspects of the extracellular environment, but the effects of mechanical stresses on such materials have not been fully investigated.

The question of how the cells yield these beneficial effects is controversial. Initially, because of the multipotency of the cells, the prevailing belief was that the cells would differentiate to a cardiac-specific lineage and even exhibit cardiomyocyte-like properties. Several studies have supported this theory. In MSCs derived from adipose tissue, it was found that increased levels of VEGF were associated with an increase in the expression of cardiomyocyte-specific markers Nkx2.5 and GATA-4 [21], although the mean rate of differentiation was low. The DNA methyltransferase inhibitor 5-azacytidine also might induce MSC differentiation into cardiomyocytes, as characterized by the expression of markers such as cardiac troponin T, beta myosin heavy chain, and alpha actinin [19]. One study of a swine infarct model presented immunofluorescence data indicating MSC expression of alpha-actinin, troponin T, tropomyosin, and phospholamban [22]. However, it is not been clearly shown that implanted MSCs can progress into terminally differentiated, functioning adult cardiomyocytes in vivo or in vitro. In fact, the benefit of differentiation to a cardiomyocyte remains questionable given the potential for arrhythmias that would arise if the newly differentiated cardiomyocytes were not aligned correctly with the existing myocardial architecture.

Several studies have provided evidence that MSCs may fuse with damaged cardiomyocytes, which may be a mechanism of reparative function [15–18]. Another proposed mode of action of implanted MSCs is the release of paracrine factors that have angiogenic and cardioprotective effects. These paracrine mechanisms include but are not limited to factors that work through the prosurvival PI3K/Akt pathway (hepatocyte growth factor, IGF-1, VEGF, adrenomedullin), the cardioprotective protein kinase C pathway (fibroblast growth factor 2 and erythropoietin), and neovascularization (VEGF) [14]. Likewise, MSCs transduced to overexpress certain signaling molecules such as Akt, myocardin, and tumor necrosis factor receptor can improve paracrine release and cell survival [46–50]. However, recent studies have yielded mixed results concerning certain metrics of cardiac function [51] and the effect of Akt overexpression on commitment to a specific lineage [52]. Studies have also investigated the paracrine effect of implanted MSCs on Kit+ cardiac stem cells (CSCs). MSCs have been associated with increased proliferation and differentiation of CSCs [53] for which the release of VEGF and stromal cell–derived factor 1 may be responsible [54]. An emerging theory is that MSCs may actually begin to express characteristics of CSCs when in the myocardium [55].

Although strong evidence exists of the benefits of using MSC for cardiac repair, there also have been suggestions that such treatments are not efficacious and can in fact be harmful. In particular, there have been questions about the value of implanting isolated MSCs into the myocardium compared with injecting the angiogenic, anti-apoptotic, or mitogenic factors they release. Several studies have shown evidence of cell homing to the damaged myocardium [1]; therefore, cytokines that induce this cell homing could be injected instead of MSCs. In fact, several recent studies indicated that injecting conditioned media from MSCs improved various metrics of cardiac function [56,57]. An in vitro model also demonstrated the cardioprotective effects of conditioned media [58]. Additionally, bone marrow–derived MSC injected into a murine model of acute infarction were found to create bonelike deposits in the myocardium [59]. The implanted MSCs were labeled, and it was found that they expressed osteocalcin, a marker of osteogenic differentiation, although other studies using similar delivery methods and injury models have not observed this effect. However, the ability of MSCs to commit to osteogenic and chondrogenic lineages is well established [60–63]. Another study found evidence that implanted MSCs may actually contribute to scar formation in the infarcted myocardium [64]. These studies suggest that perhaps acellular therapies may be preferred over those applying living cells.

A number of clinical trials involving the delivery of MSCs to the heart are currently being conducted. An early trial focused on people with severe ischemic heart failure [3]. Autologous MSCs isolated from the bone marrow of patients were injected intramyocardially using a catheter. Results from this early work suggested that the injected MSCs helped to improve heart function primarily through an angiogenic effect. Similarly, a recent clinical trial used intracoronary injection to deliver a mix of endothelial progenitor cells and MSCs to stimulate formation of new blood vessels and found an improvement in ejection fraction [65]. Other trials have also shown the benefit of intravenously injected MSCs for treating myocardial infarct patients [66]. These trials highlight the need for understanding how implanted MSCs are affected by the myocardial microenvironment.

The field of MSC transplantation would benefit greatly from a more complete understanding of how the mechanics of the myocardium affect MSC phenotype. The mechanical environment in the heart changes not only with different pathologies but also with the type of implantation technique. The remainder of this chapter focuses on the mechanical environment in the heart and discusses examples of published studies focusing on the effect of mechanical stimuli on MSC phenotype and how this relationship can be used to better control these cells for cardiac repair.

The Mechanical Environment of the Heart

Cells in the heart wall experience a multifaceted mechanical environment that includes tensile and compressive stresses, bending moments, and shear exerted by the contraction and relaxation of cardiomyocytes [67,68]. In addition to the solid mechanical stresses, cells in the myocardium are exposed to fluid pressure, and shear forces are exerted by the flow of interstitial fluid within the myocardium [69]. Heart tissue is anisotropic and dynamic; therefore, the stress state varies both spatially and temporally. Figure 3-3 illustrates several components of this complex mechanical environment. Cardiac pathologies can change the structure and composition of heart tissue, and subsequent delivery of pharmacological or surgical treatment can further alter the mechanical environment. Because of the complexity of the mechanical milieu in the heart wall, computational and analytical models are important tools in studying both the tissue and cell-level behavior of the heart. Experimental approaches to measuring strains and fluid transport in the heart also have been developed [70,71] and yield crucial insight into the mechanics of the myocardium.

The architecture of the heart is one of the primary determinants of the stress state in the myocardium as the cardiac cycle progresses. Although strongly anisotropic, mammalian heart tissue has a mostly uniform structure and order. The myocardial wall is a composite of repeating laminar sheets each approximately four myocytes thick [72]. Within the wall, myocytes branch and connect with one another through gap junctions, and their interactions with type I collagen fibers form myofibrils within the laminar sheets. Branching between laminar sheets also occurs, although to a lesser extent. This affects depolarization of the myocardium during systole because by some estimates the conduction velocity is two to three times greater along the plane of the lamina compared with the transverse direction [72]. The lamina also are connected by collagen fibers, although these tend to be thin and uncoiled [72–74]. It has been postulated that this structure facilitates a sliding movement between the laminar sheets, resulting in a physiologically important shearing component of mechanical stress.

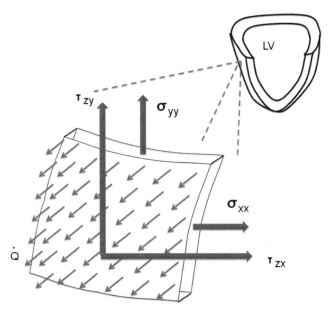

Figure 3-3. Three-dimensional mechanical stress environment in the myocardium. A section of the myocardium sustains normal stresses because of contraction and expansion during systole and diastole. Shear stress along the surface is created by slippage between laminar sheets. Moreover, interstitial fluid flow is driven by perfusion from vasculature as well as the pressure gradient between endocardium and epicardium. LV = left ventricle; $\dot{Q}$ = fluid flow rate; σ_{xx} = normal stress in the x-direction; σ_{yy} = normal stress to the y-direction; $\mathbf{T}_{zx}$ = shear stress in the z-x plane; $\mathbf{T}_{zy}$ = shear stress in the z-y plane.

During systole, the heart produces ejection fractions of 60 to 70 percent, which is accompanied by radial thickening of the heart wall of around 40 percent. However, the maximum contraction of an individual myocyte is limited to approximately 15 percent [73]. This discrepancy in dimensional changes is thought to be a result of the shear exerted by slip between lamina in the myocardium, which causes thickening of the heart wall as myocytes contract, in addition to influencing the orientation of the cells within the sheets [70,73,74]. The myocardium exhibits subtle differences in fiber orientation between areas within the sheets and the orientation of the sheets themselves, with respect to an orthogonal coordinate system. Fiber angles vary from −60 degrees at the endocardium to +60 degrees at the epicardium, creating a helical pattern to the radial direction of the wall [73]. However, the sheet angles of the lamina are restricted to either −45 or +45 degrees and alternate depending on the location of the sheet in the myocardium [73]. Because the sheet orientations are alternating, the lamina slide along one another in different directions even though the magnitude of the shear deformation is uniform across the wall [73], causing a net thickening of the wall. In addition, the orientation of these sheets has been shown to align with planes of maximum shear strain [70,74].

The importance of interstitial flow to cardiac tissue is well recognized [63,75]. Because of the large deformation of the heart wall during the cardiac cycle, the interstitial fluid undergoes substantial flux and consequently exerts a pressure and shear force on cells within the myocardium. The fluid balance within the myocardium is controlled by the perfusion of the coronary artery and corresponding microcirculation as well as by lymphatic drainage that transports the products of cell metabolism [69,76]. Moreover, the factors that control fluid balance are strongly interdependent [77]. For example, the pressure of the interstitial fluid is a regulator of the rate of perfusion. This effect is manifested during systole, when perfusion in the coronary capillaries is impeded because of the high pressure existing in the contracting myocardium. In addition, the myocardium separates two different bodies of fluid: the endocardium surrounds the blood-filled cardiac chambers, and the epicardium is surrounded by epicardial fluid. Consequently, a pressure gradient in the radial direction of the myocardium may influence interstitial fluid flow [69]. Evidence indicates that the flow of interstitial fluid affects the development of fibrosis [78].

The cardiac mechanical environment is strongly affected by and may be contributing factor to the damaging effects of various pathologies. Many of the pathologies affecting the heart, including acute infarction, dilated cardiomyopathy, and others, are associated with changes in the ECM. These conditions affect the interaction between the sheets of cardiomyocytes and consequently the stresses exerted on the resident cells. In the case of acute myocardial infarction, the heart progresses through ischemic, necrotic, fibrotic, and remodeling phases that are each characterized by different mechanical properties [79]. The necrotic phase is characterized by edema, which affects the transport of the interstitial fluid within the myocardium. During the fibrotic phase, the mechanics are influenced by excess collagen, the cross-linking of which changes the mechanical environment during remodeling [79]. Changes in the ECM have profound effects on the mechanism of contraction during systole and flexion during diastole. In a canine model of infarction, researchers found that the twisting motion of the heart during systole was significantly reduced by fibrosis [80]. Other studies have found that the wall stress increases with the size of a remodeling left ventricle, indicating that excess collagen increases the stress on cells in the myocardium [81]. Therefore, both normal and pathological tissue mechanics are of importance when examining the behavior of cardiac cells in response to mechanical stimuli.

Modeling the structural mechanics of the heart is challenging because of the tissue's complex microstructure. In addition, comprehensive models must account for the large and cyclical deformations of the tissue, as well as the interaction between the fluid mechanics of blood in the ventricle lumen with the structural mechanics of the myocardial wall. Such models necessarily require that simplifying assumptions be made, and validation of these assumptions is often made difficult by the lack of experimental data, although more empirical data are becoming available [70,74,77]. However, useful models have been constructed and applied to further our understanding of cardiac mechanics. An example of a model that has incorporated both solid and fluid elements is a finite element model that incorporates an arbitrary Lagrangian-Eulerian reference frame to track the interaction between blood and the left ventricle wall [29]. Although this study was limited to the left ventricle, it validated such key concepts as the thickening of the myocardial wall during systole. Other studies have been able to predict the planes of maximum shear strain [70], and more complex models that incorporate the complex tissue structure and solid–fluid interactions in the heart are emerging.

The Effect of the Myocardial Mechanical Environment on Mesenchymal Stem Cell Phenotype

The manner in which MSCs respond to the mechanical environment when implanted into the myocardium depends strongly on the mode, location, and timing of delivery, as well as on the pathology being treated. Because of the complexity of the in vivo environment of the heart, most studies of mechanical stimulation of MSCs to date have relied on relatively simple in vitro culture models, which provide a more controllable setting for studying specific stimuli. These experimental systems provide only an approximation of the in vivo environment, and it is difficult to recapitulate the complex combined loading regimens experienced by cells in the myocardium. Despite these limitations, in vitro experiments and modeling have proven useful for understanding both cardiomyocyte and cardiac fibroblast mechanobiology [82–84] by providing valuable and insightful information on the effects of specific loading modes on MSC phenotype. The effects that have been studied include changes in cell phenotype and proliferation, as well as the secretion of antiapoptotic, angiogenic, mitogenic, and other factors.

Two-dimensional culture of MSCs on deformable substrates has provided insight into how these cells are affected by mechanical signals. Cyclic tension has been found to have a strong effect on several aspects of MSC phenotype. Exposure to 10 percent cyclical, uniaxial tension at 1 Hz for 7 days causes the actin cytoskeleton of the cell to align, impedes proliferation, and increases expression of smooth muscle alpha-actin and calponin [31]. These results suggest differentiation into a smooth muscle cell (SMC) phenotype rather than a cardiomyocyte lineage. Such experiments have been repeated on both collagen and elastin substrates, and it was shown that exposure of MSCs to two-dimensional equiaxial strain downregulates the production of smooth muscle alpha-actin and other SMC markers [34]. In another study, equibiaxial strain caused an increase in proliferation of MSC [85]. These varying responses suggest that MSC phenotype depends on the type of mechanical loading. The observed differentiation toward the SMC phenotype in a subset of these studies suggests that the primary benefit of implanted MSCs may be formation of new vasculature, as confirmed by multiple in vivo studies.

Three-dimensional cultures of MSCs embedded in protein matrices also have been used to study mechanical effects on cell phenotype. In particular, MSCs embedded in three-dimensional collagen type I matrices have been subjected to either uniaxial or biaxial strains. One such study found that MSCs form multicellular units in response to cyclic strain [86]. In one such study, a construct seeded with MSCs was exposed to either 10 or 12 percent strain at 1 Hz for 4 hours a day for 1 week, and the cells produced significant levels of bone markers such as bone morphogenetic protein 2 [61]. An osteogenic response was also observed in another study using a similar type of construct for a wider range of strain values and lower frequency [87] and in a study in which MSCs were seeded on a synthetic polymer scaffold and exposed to cyclic compression [88]. These studies did not assess markers of the cardiomyocyte or SMC phenotype, but their results are aligned with the observed presence of bone markers in an in vivo study of implanted MSCs [59]. A recent study suggested the osteogenic response may be mediated by transforming growth factor-β [89]. These studies imply that three-dimensional culture in collagen matrices under mechanical loading promotes osteogenic differentiation in MSCs. However, it is difficult to make broad conclusions based on in vitro studies that recapitulate only selected aspects of the in vivo environment.

Fluid shear in the myocardium has been shown to affect the depolarization of neonatal cardiomyocytes [35] as well as the alignment and branching of these cells [75]. The effect of fluid stresses on MSCs in three-dimensional environments has not been extensively studied but is an important area of investigation if these cells are to be transplanted into the heart. Studies of embryonic stem cells exposed to fluid shear showed that these cells differentiate to endothelial cell types, as evidenced by the expression of von Willebrand factor [36]. In a study focused on MSCs, cells were plated on two-dimensional surfaces and exposed to pressure-dominant, shear-dominant, and combined constant fluid stresses. It was found that fluid shear and compressive stress individually and in combination led to the expression of SMC-like markers, including alpha smooth muscle actin and smooth muscle myosin heavy chain [90]. This study did not examine the presence of any cardiac-specific markers, but the resulting cell morphology resembled the smooth muscle phenotype. A recent study did analyze the effects of perfusion in a three-dimensional scaffold and found that flow affected MSC morphology and cell interactions [91].

The effects of combined fluid shear stress and cyclical tension on MSC phenotype also have been investigated. In a study aimed at developing engineered heart valves using MSCs seeded in a three-dimensional polymeric scaffold, it was found that cell response depended on the type of loading: flexure, fluid shear, or combined loading. Under combined loading, MSCs were responsible for a 75 percent increase in collagen deposition on the polymeric substrate. Moreover, the cells tested positive for such endothelial markers as CD31, laminin, and von Willebrand factor [92]. In another example of combined loading, MSCs were seeded on the lumen of a silicone tube and exposed to both 5 percent radial distention and a shear stress of 1 Pa at a frequency of 1 Hz. The MSCs on the silicone tubes aligned in the direction of the flow as endothelial cells would, but they expressed SMC markers including alpha smooth muscle actin and calponin [93].

The mechanical properties of individual MSCs also have been examined. Using a micropipette aspiration technique, it was found that these cells are inherently viscoelastic and that the mechanical properties are strongly dependent on the organization of the actin cytoskeleton [94]. The measured properties were fit to a linear viscoelasticity model of the cells for use in future modeling studies. Temperature was shown to modulate cell mechanical properties, and it is likely that the mechanics of the cells are also altered by other factors relevant to implantation into the myocardium. For example, understanding how mechanical properties change in the presence of different biochemicals or in reduced oxygen concentrations would be useful for cardiac applications. It has been shown that MSCs exposed to hypoxic conditions are more successful in implantation [95], but the mechanism behind this phenomenon is not clear. Therefore, the relationship between oxygen concentration and cell mechanics is an example of an area that could be probed to help determine how the success of cell transplantation is dependent on cell mechanics.

Conclusion

A better understanding of the mechanical environment in the myocardium and how these mechanical stimuli affect implanted MSC phenotype is critical to improving cell-based therapies for heart repair. Such therapies are currently being tested clinically for treatment of heart conditions, including dilated cardiomyopathy and acute myocardial infarction; therefore, there is an urgent need to better understand MSC behavior in this application. These efforts are complicated by the fact that the myocardium is a complex and heterogeneous environment and the mechanical stimuli exerted on its cells can be difficult to characterize. In addition, the mechanical environment will be affected by the pathology being treated, the progression of the disease, and the mode and location of delivery of the cells.

Studies on how MSCs react to mechanical stimuli have begun to illuminate the factors involved in controlling MSC differentiation. Few of these studies have focused specifically on cardiac applications, but they have provided insight into how MSCs might respond when delivered to the acutely or chronically injured myocardium and how these cells might act to improve cardiac function. In vitro studies focused directly on mechanical stimulation of MSCs have suggested that these cells respond quite differently to cyclic tension and compression when it is applied in two-dimensional systems versus a three-dimensional manner. Whereas tensile and compressive loading of MSCs in two-dimensional systems tends to promote differentiation toward the smooth muscle lineage, the same type of stimuli applied to three-dimensional constructs appears to encourage differentiation to an osteogenic lineage. However, combining tension and compression with fluid shear stress in three-dimensional systems appears to promote cardiovascular lineages. These varied responses to different combinations of mechanical stimuli applied in different systems reinforce the need for more systematic studies of the regulation of MSC phenotype by mechanical stresses, particularly in combined loading regimes.

The focus of this chapter has been on the importance of mechanical factors on MSC phenotype in cardiac applications. Clearly, MSC phenotype also is influenced by biochemical, matrix, and other environmental parameters, and these factors interact with the mechanical environment to determine cell behavior. The cardiac microenvironment is characterized by the presence of growth factors, primary and secondary messengers in both normal and pathologic states. Tissue oxygen levels, ECM content and composition, and cellularity vary with time and space in the heart and change when heart tissue is damaged. Improved knowledge of how these factors affect MSC function will allow bioengineers and surgeons to refine therapies and delivery methods to increase the probability that transplanted cells will survive, engraft, and provide therapeutic benefit.

Acknowledgments

The authors are grateful to their colleagues in the field of cardiovascular tissue engineering for their valuable insight, discussions, and support. In this chapter, we have used selected examples of published studies to illustrate key aspects of the mechanical environment in the heart, as well as mechanical control of MSC phenotype. We apologize to those whose work could not be included because of space limitations. This work was supported in part by the Microfluidics in Biomedical Sciences Training Program at the University of Michigan sponsored by the National Institute of Biomedical Imaging and Bioengineering.

References

1. Novotny N, et al. Stem cell therapy in myocardial repair and remodeling. *J Am Coll Surg* 2008; 207(3): 423–434.
2. Nagaya N, et al. Model of dilated cardiomyopathy transplantation of mesenchymal stem cells improves cardiac function in a rat. *Circulation* 2005; 112: 1128–1135.
3. Perin EC, et al. Transendocardial, autologous bone marrow cell transplantation for severe, chronic ischemic heart failure. *Circulation* 2003; 107(18): 2294–2302.
4. Yu LH, et al. Improvement of cardiac function and remodeling by transplanting adipose tissue-derived stromal cells into a mouse model of acute myocardial infarction. *Int J Cardiol* 2010; 139(2): 166–172.
5. Hu X, et al. Transplantation of hypoxia-preconditioned mesenchymal stem cells improves infarcted heart function via enhanced survival of implanted cells and angiogenesis. *J Thorac Cardiovasc Surg* 2008; 135(4): 799–808.
6. Zhou Y, et al. Marrow stromal cells differentiate into vasculature after allogeneic transplantation into ischemic myocardium. *Ann Thorac Surg* 2011; 91(4): 1206–1212.

7. Mathieu M, et al. Cell therapy with autologous bone marrow mononuclear stem cells is associated with superior cardiac recovery compared with use of nonmodified mesenchymal stem cells in a canine model of chronic myocardial infarction. *J Thorac Cardiovasc Surg* 2009; 138(3): 646–653.

8. Gnecchi M, et al. Early beneficial effects of bone marrow-derived mesenchymal stem cells overexpressing akt on cardiac metabolism after myocardial infarction. *Stem Cells* 2009; 27(4): 971–979.

9. Wang D, et al. Mesenchymal stem cell injection ameliorates the inducibility of ventricular arrhythmias after myocardial infarction in rats. *J Cardiol* 2011; 152(3): 314–320.

10. Zhou Y, et al. Direct injection of autologous mesenchymal stromal cells improves myocardial function. *Biochem Biophys Res Comm* 2009; 390(3): 902–907.

11. Meluzin J, et al. Intracoronary delivery of bone marrow cells to the acutely infarcted myocardium. *Cardiology* 2009; 112: 98–106.

12. Ohnishi S, et al. Mesenchymal stem cells attenuate cardiac fibroblast proliferation and collagen synthesis through paracrine actions. *FEBS Lett* 2007; 581: 3961–3966.

13. Segers VFM, Lee RT. Stem cell therapy for cardiac disease. *Nature* 2008; 451: 937–942.

14. Gnecchi M, et al. Paracrine mechanisms in adult stem cell signaling and therapy. *Circ Res* 2008; 103: 1204–1219.

15. Terada N, et al. Bone marrow cells adopt the phenotype of other cells by spontaneous cell fusion. *Nature* 2002; 416: 542–545.

16. Avitabile D, et al. Human cord blood CD34+ progenitor cells acquire functional cardiac properties through a cell fusion process. *Am J Physiol Heart Circ* 2011; 300(5): H1875–1884.

17. Nygren J, et al. Bone-marrow derived hematopoietic cells generate cardiomyocytes at a low frequency through cell fusion, but not transdifferentiation. *Nat Med* 2004; 10(5): 494–501.

18. Acquistapace A, et al. Human mesenchymal stem cells reprogram adult cardiomyocytes towards a progenitor-like state through partial cell fusion and mitochondria transfer. *Stem Cells* 2011; 29(5): 812–824.

19. Xu W, et al. Mesenchymal stem cells from adult human bone marrow differentiate into a cardiomyocyte phenotype in vitro. *Exp Biol Med* 2004; 229: 623–631.

20. Lu T, et al. Cardiomyocyte differentiation of rat bone marrow multipotent progenitor cells is associated with downregulation of Oct-4 expression. *Tissue Eng Part A* 2010; 16(10): 3111–3117.

21. Song Y, et al. VEGF is critical for spontaneous differentiation of stem cells into cardiomyocytes. *Biochem Biophys Res Comm* 2007; 354: 999–1003.

22. Shake J, et al. Mesenchymal stem cell implantation in a swine myocardial infarct model: engraftment and functional effects. *Ann Thorac Surg* 2002; 73: 1919–1926.

23. Berk B, Fujiwara K, Lehoux S. ECM remodeling in hypertensive heart disease. *J Clin Invest* 2007; 117(3): 568–75.

24. Wang M, et al. STAT3 mediates bone marrow mesenchymal stem cell VEGF production. *J Mol Cell Cardiol* 2007; 42 1009–1015.

25. Herrmann JL, et al. IL-6 and TGF-alpha costimulate mesenchymal stem cell VEGF production by ERK, JNK, and PI3K-mediated mechanisms. *Shock* 2011; 35(5): 512–516.

26. MacKenna D, et al. Role of mechanical factors in modulating cardiac fibroblast function and extracellular matrix synthesis. *Cardiovasc Res* 2000; 46: 257–263.

27. Engler A, et al. Matrix elasticity directs stem cell lineage specification. *Cell* 2006; 126: 677–689.

28. Batorsky A, et al. Encapsulation of adult human mesenchymal stem cells within collagen-agarose microenvironments. *Biotechnol Bioeng* 2005; 92(4): 492–500.

29. Watanabe H, et al. Multiphysics simulation of left ventricular filling dynamics using fluid-structure interaction finite element method. *Biophys J* 2004; 87: 2074–2085.
30. Oertel H, et al. *Modeling Human Cardiac Fluid Mechanics*. 2nd ed. Universitatsverlag Karlsruhe, Germany, 2006.
31. Hamilton D, et al. Characterization of the response of bone marrow-derived progenitor cells to cyclic strain: implications for vascular tissue-engineering applications. *Tissue Eng* 2004; 10(3/4).
32. Kobayashi N, et al. Mechanical stress promotes the expression of smooth muscle-like properties in marrow stromal cells. *Exp Hematol* 2004; 32: 1238–1245.
33. Park J, et al. Mechanobiology of mesenchymal stem cells and their use in cardiovascular repair. *Frontiers Biosci* 12 (2007), 5098–5116.
34. Park J, et al. Differential effects of equiaxial and uniaxial strain on mesenchymal stem cells. *Biotechnol Bioeng* 2004; 88(3).
35. Kong CR, et al. Mechanoelectrical excitation by fluid jets in monolayers of cultured cardiac myocytes. *J Appl Physiol* 2005; 98: 2328–2336.
36. Wang H, et al. Shear stress induces endothelial differentiation from a murine embryonic mesenchymal progenitor cell line. *Arterioscler Thromb Vasc Biol* 2005; 25: 1817–1823.
37. Wang X, Li Q. The roles of mesenchymal stem cells (MSC) therapy in ischemic heart diseases. *Biochem Biophys Res Comm* 359 (2007) 189–193.
38. Barallobre-Barreiro J, et al. Gene expression profiles following intracoronary injection of mesenchymal stromal cells using a porcine model of chronic myocardial infarction. *Cytotherapy* 2011; 13(4): 407–418.
39. Gyöngyösi M, et al. Hypoxia-inducible factor 1-alpha release after intracoronary versus intramyocardial stem cell therapy in myocardial infarction. *J Cardiovasc Transl Res* 2010; 3(2): 114–121.
40. Germain P, et al. Myocardial flow reserve parametric map, assessed by first-pass MRI compartmental analysis at the chronic stage of infarction. *J Magn Reson Imaging* 2001; 13(3): 352–360.
41. Gyöngyösi M, et al. Delayed recovery of myocardial blood flow after intracoronary stem cell administration. *Stem Cell Rev* 2011; 7(3): 616–623.
42. Miyahara Y, et al. Monolayered mesenchymal stem cells repair scarred myocardium after myocardial infarction. *Nat Med* 2006; 12(4): 459–465.
43. Simpson D, et al. A tissue engineering approach to progenitor cell delivery results in significant cell engraftment and improved myocardial remodeling. *Stem Cells* 2007; 25: 2350–2357.
44. Zhang GE, et al. Enhancing a PEGylated fibrin biomatrix. *Tissue Eng Part A* 2008; 14(6).
45. Wang B, et al. Fabrication of cardiac patch with decellularized porcine myocardial scaffold and bone marrow mononuclear cells. *J Biomed Mat Res A* 2010; 94A(4): 1100–1110.
46. Mangi A, et al. Mesenchymal stem cells modified with Akt prevent remodeling and restore performance of infarcted hearts. *Nat Med* 2003; 9(9): 1195–1201.
47. Mirotsou M, et al. Secreted frizzled related protein 2 (Sfrp2) is the key Akt-mesenchymal stem cell-released paracrine factor mediating myocardial survival and repair. *PNAS* 2007; 104(5): 1643–1648.
48. Grauss R, et al. Forced myocardin expression enhances the therapeutic effect of human mesenchymal stem cells after transplantation in ischemic mouse hearts. *Stem Cells* 2008; 26: 1083–1093.
49. Bao C, et al. Enhancement of the survival of engrafted mesenchymal stem cells in the ischemic heart by TNFR gene transfection. *Biochem Cell Biol* 2010; 88(4): 629–634.

50. Gnecchi M, et al. Early beneficial effects of bone marrow-derived mesenchymal stem cells overexpressing Akt on cardiac metabolism after myocardial infarction. *Stem Cells* 2009; 27(4): 971–979.

51. Noiseux N, et al. Mesenchymal stem cells overexpressing Akt dramatically repair infarcted myocardium and improve cardiac function despite infrequent cellular fusion or differentiation. *Molec Ther* 2006; 14(6): 840–850.

52. Fischer KM, et al. Cardiac progenitor cell commitment is inhibited by nuclear Akt expression. *Circ Res* 2011; 108(8): 960–970.

53. Hatzistergos KE, et al. Bone marrow mesenchymal stem cells stimulate cardiac stem cell proliferation and differentiation. *Circ Res* 2010; 107(7): 913–22.

54. Tang JM, et al. VEGF/SDF-1 promotes cardiac stem cell mobilization and myocardial repair in the infarcted heart. *Cardiovasc Res* 2011;.

55. Barile L, et al. Bone marrow-derived cells can acquire cardiac stem cells properties in damaged heart. *J Cell Mol Med* 2011; 15(1): 63–71.

56. Nguyen BK, et al. Improved function and myocardial repair of infarcted heart by intracoronary injection of mesenchymal stem cell-derived growth factors. *J Cardiovasc Transl Res* 2010; 3(5): 547–558.

57. Dai W, et al. Role of a paracrine action of mesenchymal stem cells in the improvement of left ventricular function after coronary artery occlusion in rats. *Regen Med* 2007; 2(1): 63–68.

58. Angoulvant D, et al. Mesenchymal stem cell conditioned media attenuates in vitro and ex vivo myocardial reperfusion injury. *J Heart Lung Transplant* 2011; 30(1): 95–102.

59. Breitbach M, et al. Potential risks of bone marrow cell transplantation into infarcted hearts. *Blood* 2007; 110: 1362–1369.

60. Knippenberg M, et al. Adipose tissue-derived mesenchymal stem cells acquire bone cell-like responsiveness to fluid shear stress on osteogenic stimulation. *Tissue Eng* 2005; 11(11): 1780–1788.

61. Sumanasinghe R, et al. Osteogenic differentiation of human mesenchymal stem cells in collagen matrices: effect of uniaxial cyclic tensile strain on bone morphogenetic protein (BMP-2) mRNA expression. *Tissue Eng* 2006; 12(12): 3459–3465.

62. Huang CY, et al. Effects of cyclic compressive loading on chondrogenesis of rabbit bone-marrow derived mesenchymal stem cells. *Stem Cells* 2004; 22(3): 313–323.

63. Lorenzen-Schmidt I, et al. Chronotropic response of cultured neonatal rat ventricular myocytes to short-term fluid shear. *Cell Biochem Biophys* 2006; 46(2).

64. Carlson S, et al. Cardiac mesenchymal stem cells contribute to scar formation after myocardial infarction. *Circ Res* 2011; 91(1): 99–107.

65. Lasala GP, et al. Combination stem cell therapy for the treatment of medically refractory coronary ischemia: a Phase I study. *Cardiovasc Revasc Med* 2011; 12(1): 29–34.

66. Hare JM, et al. A randomized, double-blind, placebo-controlled, dose-escalation study of intravenous adult human mesenchymal stem cells (prochymal) after acute myocardial infarction. *J Am Coll Cardiol* 2009; 54(24): 2277–2286.

67. Taber L, et al. Mechanics of ventricular torsion. *J Biomech* 1996; 29(6): 745–752.

68. Tendulkar A, Harken A. Mechanics of the normal heart. *J Card Surg* 2006; 21: 615–620.

69. Mehlhom U, et al. Myocardial fluid balance. *Eur J Cardiothorac Surg* 2001; 20: 1220–1230.

70. LeGrice IJ, et al. Transverse shear along myocardial cleavage planes provides a mechanism for normal systolic wall thickening. *Circ Res* 1995; 77: 182–193.

71. Ashikaga H, et al. Changes in regional myocardial volume during the cardiac cycle: implications for transmural blood flow and cardiac structure. *AJP Heart Circ Phys* 2008; 295(2): H610–H618.

72. LeGrice IJ, et al. Laminar structure of the heart: ventricular myocyte arrangement and connective tissue architecture in the dog. *Am J Physiol Heart Circ* 1995; 269(38): H571–H582.
73. Harrington K, et al. Direct measurement of transmural laminar architecture in the anterolateral wall of the ovine left ventricle: new implications for wall thickening mechanics. *Am J Physiol Heart Circ* 2005; 288: 1324–1330.
74. Arts T, et al. Relating myocardial laminar architecture to shear strain and muscle fiber orientation. *Am J Physiol Heart Circ* 2001; 280: H2222–H2229.
75. Dvir T, et al. Activation of the ERK1/2 cascade via pulsatile interstitial fluid flow promotes cardiac tissue assembly. *Tissue Eng* 2007; 13(9): 2185–2193.
76. Stewart RH, et al. Regulation of microvascular filtration in the myocardium by interstitial fluid pressure. *Am J Physiol Regulatory Integrative Comp Physiol* 1996; 271: 1465–1469.
77. Rabbany SY, et al. Intramyocardial pressure: interaction of myocardial fluid pressure and fiber stress. *AJP Heart Circ Physiol* 1989; 257(2): H357–H364.
78. Davis KL, et al. Effects of myocardial edema on the development of myocardial interstitial fibrosis. *Microcirculation* 2000; 7(4): 269–280.
79. Holmes J, et al. Structure and mechanics of healing myocardial infarcts. *Annu Rev Biomed Eng* 2005. 7: 223–253.
80. Wang J, et al. Left ventricular twist mechanics in a canine model of reversible congestive heart failure: a pilot study. *J Am Soc Echocardio* 2009; 22: 95–98.
81. Aikawa Y, et al. Regional wall stress predicts ventricular remodeling after anteroseptal myocardial infarction in the Healing and Early Afterload Reducing Trial (HEART): An echocardiography-based structural analysis. *Am Heart J* 2001; 141: 234–42.
82. Nishimura S, et al. Single cell mechanics of rat cardiomyocytes under isometric, unloaded, and physiologically loaded conditions. *Am J Physiol Heart Circ Physiol* 2004; 287: H196–H202.
83. Tracqui P, et al. Theoretical analysis of the adaptive contractile behaviour of a single cardiomyocyte cultured on elastic substrates with varying stiffness. *J Theor Biol* 2008; 255(1): 92–105.
84. Galie PA, et al. Reduced serum content and increased matrix stiffness promote the cardiac myofibroblast transition in 3D collagen matrices. *Cardiovasc Pathol* 2011; 20(6): 325–333.
85. Song G, et al. Mechanical stretch promotes proliferation of rat bone marrow mesenchymal stem cells. *Colloids and surfaces B: Biointerfaces* 2007; 58: 271–277.
86. Doyle AM, et al. Human mesenchymal stem cells form multicellular structures in response to applied cyclic strain. *Ann Biomed Eng* 2009; 37(4): 783–793.
87. Farng E, et al. The effects of GDF-5 and uniaxial strain on mesenchymal stem cells in 3-D culture. *Clin Orthop Relat Res* 2008; 466: 1930–1937.
88. Duty A, et al. Cyclic mechanical compression increases mineralization of cell-seeded polymer scaffolds in vivo. *J Biomech Eng* 2007; 129: 531–539.
89. Bhang SH, et al. Cyclic mechanical strain promotes transforming-growth-factor-β1-mediated cardiomyogenic marker expression in bone-marrow-derived mesenchymal stem cells in vitro. *Biotech Appl Biochem* 2010; 55(4): 191–197.
90. Kobayashi N, et al. Mechanical stress promotes the expression of smooth muscle-like properties in marrow stromal cells. *Exp Hematol* 2004; 32: 1238–1245.
91. Zhao F, et al. Perfusion affects the tissue developmental patterns of human mesenchymal stem cells in 3D scaffolds. *J Cell Physiol* 2009; 219: 421–429.

92. Engelmayr G, et al. Cyclic flexure and laminar flow synergistically accelerate mesenchymal stem cell-mediated engineered tissue formation: Implications for engineered heart valve tissues. *Biomaterials* 2006; 27: 6083–6095.

93. O'Cearbhaill ED, et al. Response of mesenchymal stem cells to the biomechanical environment of the endothelium on a flexible tubular silicone substrate. *Biomaterials* 2008; 29: 1610–1619.

94. Tan S, et al. Viscoelastic behavior of human mesenchymal stem cells. *BMC Cell Biol* 2008; 9: 40.

95. Rosová I, et al. Hypoxic preconditioning results in increased motility and improved therapeutic potential of human mesenchymal stem cells. *Stem Cells* 2008; 26(8): 2173–2182.

4

Kidney and Bladder Regeneration: Pharmacologic Methods

TIMOTHY A. BERTRAM, BELINDA J. WAGNER, AND BERT SPILKER

Regenerating human bladder and kidney has been attempted many times using multiple approaches. An early procedure for regenerating the bladder (Taguchi et al. 1977), derived from a 1970 cystoplasty approach of Orikasa and Tsuji (1970), placed a thin paper cover with a liquid synthetic resin (nobecutane) similar to a cap over the opened bladder. Within 3 to 4 weeks, the implant was covered by granulated tissue, and the artificial cap was removed transurethrally. More recent surgical approaches for regenerating bladder use autografts of gastrointestinal mucosa (Kropp et al. 2004), oral mucosa, or skin (Staack et al. 2005). Nonsurgical approaches include efforts to use growth factors (e.g., hepatocyte growth factor [HGF]) as aids to accelerate or assist in renal regeneration (Kawaida et al. 1994).

More advanced technologies for regenerating human organs have moved from bench experiments to bedside clinical successes. Clinical trials have been conducted with neo-tissues and neo-organs derived from a patient's own (autologous) cells. "Neo" is a prefix derived from the Greek word "neos" meaning new, young, or fresh. The terms "neo-tissue" and "neo-organ" are used to distinguish regenerative implants made ex vivo from cells and biomaterials from the more traditional grafts that use intact tissues or organs. A neo-tissue or neo-organ implant made as cell-scaffold combination product is also called a "construct" in this chapter. Implants of synthetic biopolymers combined with autologous urothelial and smooth muscle cells are examples of neo-tissues that have been used in humans to regenerate bladder tissue (Atala et al. 2006) as alternatives to enterocystoplasty, an autograft procedure that augments the urinary bladder with a segment of bowel tissue. Similar neo-organ constructs have been implanted into dogs to replace the entire bladder (Bertram et al. 2008a). A 24-month study that compared histologically and physiologically such construct implants with autotransplantation of reimplanted native urinary bladder in large mammals revealed that both neo-tissue or neo-organ and graft approaches yielded positive results (Jayo et al. 2008a); however, the more advanced regenerative technology platforms allowed treatment of disease states that involve the urinary

52

bladder to undergo cystectomy and bladder replacement without the need for bowel resection and exposing the gut mucosa to urine.

Regardless of the medical approach used to regenerate tissue, subsequent tissue responses and clinical outcomes are usually evaluated by histologic, physiological, and functional endpoints. Treating kidney and bladder disease by regenerative methods offers a new approach to improve diseased organ function, and the outcomes may be evaluated not only by histologic and physiologic tests of the structural and functional aspects of regenerating tissues and organs but also by using pharmacological evaluations. Pharmacological approaches to the evaluation of regenerating bladder and renal tissues and organs are the subject of this chapter.

Pharmacological studies can evaluate:

1. The relative tissue sensitivity between native and regenerated tissues
2. Differences between regenerated tissues in juvenile, adult, and elderly subjects
3. Impact of cell source and type on the regeneration process and outcome
4. Impact of pharmacological intervention on the regeneration process and outcome

Pharmacological studies are useful for investigating the presence or absence of growth factors and other molecules of interest (e.g., hormones). For example, during bladder or kidney regeneration, pharmacological studies can help determine if native pharmacological responsiveness has been restored or whether a disease state has been attenuated. In the bladder, measuring dose responses to parasympathomimetic agents can evaluate hypersensitivity. In the kidney, measuring hormone level changes (e.g., vitamin D_3) or blood pressure can evaluate the status of the renin–angiotensin system during renal regeneration. Additionally, levels of growth factors may potentially be also used to monitor the regeneration process and status of a regenerated tissue.

Regeneration versus Repair

The process of **regeneration** is associated with maintenance or restoration of the original structure and function of a tissue or organ (Stocum, 2002). However, an injury that exceeds the regenerative capacity of a tissue triggers another mechanism – healing by **repair and fibrosis** – a process that covers a wound with dense fibrous or scar tissue and structural elements that are different from the original (Stocum, 2002). The body's response to injury is the sum of several factors including age, site of injury, and the urgency of restoring homeostasis (Stanger et al. 2007; Stocum, 2002). Kidney and bladder tissues may be prompted to regenerate if assisted by regenerative medical products (Atala et al. 2006; Bertram et al. 2008a; Jayo et al. 2008a; Jayo et al. 2008b; Oberpenning et al. 1999). One goal of regenerative medicine is to identify and develop products that consistently trigger regenerative healing and effectively restore function and structure to damaged tissues and organs.

Table 4-1. *Summary of basic pharmacologic tools and approaches*

Tool	Question answered
Single-dose effect	Does the agent stimulate, block, or potentiate a biochemical, cellular, histologic, physiological, embryologic, or clinical endpoint?
Dose-response relationship	How is an endpoint influenced by different doses or at different times after administration of an agent?
Structure–activity relationships	How do different chemical structures or forms of an agent affect an endpoint?
Chronopharmacology	At what point in the regenerative process does an agent deliver its maximal effect on an endpoint?

Definition of Regenerative Pharmacology

The field of pharmacology overlaps with a variety of other biologic sciences, including but not limited to physiology, biochemistry, embryology, pathology, microbiology, virology, immunology, and pharmacokinetics. Pharmacology encompasses both preclinical and clinical phases of product development and involves both in vitro and in vivo evaluations. The working definition of regenerative pharmacology used in this chapter is "any study that evaluates a chemical, biologic, or drug that may be involved in promoting regeneration, or any evaluation of the pharmacological characterization of regenerated tissues resulting from the use of regenerative medicine technologies."

Basic Pharmacological Tools and Approaches

Evaluating the Effect of a Single Dose of an Agent on the Activity of a Biologic System

This is the most basic pharmacological tool in which the effect (i.e., activity) of an agent, usually a chemical product, on an in vitro, in situ, in silico, or in vivo system is studied (Table 4-1). Endpoints are defined for one or more biochemical, cellular, histologic, physiologic, embryologic, or clinical systems. The agent is delivered, and its stimulating, blocking, or potentiating effect on the endpoint(s) is measured.

Agents may be evaluated in models of regeneration as well as other systems. Note that clinical endpoints may be evaluated in animals as well as humans. For example, behavior, morbidity, and mortality are endpoints that are often studied in both animals and humans.

Single dose effect studies can also provide information about whether an agent has potential to act as a **preventive** or as a **treatment**. A preventive effect would block, delay, or attenuate the onset or effects of a disease or problem in a naïve organism that might be at risk of developing a medical problem. A treatment effect would arrest or reverse the progression of a disease or its symptoms in an affected organism. Diseases or problems in a tissue (or organ) can arise naturally through congenital or acquired circumstances or be the result of human intervention (e.g., chemically, biologically, or surgically induced animal models or an iatrogenic condition in humans).

The status of organ or tissue regeneration can be monitored using biomarkers indicative of native tissue function (e.g., creatinine in the case of renal regeneration) in samples obtained from blood, urine, or tissues to evaluate and track the development of regeneration, need for therapeutic intervention, or changes in disease progression. Both acute assessment and long-term monitoring of hormone levels or other biomarkers can involve evaluating the response to pharmacological agents administered as part of the evaluation or quantifying the endogenous levels of specific molecules (e.g., growth factors) presumed to be influenced by the regenerative process or that might influence its outcome.

Dose-Response Relationships

Dose-response relationships refer to studies in which the impacts of different doses of an agent (e.g., chemical, biologic, biomaterial, or combination) on a biologic system or the response of a regenerated biologic system to known pharmacological agents are evaluated (Table 4-1). The relationship of dose and response is often illustrated (i.e., plotted) as the range of doses tested on the "x" axis versus the effect observed at each of the doses on the "y" axis. The dimension of time may also be an important component of the relationship; this is especially true when evaluating regenerative processes and outcomes. The time dimension of dose-response relationships is not only important for characterizing the regenerated tissue and the regenerative process but can also help guide the discovery, development, and therapeutic use of pharmacological agents that could be used to promote or modify regenerative healing.

In many cases, a log scale for plotting doses is used, particularly for in vitro experiments in which several log ranges of doses are tested. Such curves often show sigmoid-shaped dose-response relationships and allow one to learn the threshold dose needed to evoke a response (e.g., contractile strength of regenerated bladder tissue), the doses at which a near-linear relationship between dose and response (i.e., a rapid change in response to relatively small changes in dosage) exists, and the dose at which the response plateaus. In many cases, high doses of a pharmacological agent elicit a reduced effect (i.e., toxicity), and the plots of such relationships are referred to as U-shaped dose-response curves.

Structure–Activity Relationships

Structure–activity relationships (SARs) refer to studies in which a series of different agents that are closely related at the chemical level are evaluated to determine the effect of making minor modifications in chemical structure on endpoints (Table 4-1). During regeneration, the topography, concentration, or distribution of receptors might be different than those seen in native tissues or organs. SAR studies comparing regenerated tissue responses with native tissues provide way of monitoring the influence of chemical structure on functional effects. Altered SAR may be a signal that receptor expression, distribution, receptor–ligand interaction, intracellular signaling pathways, or other biologic response capabilities are different in the regenerated tissue or organ. Again, the SAR might need to be evaluated at different time periods in the regenerative process to fully understand whether the SAR changes over time.

Chronopharmacology

Chronopharmacology refers to studies that evaluate the temporal relationship between agents (e.g., regenerative technologies, drugs, growth factors) and endpoints. The age of a subject and the duration of the target condition that a product is designed to address can affect an agent's ability to elicit a response or outcome (Table 4-1). For regenerative medical products that use cell or tissue components that must be harvested, these same conditions might also affect potency. Regeneration is a dynamic process that occurs over time, and chronopharmacology is of particular relevance when the regenerative process occurring in a tissue or organ is incomplete. Chronopharmacological studies of traditional pharmaceutical agents typically span a 24-hour time period; however, new approaches over longer time frames might be required to evaluate temporal relationships in a regenerative process. The goal of such chronopharmacological studies would be to characterize the temporal process of regeneration in different tissues, organs, and populations and help identify the point in time when maximal responses are achieved or native responses are restored in a regenerating tissue or organ. The influence of various agents (e.g., growth factors or pharmacological agents, singly or in combination) on the time needed to achieve a regenerative outcome could also be tested using chronopharmacological experiments.

Regenerative Medicine's Basic Tools and Approaches

The field of regenerative medicine has introduced its own set of tools and approaches with which pharmacological tools and approaches must interact.

Cell- and Tissue-Based Therapies

Some regenerative medical products use cells or tissue components that must be obtained from a subject:

- Autologous cells or tissues are obtained from the same individual who receives the resulting product.
- Allogenic cells or tissues are obtained from someone other than the product recipient.

- Xenogenic sources refer to cells or tissues that are harvested from other species (e.g., a pig) and incorporated into products for humans.

Another characteristic of cells or tissues used in regenerative medical products is whether they originate from the same tissue or organ as that being regenerated (homologous) or a different tissue or organ (heterologous). Therefore, in terms of cell and tissue sources for regenerative medical products, these six basic categories encompass all of the available combinations of the originating source of cell and tissue components (Bertram and Jayo, 2008; Russell and Bertram, 2007).

Autologous (Jayo et al. 2008a; Jayo et al. 2008b; Oberpenning et al. 1999; Presnell et al. 2009) and allogenic (Bertram et al. 2009; Bertram et al. 2008b) homologous cells have been used to successfully regenerate bladder and kidney tissues and organs. Autologous and homologous approaches have been successfully translated into clinical trials with demonstrated clinical benefits (Atala et al. 2006; Joseph et al. 2009; Seltzer et al. 2009). Approaches using allogenic and heterologous cells are in development. Autologous approaches avoid an immune response that may be elicited when cell or tissue sources are allogenic or xenogenic (Atala et al. 2006). Such an immune response has the potential for influencing the regenerative outcome, and products using allogenic or xenogenic material must be evaluated for that potential (Bertram and Jayo, 2008; Russell and Bertram, 2007).

Scaffolds Used in Regenerative Medicine

Various synthetic and natural agents are used to support a regenerative tissue outcome (Table 4-2). Scaffold materials may be combined with cells or impregnated with pharmacologically active molecules to promote regeneration of tissues or organs (Jayo et al. 2008c).

Biomaterials without cells have been used to promote regeneration, particularly in the bladder and lower urologic systems (Cheng and Kropp, 2000; Kropp et al. 2004; Landman et al. 2004). Pharmacological characterization of the neo-tissues resulting from scaffold-only approaches has not been reported. Other work comparing seeded and unseeded synthetic biomaterials in bladder regeneration demonstrated that neo-tissues formed after unseeded scaffold implantation healed by repair, not regeneration, and lacked long-term durability (Jayo et al. 2008a; Jayo et al. 2008b). Further characterization of neo-tissues resulting from cell-seeded implants used for bladder augmentation revealed pharmacological responsiveness similar to native bladder at 6 months after implantation (Bertram et al. 2008a).

Regenerative pharmacology studies will likely provide an important component for understanding the long-term durability and functionality of regenerative medical products. Of particular utility to new product development and testing will be pharmacological assessments that can provide insight into neo-organ and neo-tissue

Table 4-2. *Scaffolds used in regenerative medicine*

Classification or composition	Materials	Form of material
Polyester family	Poly(lactic-co-glycolic acid) (PLGA)	Film, foam, fiber
	PGA	Films, fibers
	PLA-polydioxanone	Fibers
	Poly(caprolactone)	Foam
Polyurethane family	Poly(ether urethane) (PEU)	Foam
	Poly(ester-urethane)urea (PEUU)	Nanofiber
Polyaminoacids	Poly(alpha-amino acid) membrane	
	Branched peptide-amphiphile coating	Coating on PGA fibers
Natural polymers	Collagen	Sponge, fiber, membrane
	Collagen/elastin	Fiber/mesh, membrane
	Fibrinogen	Nanofiber
	Cellulose	Fleece
	Poly(ethylene glycol) (PEG) hydrogel	
Gels	Alginate	Gel
	Hyaluronic acid or dextran gel	

regeneration. Assessments that can evaluate the status of regeneration without disrupting the healing process will be important for clinical evaluation in humans.

Growth Factors

Although many growth factors are believed to participate in some way with regeneration, the role(s) of specific growth factors in the regenerative process are not yet fully characterized or understood (Matsumoto and Nakamura, 2001). We have summarized studies of several growth factors that have been evaluated in the context of kidney regeneration.

1. **Activins** consist of multifunctional cytokines and are members of the transforming growth factor-β (TGF-β) super-family whose role in the regeneration of kidney has been studied (Maeshima et al. 2001). In kidney organogenesis and regeneration, a combination of activin and follistatin has been shown to mediate tubule formation. Follistatin is a single-chain polypeptide that binds to activins and blocks their actions.
2. **HGF** is expressed in interstitial cells, endothelial cells, and macrophages in the normal kidney, and its receptors are present on the surfaces of the proximal tubular cells (Schena, 1998). HGF's role as an endogenous renoprotective factor that inhibits renal fibrosis in part by inhibiting the profibrotic activity of TGF-β (see below) is beginning to be elucidated at a molecular level (Liu, 2004).
3. **Epidermal growth factor (EGF)** binds to a receptor that initiates a complicated cascade of intracellular signals triggered by the formation of a ligand-receptor complex at the cell surface. Recent work out of Safirstein's lab (Arany et al. 2008; Arany et al. 2006) has

begun to elucidate the intricacies of how the different molecules that interact with the EGF receptor either promote or inhibit kidney regeneration following acute renal failure (ARF). Many of these effects are modulated by pharmacological agents, emphasizing regenerative pharmacology's potential for contributing to regenerative medical product development.

4. **Transforming growth factor-α (TGF-α)** has been shown to have a renoprotective role during oxidative stress in the kidneys and functions by interacting with the EGF receptor–mediated signaling pathway discussed earlier (Kuper et al. 2007).

5. **Transforming growth factor-β 1 (TGF-β 1)** is presumed to have a detrimental effect on kidney regeneration by promoting fibrosis (Liu, 2004); however, recent work suggests that TGF-β 1 may contribute to kidney regeneration by modulating an epithelial-to-mesenchymal transition, in which tubular epithelial cells have been observed to acquire a mesenchymal phenotype in response to ischemic or toxic injury (Campanaro et al. 2007).

Note that the kidney disease models studied used to study the roles of growth factors in kidney regeneration are models of ARF. In these models, kidney regeneration occurs within 3 to 4 weeks after injury if the reduction in glomerular filtration rate can be supported during the ARF episode (Anglani et al. 2008). These preclinical models of kidney regeneration after ARF reveal a native pathway of regeneration and are useful for elucidating the roles of growth factors in promoting or hindering regeneration. However, the relationship between the regeneration process after ARF and the components required to promote kidney regeneration in cases of chronic renal failure is as yet unknown.

Bladder and Kidney Regeneration

Basic pharmacology tools may be applied to native, repaired, or regenerated urinary tract tissues or organs as a means to identify:

- The extent of regeneration and characterization of the pharmacological status of regenerated urinary tissues (e.g., bladder or kidney)
- Novel pathways suitable for cell-based, scaffold, growth factor, or pharmacological intervention to promote regeneration of urinary tissues
- Novel compounds or applications of such compounds to promote tissue healing and regeneration of the bladder, kidney, or other portions of the genitourinary system
- Identification of new therapeutic targets (e.g., molecular, cellular, or receptors) that may useful in the treatment of organ and tissue failure.

Bladder Regeneration

Most therapeutic approaches for the bladder are related to:

- Control of continence
- Decreasing bladder hyperactivity

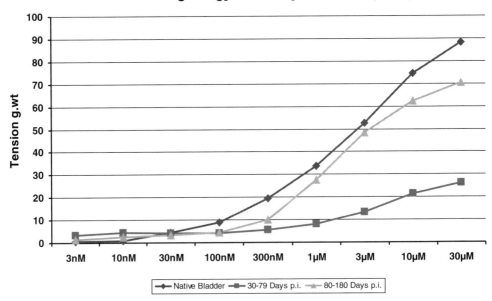

Figure 4-1. Carbachol stimulation of regenerated versus native bladder tissue in large mammals. Chronopharmacological evaluation of bladder tissues retrieved from canines at necropsy demonstrates that the receptor–ligand pathway is restored by 6 months after initiating the regenerative process (compare the *green line* with the *red line*). The lower concentrations represent physiological and pharmacological conditions. (See color plate 5.)

- Increasing bladder capacity (i.e., volume)
- Replacing the urine elimination function of bladders that have been removed because of cancer or other maladies

Detrusor muscle activity is studied using pharmacological agents (e.g. carbachol, phenylephrine) to evaluate pharmacological receptor-mediated smooth muscle stimulation. The extent of bladder regeneration can be evaluated by measuring the contractile response of regenerated tissue to these pharmacological agents. Such information not only provides a useful comparison between regenerated and native tissues but can also be used to determine the temporal pattern of an organ's regenerative capacity. When a chronopharmacological analysis is done on regenerating urinary bladder, response to a cholinergic agonist can be seen as early as 3 months after initiation of the regeneration process (Fig. 4-1). At 3 months, the response is usually attenuated relative to that of native bladder but attains near normal dose and strength responses by 6 months. The timing of acquiring near-native pharmacological response to cholinergic stimulation coincides with the regeneration of a full-thickness bladder wall composed of all tissue constituents (Bertram et al. 2008b; Jayo et al. 2008a).

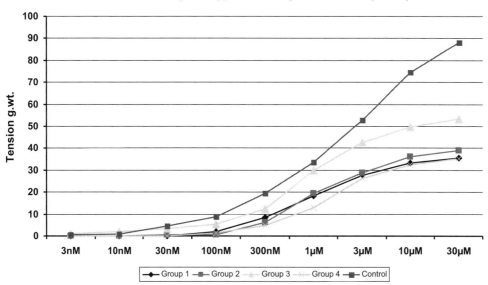

Figure 4-2. Influence of cell number on carbachol stimulation of regenerated versus native bladder in large mammals. The regenerative process is primed by including more cells in the cell–biomaterial scaffold regenerative template (i.e., construct). Force generated by the regenerated bladder tissue retrieved from group 3 dogs that received a higher number of cells than groups 1 and 3 is most similar to that of native canine bladder tissue at the lower agonist concentrations that are closer to physiological and pharmacological conditions. At higher carbachol concentrations, the force generated by neo-tissues retrieved from group 3 dogs was also greater than that generated by neo-tissues from constructs having fewer cells and approached the response seen from native tissue. (See color plate 6.)

Pharmacological evaluation can also be used to define optimal product characteristics for selecting the most appropriate regenerative product prototype to develop. Adding different cell numbers to a regenerative template (e.g., biomaterial scaffold) can yield regenerated organs with different levels of pharmacological responsiveness (Fig. 4-2). In the long term, such differences may allow for development of regenerated organs with differing levels of pharmacological receptivity. The results of as yet unpublished experiments summarized in Figures 4-1 and 4-2 demonstrate that both the number of cells seeded onto a biomaterial matrix and the time allowed for regeneration after construct implantation influence the characteristics of the regenerated bladder, development of intrinsic nerves within the bladder wall, and receptor-mediated transduction between the regenerated detrusor muscle and bladder wall nerves.

Histologic evaluation of regenerated bladder tissue that has pharmacological responsiveness reveals a complete muscle, mucosal, and stroma layering with Fura-2 analysis demonstrating the syncytial response of the muscle layers after calcium ionophore stimulation (Fig. 4-3, unpublished data).

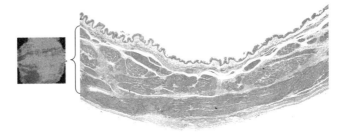

Figure 4-3. Histologic evaluation of regenerated bladder demonstrates a full-thickness multilayer structure. When stimulated with the calcium ionophore (A23187), the detrusor muscle mobilizes calcium as a syncytial tissue as would be observed in a native bladder detrusor muscle. (See color plate 7.)

Kidney

Kidney regeneration may be viewed in terms of the overall kidney or specific anatomical areas. As organs, kidneys have an intrinsic ability to regenerate in response to injury. Kidney damage also appears to activate bloodborne signals that are communicated to distal organs via what is called the "renotropic system" (Matsumoto and Nakamura, 2001), whose components have yet to be fully elucidated. The growth factors listed earlier are believed to participate in the renotropic system and its regulation.

Evidence supports two distinct routes for kidney regeneration. Neither route completely excludes the other. The two routes may be redundant mechanisms, each leading to regeneration, or it is possible that a combination of both is necessary for successful kidney regeneration. One route is endogenous to the kidney tissue. The other route involves the mobilization of stem cells from distal organs (e.g., bone marrow) localizing to the kidney (Anglani et al. 2008; Cantley, 2005; Huls et al. 2008; Humphreys and Bonventre, 2008; Lin, 2006).

Proliferation of endogenous tubular epithelial cells is observed early in ARF, and some epithelial cells have been observed to acquire a mesenchymal cell phenotype, the epithelial-to-mesenchymal transition (EMT) that TGF-β 1 appears to modulate (see earlier discussion). It is also possible that a reservoir of stem cells resides in kidney tissue that is activated to expand by injury (Humphreys et al. 2008; Kinomura et al. 2008; Oliver et al. 2004). Other researchers have demonstrated that stem cells from outside the kidney can localize in regenerating kidney tissue in ARF (Kirpatovskii et al. 2007; Morigi et al. 2008; Patschan et al. 2006; Prodromidi et al. 2006).

Regardless of whether kidney regeneration occurs via endogenous, exogenous, or a combination of both mechanisms, what is clear from the research to date is that kidney regeneration is a complex process with multiple, interacting pathways of activation and inhibition of cell–cell, cell–matrix, and intracellular signaling events. The potential contribution that regenerative pharmacology can make to the development of products that promote or sustain kidney regeneration is clear.

Pharmacological evaluation of kidney regeneration is usually done by monitoring blood urea nitrogen and creatinine levels because these indicators provide insight into the overall process and are relatively inexpensive and easy assays to conduct. However, other targets provide additional insight into the status of structural or functional components of the kidney. Two examples are blood pressure, which provides information on the glomerular and interstitial functions that interact with the renin–angiotensin system, and erythropoietin production, which provides information on hematologic homeostasis. As regenerative medical products progress through the discovery and development pipelines, additional pharmacological evaluations will be needed to assess product-specific safety and efficacy parameters.

Animal Models

Pharmacologically oriented animal models may be classified based on their level of organization (i.e., as tissue, organ, or organism). These models can also be categorized by species and by whether testing occurs in vitro, in situ, or in vivo. The majority of pharmacological models related to regenerative medicine involve in vivo or whole-organism studies because regeneration of an organ or tissue requires an intact, homeostatically balanced organism for evaluating the safety and efficacy potential for clinical application.

Physiologically, the canine model has been useful in the investigation of micturition, continence, and neural control bladder function (Van der Werf and Creed, 2002; Van der Werf et al. 2000). Pharmacological and electrophysiologic studies conducted in dogs or their tissues ex vivo have provided clinically applicable information on biomechanical and functional properties of the urinary bladder (Koraitim et al. 1977; Van der Werf and Creed, 2002; Van der Werf et al. 2000). Ultimately, in dogs and humans, normal micturition requires the proper coordination between the bladder's detrusor muscle, internal bladder neck, and external urethral sphincters. Koratim (1977) used electromyography in anesthetized dogs to study the bladder neck region during bladder filling and emptying. The advantages of the canine model include body size, ease of surgical manipulation and tissue sampling, and a well-understood comparative physiology between dogs and humans (Tibbitts, 2003).

Disease-specific models are also useful for studying the regeneration of pharmacological responses in regenerating bladder and kidney tissues and organs. Models that mimic physiological parameters of human disease can be important and critical for evaluating the potential clinical utility of new therapeutic agents.

Animal Models for Studying Bladder Regeneration

The dog has been used extensively for comparative safety studies of the urologic system. Results from studies evaluating bladder regeneration (Yoo et al. 1998) showed that bladder augmentation with cell-seeded scaffolds could be achieved in vivo; however, it could not be determined whether the improved functional parameters noted were attributable to the augmented segment or to the intact native bladder tissue (Oberpenning et al. 1999).

Cell-seeded scaffolds have been repeatedly demonstrated to regenerate normal bladder tissue with normal bladder wall structure and a return to normal or near-normal function in a 6- to 9-month period in dogs undergoing partial cystectomy (Jayo et al. 2008a; Jayo et al. 2008b; Oberpenning et al. 1999). Similar results have been demonstrated in dogs that have undergone total cystectomy (Bertram et al. 2008b). The long-term durability of the regenerated bladder tissue, bioresponsive nature of the regenerated organ (Jayo et al. 2008a), and the fundamental mechanisms of tissue regeneration (Jayo et al. 2008b) have revealed that pharmacological, physiological, and anatomic regeneration occur within similar time frames (Bertram et al. 2008b).

Models of bladder disease have largely been limited to partial or complete removal of the bladder with de novo regeneration serving as evidence of clinical utility (Oberpenning et al. 1999). Although animal models of interstitial cystitis and bladder cancer are available, the translation of these diseases to humans has not yet been demonstrated.

Animal Models for Studying Kidney Regeneration

Renal regeneration, similar to bladder regeneration, can be studied using intact animals that have had partial to complete organ removal. The 5/6 nephrectomy model has been used to study pathogenic mechanisms underlying chronic renal failure by inducing tubulointerstitial fibrosis, a common symptom that precedes end-stage renal failure (Kliem et al. 1996; Schwartz et al. 1987). The severity of tubulointerstitial inflammation and fibrosis has long been considered as a crucial determinant in progressive renal injury and long-term prognosis in both human and experimental glomerulonephritis (Cameron, 1992; Eddy, 1996; Nath, 1992). Less severe ablation (e.g., unilateral nephrectomy) induces compensatory renal regeneration and is useful for studying regeneration in a more ARF-like context and assessing the effect of agents (e.g., growth factors, local or systemic medications) on the regenerative process (Nagaike et al. 1991).

Nonsurgically induced disease models are also available for evaluating regenerative pharmacology of the kidney. Glomerulonephritis that mimics crescentic glomerulonephritis in humans can be induced in rodents by administering antibodies against the glomerular basement membrane. Antibodies to Thy-1 in rodents induce glomerulonephritis that mimics human mesangial proliferative glomerulonephritis. Yamada et al. (2005) used these two rodent models to compare the renoprotectiveness of two pharmacological agents, protein kinase CK2 inhibitor and prednisolone.

A genetic model of glomerulonephritis (imprinting control region [ICR] strain-derived glomerulonephritic mice, or imprinting control region glomerulonephritis [ICGN] mice) mimics the chronic glomerulonephritis seen in humans. In this model, glomerular injury is detectable from 3 weeks postnatally, and renal dysfunction occurs from 12 to 14 weeks, a dysfunction that coincides with tubular destruction and tubulointerstitial fibrosis. Indeed, researchers have found the same reciprocal activities of HGF and TGF-β 1 in both the ICGN and 5/6 nephrectomy rodent models, supporting the use of ICGN mice as a model for chronic renal disease (Matsumoto and Nakamura, 2001).

Acute renal failure can be produced in animals by nephrotoxic agents, ischemia, or unilateral nephrectomy; however, each model has similarities and differences with clinical ARF (Table 4-3). These patterns of similarities and differences between the experimental models and clinical presentations of ARF may influence the choice of model for studying a particular pharmacological agent or aspect of renal function (Ghielli et al. 1996).

In addition to using pharmacological agents to produce models of ARF, pharmacological agents can be used as probes for studying the regenerative process and the effect of regenerative medical products in two primary ways. First, the potential of a product for preventing development of ARF can be evaluated by applying the regenerative product before or concurrent with induction of ARF. The degree to which ARF occurs in the presence or absence of the regenerative product is the outcome measure. If a product has a demonstrated preventive effect, pharmacological agents can be used to probe the mechanism of renoprotection.

Second, a regenerative product can be applied after a disease state is established to evaluate the extent to which a product can restore renal function. One challenge in evaluating regenerative products applied after the onset of ARF is the relatively short time period of the ARF disease state in which the regenerative process can be studied. In some ARF models, renal parameters rapidly return to normal in the no-treatment control animals (e.g., ischemia model) and reduce the magnitude of difference between treatment and no treatment outcomes. The short time period of the disease window affects the number of animals needed to conduct such experiments available. Pharmacological agents can play a vital role in modulating this time frame.

Chronic disease models (e.g., 5/6 nephrectomy and ICGN mice) offer a longer period of time for preclinical evaluation of regenerative products. Pharmacological tests can be used to evaluate the effects of renal regeneration; elucidate mechanisms of regeneration; and quantify the extent of regeneration at the biochemical, cellular, or physiological level. For example, applying the experimental designs used to investigate the reciprocal pattern of HGF and TGF-β 1 expression in chronic renal disease (Matsumoto and Nakamura, 2001) to evaluating potential regenerative products would help elucidate the roles of these growth factors in the regenerative process and

Table 4-3. *Interstitial leukocytes in experimental animal models of acute renal failure and acute renal failure in humans*

Animal models of ARF	Macrophages	T Lymphocytes	B Lymphocytes	Neutrophils	Reference
Pyelone-phritis	P	P	?	+	Glauser et al. 1987
Ischemia	P	P	?	+	Klausner et al. 1989
Urethral obstruc-tion	+	+	?	+	Rovin et al. 1990
Mercuric chloride	+	+	?	–	Cuppage and Tate, 1967
PAN nephrosis	+	+	+	–	Eddy, 1989; Eddy and Michael, 1988
Aminogly-cosides	+	+	?	–	Giuliano et al. 1984
Cisplatin	?	?	?	–	Laurent et al. 1988
Clinical ARF in Humans					
Acute inter-stitial necrosis (AIN) – general	+	+	P	?	Neilson, 1989
NSAID-induced AIN	–	+	+	?	Bender et al. 1984
ATN	+	+	–	–	Boucher et al. 1986

+, present; –, not present; P, probably present; ?, not investigated; AIN = acute interstitial necrosis; ARF = acute renal failure; ATN = acute tubular necrosis; NSAID = nonsteroidal anti-inflammatory drug; PAN = polyarteritis nodosa
Adapted from Ghielli et al. 1996.

provide clues as to potential therapeutic targets that may be studied for pharmacological intervention of the regenerative process.

Summary

Cell-based products, growth factors, scaffolds, and other agents have been evaluated after implantation or injection into mammalian species using histologic, biochemical, and physiological studies, but relatively few have been extensively evaluated pharmacologically. Despite the paucity of pharmacological studies of regenerative healing models to date, pharmacological responsiveness represents a key modality for determining the extent of regenerative outcome and characterizing the pharmacological potential of the neo-organ. In addition, regenerative pharmacology has the potential for identifying additional agents that might be used in conjunction with regenerative technologies to yield optimal clinical outcomes.

Although most of the regeneration literature is reports of studies conducted in animals, some technologies are now being tested in clinical trials. There are relatively few pharmacology studies in the literature that focus on regenerated urinary tract tissue. As regenerative medical technologies advance in their clinical application, the need to understand the pharmacological response, the role of pharmacological agents, and the impact of regenerated tissues on homeostasis will promote the conduct and reporting of such studies. Incorporating pharmacological agents into scaffolds is also expected to become an active area of research and development.

The field of regenerative pharmacology is beginning to expand into testing of regenerative medical products that target the kidney and urinary bladder. Awareness of the breadth of application and value of regenerative pharmacology is growing. Applying pharmacological tools and approaches to regenerative medicine will yield greater understanding of the regenerative process and help move regenerative technologies out of the laboratory and into the clinics to address unmet medical needs.

References

Anglani, F., Ceol, M., Mezzabotta, F., Torregrossa, R., Tiralongo, E., Tosetto, E., Del Prete, D., and D'Angelo, A. (2008). The renal stem cell system in kidney repair and regeneration. *Front Biosci*, *13*, 6395–6405.

Arany, I., Faisal, A., Nagamine, Y., and Safirstein, R. L. (2008, Mar 7). p66shc inhibits pro-survival epidermal growth factor receptor/ERK signaling during severe oxidative stress in mouse renal proximal tubule cells. *J Biol Chem*, *283*(10), 6110–6117.

Arany, I., Megyesi, J. K., Nelkin, B. D., and Safirstein, R. L. (2006, Aug). STAT3 attenuates EGFR-mediated ERK activation and cell survival during oxidant stress in mouse proximal tubular cells. *Kidney Int*, *70*(4), 669–674.

Atala, A., Bauer, S. B., Soker, S., Yoo, J. J., and Retik, A. B. (2006, Apr 15). Tissue-engineered autologous bladders for patients needing cystoplasty. *Lancet*, *367*(9518), 1241–1246.

Bender, W. L., Whelton, A., Beschorner, W. E., Darwish, M. O., Hall-Craggs, M., and Solez, K. (1984, Jun). Interstitial nephritis, proteinuria, and renal failure caused by nonsteroidal anti-inflammatory drugs. Immunologic characterization of the inflammatory infiltrate. *Am J Med*, *76*(6), 1006–1012.

Bertram, T. A., Christ, G. J., Aboushwareb, T., Wagner, B. J., Jain, D., Ludlow, J. W., Payne, R., Jarapu, Y., Turner, C., and Jayo, M. J. (2008a). Total regenerated urinary bladders are structurally and pharmacologically similar to native canine bladder tissue. *J Urol*, *179*(4, Suppl 1), 76.

Bertram, T. A., Christ, G. J., Andersson, K. E., Aboushwareb, T., Fuellhase, C., Solex, R., Wagner, B. J., Jain, D., Ludlow, J. W., Payne, R., and Jayo, M. J. (2009, April 18–22). *Pharmacologic response of regenerated bladders in a preclinical model*. Poster presented at Experimental Biology, New Orleans, LA.

Bertram, T. A., Christ, G. J., Wagner, B. J., Jain, D., Aboushwareb, T., Ludlow, J. W., Payne, R., Jarapu, Y., Turner, C., and Jayo, M. J. (2008b, April 6). *Total urinary bladder regeneration with restoration of native structure and pharmacological response*. Poster presented at the 2008 Experimental Biology Meeting, San Diego, CA.

Bertram, T. A., and Jayo, M. J. (2008). Tissue engineered products: Preclinical development of neo-organs. In J. Cavagnero (Ed.), *Preclinical safety evaluation of biopharmaceuticals: A science-based approach to facilitating clinical trials* (pp. 799–826). New York: John Wiley and Sons.

Boucher, A., Droz, D., Adafer, E., and Noel, L. H. (1986, May). Characterization of mononuclear cell subsets in renal cellular interstitial infiltrates. *Kidney Int, 29*(5), 1043–1049.

Cameron, J. S. (1992, May). Tubular and interstitial factors in the progression of glomerulonephritis. *Pediatr Nephrol, 6*(3), 292–303.

Campanaro, S., Picelli, S., Torregrossa, R., Colluto, L., Ceol, M., Del Prete, D., D'Angelo, A., Valle, G., and Anglani, F. (2007). Genes involved in TGF beta1-driven epithelial-mesenchymal transition of renal epithelial cells are topologically related in the human interactome map. *BMC Genomics, 8*, 383.

Cantley, L. G. (2005, Nov). Adult stem cells in the repair of the injured renal tubule. *Nat Clin Pract Nephrol, 1*(1), 22–32.

Cheng, E. Y., and Kropp, B. P. (2000, Feb). Urologic tissue engineering with small-intestinal submucosa: potential clinical applications. *World J Urol, 18*(1), 26–30.

Cuppage, F. E., and Tate, A. (1967, Sep). Repair of the nephron following injury with mercuric chloride. *Am J Pathol, 51*(3), 405–429.

Eddy, A. A. (1989, Oct). Interstitial nephritis induced by protein-overload proteinuria. *Am J Pathol, 135*(4), 719–733.

Eddy, A. A. (1996, Dec). Molecular insights into renal interstitial fibrosis. *J Am Soc Nephrol, 7*(12), 2495–2508.

Eddy, A. A., and Michael, A. F. (1988, Jan). Acute tubulointerstitial nephritis associated with aminonucleoside nephrosis. *Kidney Int, 33*(1), 14–23.

Ghielli, M., Verstrepen, W. A., Nouwen, E. J., and De Broe, M. E. (1996, May). Inflammatory cells in renal regeneration. *Ren Fail, 18*(3), 355–375.

Giuliano, R. A., Paulus, G. J., Verpooten, G. A., Pattyn, V. M., Pollet, D. E., Nouwen, E. J., Laurent, G., Carlier, M. B., Maldague, P., Tulkens, P. M., et al. (1984, Dec). Recovery of cortical phospholipidosis and necrosis after acute gentamicin loading in rats. *Kidney Int, 26*(6), 838–847.

Glauser, M. P., Meylan, P., and Bille, J. (1987, Oct). The inflammatory response and tissue damage. The example of renal scars following acute renal infection. *Pediatr Nephrol, 1*(4), 615–622.

Huls, M., Russel, F. G., and Masereeuw, R. (2008). Insights into the role of bone marrow-derived stem cells in renal repair. *Kidney Blood Press Res, 31*(2), 104–110.

Humphreys, B. D., and Bonventre, J. V. (2008). Mesenchymal stem cells in acute kidney injury. *Annu Rev Med, 59*, 311–325.

Humphreys, B. D., Valerius, M. T., Kobayashi, A., Mugford, J. W., Soeung, S., Duffield, J. S., McMahon, A. P., and Bonventre, J. V. (2008, Mar 6). Intrinsic epithelial cells repair the kidney after injury. *Cell Stem Cell, 2*(3), 284–291.

Jayo, M. J., Jain, D., Ludlow, J. W., Payne, R., Wagner, B. J., McLorie, G., and Bertram, T. A. (2008a, Sep). Long-term durability, tissue regeneration and neo-organ growth during skeletal maturation with a neo-bladder augmentation construct. *Regen Med, 3*(5), 671–682.

Jayo, M. J., Jain, D., Wagner, B. J., and Bertram, T. A. (2008b, July). Early cellular and stromal responses in the regeneration of a functional mammalian bladder. *J Urol, 180,* 392–397.

Jayo, M. J., Watson, D. D., Wagner, B. J., and Bertram, T. A. (2008c). Tissue engineering and regenerative medicine: role of toxicologic pathologists for an emerging medical technology. *Toxicol Pathol, 36*(1), 92–96.

Joseph, D., Borer, J., De Filippo, R., McLorie, G., Goldberg, L., Tillinger, M., and Seltzer, E. (2009, April 25–30). *A phase 2 study – Autologous Neo-Bladder Construct (NBC) for augmentation cystoplasty in subjects with neurogenic bladder secondary to spina bifida.* Poster presented at the American Urology Association Annual Meeting, Chicago, IL.

Kawaida, K., Matsumoto, K., Shimazu, H., and Nakamura, T. (1994, May 10). Hepatocyte growth factor prevents acute renal failure and accelerates renal regeneration in mice. *Proc Natl Acad Sci U S A, 91*(10), 4357–4361.

Kinomura, M., Kitamura, S., Tanabe, K., Ichinose, K., Hirokoshi, K., Takazawa, Y., Kitayama, H., Nasu, T., Sugiyama, H., Yamasaki, Y., Sugaya, T., Maeshima, Y., and Makino, H. (2008). Amelioration of cisplatin-induced acute renal injury by renal progenitor-like cells derived from the adult rat kidney. *Cell Transplant, 17*(1–2), 143–158.

Kirpatovskii, V. I., Kazachenko, A. V., Plotnikov, E. Y., Marei, M. V., Musina, R. A., Nadtochii, O. N., Kon'kova, T. A., Drozhzheva, V. V., and Sukhikh, G. T. (2007, Jan). Experimental intravenous cell therapy of acute and chronic renal failure. *Bull Exp Biol Med, 143*(1), 160–165.

Klausner, J. M., Paterson, I. S., Goldman, G., Kobzik, L., Rodzen, C., Lawrence, R., Valeri, C. R., Shepro, D., and Hechtman, H. B. (1989, May). Postischemic renal injury is mediated by neutrophils and leukotrienes. *Am J Physiol, 256*(5 Pt 2), F794–802.

Kliem, V., Johnson, R. J., Alpers, C. E., Yoshimura, A., Couser, W. G., Koch, K. M., and Floege, J. (1996, Mar). Mechanisms involved in the pathogenesis of tubulointerstitial fibrosis in 5/6-nephrectomized rats. *Kidney Int, 49*(3), 666–678.

Koraitim, M., Schafer, W., Melchior, H., and Lutzeyer, W. (1977, Oct). Vesicourethral continuity in bladder neck activity. *Urology, 10*(4), 363–365.

Kropp, B. P., Cheng, E. Y., Lin, H. K., and Zhang, Y. (2004, Oct). Reliable and reproducible bladder regeneration using unseeded distal small intestinal submucosa. *J Urol, 172*(4 Pt 2), 1710–1713.

Kuper, C., Bartels, H., Fraek, M. L., Beck, F. X., and Neuhofer, W. (2007, Dec). Ectodomain shedding of pro-TGF-alpha is required for COX-2 induction and cell survival in renal medullary cells exposed to osmotic stress. *Am J Physiol Cell Physiol, 293*(6), C1971–1982.

Landman, J., Olweny, E., Sundaram, C. P., Andreoni, C., Collyer, W. C., Rehman, J., Jerde, T. J., Lin, H. K., Lee, D. I., Nunlist, E. H., Humphrey, P. A., Nakada, S. Y., and Clayman, R. V. (2004, Jun). Laparoscopic mid sagittal hemicystectomy and bladder reconstruction with small intestinal submucosa and reimplantation of ureter into small intestinal submucosa: 1-year followup. *J Urol, 171*(6 Pt 1), 2450–2455.

Laurent, G., Yernaux, V., Nonclercq, D., Toubeau, G., Maldague, P., Tulkens, P. M., and Heuson-Stiennon, J. A. (1988). Tissue injury and proliferative response induced in rat kidney by cis-diamminedichloroplatinum (II). *Virchows Arch B Cell Pathol Incl Mol Pathol, 55*(3), 129–145.

Lin, F. (2006, Apr). Stem cells in kidney regeneration following acute renal injury. *Pediatr Res, 59*(4 Pt 2), 74R–78R.

Liu, Y. (2004, Jul). Hepatocyte growth factor in kidney fibrosis: therapeutic potential and mechanisms of action. *Am J Physiol Renal Physiol, 287*(1), F7–16.

Maeshima, A., Nojima, Y., and Kojima, I. (2001, Dec). The role of the activin-follistatin system in the developmental and regeneration processes of the kidney. *Cytokine Growth Factor Rev, 12*(4), 289–298.

Matsumoto, K., and Nakamura, T. (2001, Jun). Hepatocyte growth factor: renotropic role and potential therapeutics for renal diseases. *Kidney Int, 59*(6), 2023–2038.

Morigi, M., Introna, M., Imberti, B., Corna, D., Abbate, M., Rota, C., Rottoli, D., Benigni, A., Perico, N., Zoja, C., Rambaldi, A., Remuzzi, A., and Remuzzi, G. (2008, Aug). Human bone marrow mesenchymal stem cells accelerate recovery of acute renal injury and prolong survival in mice. *Stem Cells, 26*(8), 2075–2082.

Nagaike, M., Hirao, S., Tajima, H., Noji, S., Taniguchi, S., Matsumoto, K., and Nakamura, T. (1991, Dec 5). Renotropic functions of hepatocyte growth factor in renal regeneration after unilateral nephrectomy. *J Biol Chem, 266*(34), 22781–22784.

Nath, K. A. (1992, Jul). Tubulointerstitial changes as a major determinant in the progression of renal damage. *Am J Kidney Dis, 20*(1), 1–17.

Neilson, E. G. (1989, May). Pathogenesis and therapy of interstitial nephritis. *Kidney Int, 35*(5), 1257–1270.

Oberpenning, F., Meng, J., Yoo, J. J., and Atala, A. (1999, Feb). De novo reconstitution of a functional mammalian urinary bladder by tissue engineering. *Nat Biotechnol, 17*(2), 149–155.

Oliver, J. A., Maarouf, O., Cheema, F. H., Martens, T. P., and Al-Awqati, Q. (2004, Sep). The renal papilla is a niche for adult kidney stem cells. *J Clin Invest, 114*(6), 795–804.

Orikasa, S., and Tsuji, I. (1970, Jul). Enlargement of contracted bladder by use of gelatin sponge bladder. *J Urol, 104*(1), 107–110.

Patschan, D., Krupincza, K., Patschan, S., Zhang, Z., Hamby, C., and Goligorsky, M. S. (2006, Jul). Dynamics of mobilization and homing of endothelial progenitor cells after acute renal ischemia: modulation by ischemic preconditioning. *Am J Physiol Renal Physiol, 291*(1), F176–185.

Presnell, S., Bruce, A., Wallace, S., Choudhury, S., Kelley, R., Tatsumi, P., Werdin, E., Rivera, E., Merricks, E., Nichols, T. C., Jennette, J. C., Jayo, M. J., and Bertram, T. A. (2009, April 18–22, 2009). *Isolation and characterization of bioresponsive renal cells from human and large mammal with chronic renal failure.* Submitted November 13, presented at Experimental Biology, New Orleans, LA.

Prodromidi, E. I., Poulsom, R., Jeffery, R., Roufosse, C. A., Pollard, P. J., Pusey, C. D., and Cook, H. T. (2006, Nov). Bone marrow-derived cells contribute to podocyte regeneration and amelioration of renal disease in a mouse model of Alport syndrome. *Stem Cells, 24*(11), 2448–2455.

Rovin, B. H., Harris, K. P., Morrison, A., Klahr, S., and Schreiner, G. F. (1990, Aug). Renal cortical release of a specific macrophage chemoattractant in response to ureteral obstruction. *Lab Invest, 63*(2), 213–220.

Russell, A. J., and Bertram, T. A. (2007). Moving into the clinic. In R. Lanza, R. Langer and J. P. Vacanti (Eds.), *Principles of tissue engineering* (3rd ed., pp. 15–32). Burlington, MA: Elsevier Academic Press.

Schena, F. P. (1998, May). Role of growth factors in acute renal failure. *Kidney Int Suppl, 66*, S11–15.

Schwartz, M. M., Bidani, A. K., and Lewis, E. J. (1987, Feb). Glomerular epithelial cell function and pathology following extreme ablation of renal mass. *Am J Pathol, 126*(2), 315–324.

Seltzer, E., Tillinger, M., Jayo, M. J., and Bertram, T. A. (2009, April 25–30). *Role of biomechanical stimulation (cycling) in neo-bladder regeneration – translational basis for clinical outcomes.* Poster presented at the American Urology Association Annual Meeting, Chicago, IL.

Staack, A., Hayward, S. W., Baskin, L. S., and Cunha, G. R. (2005, Apr). Molecular, cellular and developmental biology of urothelium as a basis of bladder regeneration. *Differentiation*, *73*(4), 121–133.

Stanger, B. Z., Tanaka, A. J., and Melton, D. A. (2007, Feb 22). Organ size is limited by the number of embryonic progenitor cells in the pancreas but not the liver. *Nature*, *445*(7130), 886–891.

Stocum, D. L. (2002). *Regenerative biology and medicine*. Burlington, MA: Academic Press.

Taguchi, H., Ishizuka, E., and Saito, K. (1977, Nov). Cystoplasty by regeneration of the bladder. *J Urol*, *118*(5), 752–756.

Tibbitts, J. (2003, Jan-Feb). Issues related to the use of canines in toxicologic pathology–issues with pharmacokinetics and metabolism. *Toxicol Pathol*, *31* Suppl, 17–24.

Van der Werf, B. A., and Creed, K. E. (2002, Oct). Mechanical properties and innervation of the smooth muscle layers of the urethra of greyhounds. *BJU Int*, *90*(6), 588–595.

Van der Werf, B. A., Hidaka, T., and Creed, K. E. (2000, Feb). Continence and some properties of the urethral striated muscle of male greyhounds. *BJU Int*, *85*(3), 341–349.

Yamada, M., Katsuma, S., Adachi, T., Hirasawa, A., Shiojima, S., Kadowaki, T., Okuno, Y., Koshimizu, T. A., Fujii, S., Sekiya, Y., Miyamoto, Y., Tamura, M., Yumura, W., Nihei, H., Kobayashi, M., and Tsujimoto, G. (2005, May 24). Inhibition of protein kinase CK2 prevents the progression of glomerulonephritis. *Proc Natl Acad Sci U S A*, *102*(21), 7736–7741.

Yoo, J. J., Meng, J., Oberpenning, F., and Atala, A. (1998, Feb). Bladder augmentation using allogenic bladder submucosa seeded with cells. *Urology*, *51*(2), 221–225.

Section II

Enabling Technologies for Regenerative Pharmacology

5

Stem and Progenitor Cells in Regenerative Pharmacology

MARK E. FURTH, MARTIN K. CHILDERS, AND LOLA M. REID

To achieve its goal of promoting the development, maturation, and function of bioengineered or regenerating tissue (Andersson and Christ, 2007; Furth and Christ, 2009), regenerative pharmacology must modulate the behavior of stem and progenitor cells. These constitute immature precursor cells, whether in an early embryo, a fetus, or an adult, capable of both sustained proliferation and differentiation into various types of specialized cells (Weissman et al. 2001). The crucial defining distinction of stem cells is their ability to self-renew (i.e., to maintain indefinitely a population with identical properties, through either symmetric or asymmetric cell divisions) (Morrison and Kimble, 2006; Simons and Clevers, 2011). Progenitors, by contrast, serve a transitory role in the amplification of a cell population during development or regeneration. When the self-renewal capacity of precursors cannot be rigorously ascertained, investigators sometimes use the terminology "stem/progenitor cells."

The unmet medical needs that might be addressed by harnessing the regenerative capacity of stem and progenitor cells are enormous (Perry, 2000). However, stem cell technologies generally, and regenerative pharmacology in particular, have only begun to scratch the surface of their potential to improve human health. Stem cell biology and pharmacology will intersect in three distinct ways (Xu et al. 2008b). First, they will partner in the traditional development of new pharmaceutical entities, both small molecules and biologicals such as cytokines, to mobilize the body's endogenous stem and progenitor cells for regeneration. Second, pharmacology will help to drive safe, cost-effective implementation of cell-based therapies and tissue engineering by optimizing the expansion, differentiation, and in some instances even the creation of stem cell populations ex vivo before implantation of the therapeutic product into patients (Li and Ding, 2010). Finally, stem cell biology will enable the creation of novel models of human disorders, "diseases in a petri dish," enabling a new generation of drug discovery (Saha and Jaenisch, 2009; Unternaehrer and Daley, 2011).

Stem Cell Overview

Stem cells in the first stages of the developing mammalian embryo, along with primordial germ cells at later stages, have the remarkable capacity to give rise to all of the body's cell types, and are therefore termed *pluripotent* (Solter, 2006). Embryonic stem (ES) and embryonic germ (EG) cells retain pluripotency during extensive expansion as established cell lines (Evans and Kaufman, 1981; Martin, 1981; Shamblott et al. 1998; Thomson et al. 1998). The self-renewal potential of ES cells appears virtually unlimited, although the accumulation of spontaneous mutations and chromosomal rearrangements eventually degrades their practical utility (Maitra et al. 2005). A remarkable finding with enormous implications for regenerative medicine and human genetics is that comparable pluripotent stem cells can be generated through the reprogramming of mature somatic cells by the introduction of small sets of defined genetic factors (Takahashi and Yamanaka, 2006; Yu et al. 2007). These are termed *induced pluripotent stem* (iPS) cells.

Adult stem cells, so named even at prenatal stages, are restricted to specific lineages (Weissman et al. 2001). Tissue-specific stem cells replenish mature cells that are lost through normal turnover or injury and disease. Some mature cell types, such as blood cells and those lining the gut or the outer layer of the skin, have a limited lifespan and must be replaced rapidly. Other mature cells, such as cardiomyocytes and certain neurons, can persist for the entire human lifespan (Spalding et al. 2005). The proliferation and differentiation of stem cells must be regulated tightly to ensure lifelong maintenance of appropriate numbers of specialized cells and of the stem cell compartment itself under normal conditions and when cells are replaced because of disease or injury.

The behavior of stem cells is controlled both by intrinsic genetic programs and by extrinsic cues from hormones, growth factors, and cytokines and from the surrounding cells and extracellular matrix (ECM) that comprise the niche in which stem cells reside (Li and Xie, 2005; Scadden, 2006). Signals from the niche help to maintain stem cells in a quiescent state, sometimes designated G_0 (Yamazaki and Nakauchi, 2009). That is, many adult stem cells are rarely engaged in the cell cycle except when there is a physiological demand to replace mature cells. However, there are important exceptions to this generalization. In the intestinal epithelium, which turns over every 3 to 5 days, a significant fraction of the stem cells located in the crypts of Lieberkühn remain actively cycling (Barker et al. 2010a).

Although often described as having lesser expansion capacity than pluripotent ES cells, many types of adult stem cells can self-renew extensively; a number have been maintained in culture for more than 40 population doublings, corresponding to greater than one trillion-fold (1×10^{12}) potential expansion (Bruder et al. 1997; D'Ippolito et al. 2004; De Coppi et al. 2007; Gupta et al. 2006; Jiang et al. 2002; Loo et al. 2008; McClelland et al. 2008b; Mitchell et al. 2003; Papini et al. 2003;

Rodriguez et al. 2005; Schmelzer et al. 2007; Untergasser et al. 2006). In some cases, adult stem cells, similar to ES cells, actually can propagate for hundreds of population doublings. For example, the stem cells in mouse intestinal crypts divide on average faster than once per day and may persist for the animal's 2-year lifespan (Schepers et al. 2011). A recent synthesis posits that in several tissues, exchangeable quiescent and active stem cell subpopulations coexist in adjacent zones (Li and Clevers, 2010). This may serve the dual purpose of preventing exhaustion of the active stem pool while decreasing the risk of accumulating mutations that predispose to cancer.

Hematopoiesis as a Model for Regenerative Pharmacology

Among adult stem cells, those for the blood system have been the most exhaustively characterized. Hematopoietic stem cells (HSCs) give rise to at least 10 specialized types of mature blood cells, including erythrocytes, megakaryocytes, and all the white blood cells of the innate and adaptive immune systems (Bryder et al. 2006; Seita and Weissman, 2010). HSCs maintain their own population (self-renew) and give rise to progenitors that, through a series of cell divisions, become progressively restricted to specific blood cell types and gradually lose the ability to proliferate (Bryder et al. 2006). The system can be depicted as an elaborate branching structure, with the stem cell compartment as the base of a short-trunked tree and terminally differentiated cells as the leaves, which regularly die and must be replaced (Sell, 2004). A single HSC from murine bone marrow, after intravenous injection, can reconstitute the entire blood-forming capacity of a lethally irradiated mouse (Cao et al. 2004; Osawa et al. 1996). Single human HSCs, likewise, are able to reconstitute the complete hematopoietic system, shown by long-term engraftment in immune-deficient mice (Notta et al. 2011). Serial transplantation studies indicate that murine HSCs can continue to function through at least 15 to 50 normal lifespans, a striking demonstration of self-renewal (Gazit et al. 2008). The reconstituting HSCs are rare; a recent statistical analysis calculates about one per 5,400 cells in normal mouse bone marrow (Bonnefoix and Callanan, 2010).

The powerful capacity of limited numbers of HSCs to restore hematopoiesis long term provides the basis for human bone marrow transplantation, a medical procedure dating back more than half a century (Thomas et al. 1975a; Thomas et al. 1975b). Intensive research focus on the blood-forming lineages also led to the first "blockbuster" products of regenerative pharmacology, namely, the recombinant human cytokines erythropoietin (EPO; epoetin) (Faulds and Sorkin, 1989) and granulocyte colony-stimulating factor (G-CSF; filgrastim, lenograstim) (Frampton et al. 1994). These molecules target lineage-specific hematopoietic progenitors to drive rapid increases in the populations of specific sets of blood cells in individuals with anemia or neutropenia, respectively.

Hematopoietic Cytokines

Compelling evidence for the existence of a circulating hormone-like factor capable of stimulating erythropoiesis (the production of red blood cells) came from the demonstration of such activity in the plasma and urine of anemic animals (Fried, 2009). Purification of sufficient EPO for partial amino acid sequence determination enabled molecular cloning of the corresponding human cDNA and efficient expression of the glycoprotein in engineered mammalian cells. EPO acts on a specific receptor (EPO-R) that is most prominently expressed by committed precursor cells relatively late in the red blood cell lineage. EPO promotes the survival and limited proliferation of these cells. Pharmacologically, EPO particularly benefits renal failure patients because the kidneys are the major endogenous source of the cytokine. This approach is analogous to the use of insulin to treat type 1 diabetes in compensation for the loss of pancreatic β cells. Ultimately, regenerative medicine seeks to provide a definitive cure for such hormone deficiencies by restoring functional tissue able to produce the missing factor in a regulated manner, thereby obviating the need for frequent injections of a protein drug (Furth and Christ, 2009).

The commercial success of EPO encouraged efforts to develop additional recombinant cytokines able to increase the specification, number, or activity of particular subsets of hematopoietic cells. The discovery of several cytokines active on the myeloid (granulocyte and macrophage) cell lineages initially emerged from observations in the mid-1960s of colony formation in semisolid culture media initiated by rare hematopoietic progenitor cells present in bone marrow. The clonal growth and differentiation of these progenitors required specific colony-stimulating factors (CSFs), initially found in sources such as urine from leukemia patients or fibroblast-conditioned medium (Metcalf, 2008). Many distinct CSF activities were identified and eventually manufactured in pure form using recombinant DNA technology. At least five recombinant CSFs active on subsets of myeloid progenitors via different receptors have been tested in human subjects (Antman, 1990; Demetri and Antman, 1992; Frampton et al. 1994; Vadhan-Raj, 1994). Among these, both G-CSF and granulocyte-macrophage CSF (GM-CSF; sargramostim) (Grant and Heel, 1992) received U.S. Food and Drug Administration (FDA) approval in 1991. G-CSF and GM-CSF elevate granulocyte (neutrophil) levels in cancer patients with chemotherapy-induced myelosuppression, helping to restore innate immunity against bacterial infections (Fennelly et al. 1994; Volkers, 1999). The monocyte/macrophage lineage-specific CSF, called M-CSF or CSF-1 (Chitu and Stanley, 2006), also enhances immune function after chemotherapy (Hidaka et al. 2003).

Another important activity of G-CSF and GM-CSF is the recruitment of HSCs from niches in the bone marrow into the circulation. These cytokines are used as mobilizing agents so that peripheral blood rather than bone marrow can be used as the donor stem cell source for transplantation (Damon, 2009). The pharmacology of

HSC mobilization is an active research area (Pusic and DiPersio, 2008), and synthetic compounds have been identified that augment stem cell trafficking by several mechanisms (Gertz, 2010; Hoggatt and Pelus, 2011). These agents may be administered together with a myeloid CSF or independently. Plerixafor (Mozobil; AMD3100) accomplishes mobilization by interfering with the action of stromal cell-derived factor-1 (SDF-1) at the CXCR4 alpha-chemokine receptor, which helps to regulate both HSC quiescence and homing to bone marrow niches. This drug has received regulatory approval from the FDA and the European Committee for Medicinal Products for Human Use (Brave et al. 2010). By displacing leukemia stem cells from protected niches, plerixafor also has the potential to improve outcomes of chemotherapy in patients with hematologic malignancies (Pusic and DiPersio, 2010).

The pharmacology of the hematopoietic cytokines is complex. These molecules are obligatory for cell proliferation within specific lineages. They also promote survival, lineage commitment, and differentiation of stem and progenitor cells and the specialized functionality of mature cells (Metcalf, 2008). Furthermore, cytokines that initially were thought to be specific to a particular class of blood cells often have broader activity because cells of unrelated lineages can express cognate receptors. This may have clinical value. For example, in addition to their actions on hematopoietic cells, EPO, G-CSF, and GM-CSF all bind specifically to receptors on certain neural cell precursors (Maurer et al. 2008; Sizonenko et al. 2007; Studer et al. 2000; Vitellaro-Zuccarello et al. 2007; Wang et al. 2010c). These cytokines, therefore, are now being assessed in the treatment of central nervous system disorders, including stroke, neurodegeneration, and spinal cord injuries.

Off-target activities of cytokines or growth factors, because of activity on multiple receptors or expression of receptors on multiple cell lineages, may entail risks as well as benefits. A case in point is the wide use of EPO to alleviate chemotherapy-induced anemia, which has come under scrutiny because this cytokine may stimulate tumor progression and shorten the lives of some cancer patients (Blau, 2007; Fandrey and Dicato, 2009). Mechanisms underlying this side effect include enhancement of angiogenesis and direct stimulation of cancer cell proliferation by binding to EPO-R expressed by tumors (Dicato and Plawny, 2010; Glaspy, 2009; Kuster et al. 2009; Lei et al. 2011; Tovari et al. 2008). As an example, consistent with the EPO responsiveness of normal neural stem and progenitor cells, recent reports document elevated EPO-R levels in putative stem cells of glioblastomas (Cao et al. 2010; Chen et al. 2007; Giese et al. 2010; Tsai et al. 2006).

Stem Cell Expansion

Erythropoietin and G-CSF achieved clinical success based on relatively short-term effects, rapidly boosting the level of mature end cells or of circulating HSCs. This occurs without expanding the pool of the earliest HSC or progenitor cells that are endowed with true regenerative capacity. In fact, despite the intense focus over many years on factors that regulate hematopoiesis, pharmacological manipulation of the rare population of HSCs capable of long-term reconstitution of the blood-forming and immune systems has proved a formidable challenge (Kent et al. 2008; Veiby et al. 1997; Zhang and Lodish, 2008).

Various factors have been identified that promote the survival, proliferation, and/or lineage commitment of early stage, multipotent hematopoietic stem/progenitors. Examples include the "multi-CSF" interleukin-3 (IL-3) (Ihle, 1992; Ivanovic, 2004; Lindemann and Mertelsmann, 1995) and the ligands for the protein tyrosine-kinase receptors c-Kit (CD117) and flt3/flk-2. The latter cytokines are termed, respectively, stem cell factor (SCF) and flt-3 ligand (FL or TSF) (Kent et al. 2008; Lyman and Jacobsen, 1998; Zhang and Lodish, 2008). Thrombopoietin (TPO), the main protein factor regulating development of megakaryocytes and platelets, also binds to HSCs via the Mpl receptor (Ninos et al. 2006). Genetic studies in mice provide convincing evidence that SCF, FL, and TPO play important roles in the production or maintenance of HSCs and early progenitors, and IL-3 can enhance expansion of these cells in culture (Seita and Weissman, 2010; Veiby et al. 1997; Zhang and Lodish, 2008). Nevertheless, to date, none of these four factors has been developed successfully for clinical use (Eder et al. 1997; Smith et al. 2001; Veiby et al. 1997). One limitation to the medical application of SCF, in particular, is the wide distribution of the c-Kit receptor on stem and progenitor cells of many lineages. Likewise, although the Wnt, Notch, and Hedgehog (Hh) pathways contribute to the regulation of HSC self-renewal (Cerdan and Bhatia, 2010; Duncan et al. 2005; Nemeth and Bodine, 2007) and Wnt signaling is activated during hematopoietic regeneration (Congdon et al. 2008), these factors are involved in so many aspects of normal development and tissue homeostasis, and also oncogenesis, that off-target effects would likely preclude their systemic administration to stimulate hematopoiesis.

A fallback strategy to enhance hematopoietic regeneration is the expansion in culture (termed ex vivo or in vitro) of HSCs from bone marrow or umbilical cord blood. The goal would be to provide enough stem cells for more successful, rapid engraftment or to allow more than one recipient to receive stem cells from a single donor. The prevalence of umbilical cord blood banking and the limited number of cells obtained from each cord make it especially attractive to amplify HSCs from this source (Wagner et al. 2009). Surprisingly, in light of the great self-renewal capacity of HSCs in the living organism, only modest expansion has been achieved ex vivo using expensive growth factor and cytokine cocktails (Ivanovic, 2004; Smith et al. 2001; Suzuki et al. 2006; Zhang et al. 2008a; Zhang and Lodish, 2008). A major difficulty is that differentiation of HSCs to more restricted progenitors generally overbalances stem cell self-renewal. However, a recent report using stringent criteria to enumerate stem cells capable of hematopoietic reconstitution in immune-deficient mice demonstrated approximately 20-fold expansion of HSCs in a defined medium containing angiopoietin-like protein 5 (Angptl5), SCF, TPO, fibroblast growth factor 1 (FGF1), and insulin-like growth factor binding protein 2 (IGFBP2) (Drake et al. 2011).

A potent new candidate molecule to expand HSCs emerged recently from the analysis of factors secreted by stromal and endothelial cells that promoted self-renewal of the stem cells in co-cultures. Pleiotrophin, a small (17-kDa) heparin-binding cytokine, acts on the receptor protein tyrosine phosphatase-β/ζ (RPTP-β/ζ or Rptpz1), which is expressed by bone marrow cells, including those at early stages in the hematopoietic lineage (Himburg et al. 2010). RPTP-β/ζ is present in many lineages, and, as implied by its name, pleiotrophin shows activity on diverse cell types. It enhances neurite outgrowth and promotes proliferation or differentiation of various cells, including fibroblasts, endothelial and epithelial cells, neural stem cells, osteogenic progenitors, and ES cells (Deuel et al. 2002). Genetic knockout of pleiotrophin did not cause a significant deficiency in hematopoiesis and led to relatively subtle changes in the balance of HSCs and hematopoietic progenitors ex vivo and in regeneration after transplantation (Istvanffy et al. 2011). However, when added ex vivo along with a standard set of HSC growth factors (e.g., TPO, SCF, and FL), pleiotrophin substantially increased the production of HSC with long-term repopulating activity in cultures from mouse bone marrow or human cord blood (Himburg et al. 2010). Most remarkably, the daily administration of recombinant pleiotrophin to mice that had received whole-body irradiation led to a robust increase in total bone marrow cells, and at 2 weeks, augmented by more than 20-fold the number of long-term reconstituting HSCs (Himburg et al. 2010). This suggests potential clinical value for pleiotrophin in hematopoietic regeneration after chemotherapy or radiotherapy.

Small Molecule Stem Cell Modulators

Small molecules also have emerged as candidates for regenerative pharmacology targeting HSC. Following the rationale that the expression of genes associated with "stemness" must be maintained to enable ex vivo self-renewal of HSC and that these are downregulated by DNA methylation and deacetylation of histones, investigators tested compounds known to interfere with the epigenetic silencing of gene expression. They found that both the DNA methyl transferase inhibitor 5-aza-2′-deoxycytidine, and the histone deacetylase (HDAC) inhibitor trichostatin A, when added to a cytokine cocktail, enhanced the production of multipotent hematopoietic progenitors and HSCs in cultures of human cord blood cells (Araki et al. 2006).

Another small molecule approach to promote HSC expansion sprang from the observation that the activity of p38 mitogen-activated protein kinase (MAPK p38) was associated with bone marrow suppression in certain pathological conditions (e.g., aplastic anemia and myelodysplastic syndromes) and with the premature exhaustion and senescence of HSCs under oxidative stress. Routine culturing of HSCs leads to specific activation of p38 (Wang et al. 2011d). The response may be linked to oxidative stress because the level of oxygen to which cells are typically exposed in culture (corresponding to ambient air with 20 percent O_2; $pO_2 \approx 152$ mm Hg) is far higher than in vivo (Csete, 2005). Indeed, normal HSCs are concentrated in the most hypoxic region of the bone marrow (estimated at ≈ 1.5 percent O_2; $pO_2 \approx 10$ mm Hg) (Chow et al. 2001; Parmar et al. 2007). A specific p38 inhibitor, SB203580, added to serum-free medium with a standard cytokine cocktail, substantially improved the self-renewal and expansion of HSCs (Wang et al. 2011d).

Large-scale screening provides an additional means to find molecules that promote stem cell expansion ex vivo. Investigators recently used a high content assay to screen for compounds able to enhance the proliferation of cells expressing CD34, a surface marker of hematopoietic stem cells, over 5 to 7 days in bone marrow cells cultured with standard cytokines. From a library of 100,000 heterocyclic molecules, they identified a purine derivative with the desired activity and named it StemRegenin 1 (SR1) (Boitano et al. 2010). Mechanistic studies indicated that SR1 inhibits signaling through the aryl hydrocarbon receptor (AHR), a ligand-dependent transcription factor best known for mediating the toxicity of xenobiotics such as dioxin. HSCs are known to express this receptor. Other AHR antagonists also induced dose-dependent increases in the number of CD34-positive cells. At an optimal dose SR1 induced more than a 1,000-fold increase in this population. However, only a fraction of CD34-positive cells constitute "early" HSCs. The actual expansion of stem cells capable of in vivo reconstitution was only about 16-fold, several-fold less than in co-cultures of HSC with support cells engineered to secrete Angpl5 (Drake et al. 2011; Khoury et al. 2011).

The studies of HSC expansion demonstrate that signaling pathways responsive to cues such as oxygen level or the presence of planar aromatic hydrocarbons can profoundly influence stem cell proliferation, self-renewal, and differentiation. The AHR belongs to the Per-Arnt-Sym (PAS) superfamily, proteins with modular domains that monitor environmental changes in oxygen, redox levels, light, and ion flow (Gu et al. 2000; Taylor and Zhulin, 1999). The family also includes the hypoxia-inducible factors (HIFs), which have been implicated in regulating the stemness of HSC and other stem cell populations (Fatrai et al. 2011; Forristal et al. 2010; Simsek et al. 2010; Takubo et al. 2010). Regulation of the transcription factor HIF-1α, in particular, appears essential for correct balancing between HSC quiescence and activation (Takubo et al. 2010). Consistent with their location in a hypoxic niche, HSCs derive energy primarily from glycolysis rather than mitochondrial oxidative phosphorylation (Simsek et al. 2010). Thus, in addition to cytokines or matrix molecules present in stem cell niches, targets for regenerative pharmacology may be derived from understanding the broader environmental parameters and signaling mediated by PAS-domain proteins. These reflect such fundamental properties of stem cells as utilization of specific metabolic pathways, response to oxidative stress (Hosokawa et al. 2007), and regulation by circadian oscillations (Mendez-Ferrer et al. 2008).

Hepatic Stem Cells

To what extent can lessons learned from hematopoietic biology be extended to other cell lineages? Most adult organs contain a pool of undifferentiated progenitor or stem cells (or both) that serve as precursors to specific parenchymal cell types (Alison and Islam, 2009; Anversa et al. 2006; Barker et al. 2010a; Gage, 2000; Katsumoto et al. 2010; Turner et al. 2011; Verstappen et al. 2009; Weissman et al. 2001). In general, neither the characterization of these rare cells nor their mobilization for the therapy of injuries and degenerative diseases has advanced so far as for HSCs. Nevertheless, several cases support the feasibility of promoting regeneration either through the delivery of stem and progenitor cells expanded and, in some instances, induced to differentiate ex vivo or through local delivery of drugs to enhance activity of the endogenous precursor cells. Liver and bone serve as examples.

Those familiar with the myth of Prometheus will recall that the liver possesses a considerable capacity for regeneration (Michalopoulos and DeFrances, 2005). Even so, liver diseases potentially leading to organ failure, caused by factors such as hepatitis viruses, alcohol consumption, diet, and metabolic disorders, constitute a major medical burden (Beier et al. 2011; Cohen et al. 2011; Masarone and Persico, 2011; Said, 2011). Cell-based therapies and tissue engineering represent possible approaches to address the need (Baptista et al. 2011; Fukumitsu et al. 2011; Muraca, 2011; Russo and Parola, 2011; Shupe and Petersen, 2011). Sourcing of cells for such applications is a significant challenge. Here we will focus specifically on stem and progenitor cells of the liver and biliary tree. The role of stem cells in the normal maintenance of the liver and in regeneration from various types of insults remains a subject of active research and debate (Duncan et al. 2009; Michalopoulos, 2011; Tanaka et al. 2011). The discussion in this section derives from our view that throughout life the liver contains stem cells that give rise to the organ's two specialized epithelial cell types, hepatocytes and cholangiocytes (bile duct cells), via an organized maturational lineage system (Turner et al. 2011). Given this premise, a role for regenerative pharmacology is to help provide sufficient hepatic stem/progenitor cells and to promote differentiation to the mature liver cell types.

Stem Cell Isolation and Expansion

We (Reid, Furth, and colleagues) reported the isolation of hepatic stem cells (HpSCs) from fetal, neonatal, and adult human livers by selection with a monoclonal antibody for the cell surface marker CD326 (epithelial cell adhesion molecule [EpCAM]) (Schmelzer et al. 2007). These cells constitute approximately 1 percent of the total

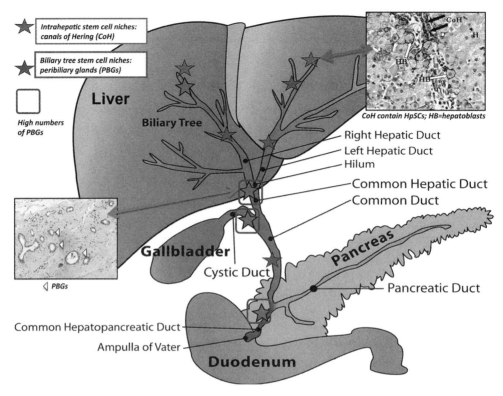

Figure 5-1. Schematic diagram of stem cell niches in the liver and biliary tree. *Hepatic stem cells* (HpSCs) are found within the liver in canals of Hering (CoH). *Inset top right* shows immunohistochemical staining (*brown*) for CD326 (EpCAM). HpSCs are small, strongly stained cells within CoH. *Hepatoblasts* (HBs), progenitors derived from HpSCs, are larger and characteristically show distinct staining of the cell membrane. *Inset left*, hematoxylin and eosin staining shows the location of *biliary tree stem cells in peribiliary glands* (PBGs). The pancreas contains committed progenitors but appears to lack stem cells capable of extended self-renewal. (See color plate 8.)

liver population from early childhood onward. Unlike mature hepatocytes, they survive extended periods of ischemia, allowing collection even several days after cardiac arrest (Stachelscheid et al. 2009). The HpSCs express additional surface markers often found on stem cells, such as CD133 (prominin), CD56 (neural cell adhesion molecule [NCAM]), and CD44 (the hyaluronan receptor), and express characteristic endodermal transcription factors SOX9, SOX17, and HES1. They are small (diameter of 7–9 μm, less than half that of mature parenchymal cells) and express negligible levels of adult liver-specific functions such as albumin, cytochrome P450s, and transferrin (TF). The stem cells display far greater capacity to proliferate in culture than hepatocytes or cholangiocytes and can continue to expand for months with a doubling time of 36 to 40 hours (McClelland et al. 2008b).

The HpSCs serve as the immediate precursors of a progenitor population known as hepatoblasts (HBs, Fig. 5-1, *inset top right*). Although also positive for CD326, the HBs are readily distinguished by the expression of α-fetoprotein and intercellular adhesion molecule-1 (ICAM-1), for which the HpSCs are negative (Schmelzer et al. 2007; Zhang et al. 2008b). The HBs, in turn, are precursors of committed unipotent progenitors for hepatocytes and cholangiocytes. When injected into livers of immune-deficient mice, the HpSCs give rise to cells expressing characteristic human liver and bile duct proteins, especially after the hosts' own liver cells have been damaged by treatment with carbon tetrachloride.

We noted earlier the requirement for complex mixtures of cytokines or small molecules and the limited success that has been achieved to date in ex vivo expansion of HSCs. The problems and the role for regenerative pharmacology are rather different for the hepatic lineage. Remarkably, the human HpSCs proliferate rapidly and for a sustained period in a defined serum-free culture medium (Kubota's medium; Kubota and Reid, 2000) containing insulin (needed for glucose uptake), TF (for iron transport), and a mixture of free fatty acids bound to albumin (McClelland et al. 2008b; Schmelzer et al. 2007; Wang et al. 2010b; Wauthier et al. 2008). No additional growth factor or cytokine is required. Conceivably, pathways important for hepatic stem/progenitor cell survival in vivo, such as Hh signaling (Sicklick et al. 2006), are activated through autocrine loops. The expanded HpSCs maintain a stable marker phenotype and express the enzyme telomerase, localized to the nucleus, consistent with a capacity for self-renewal (Schmelzer and Reid, 2009).

It appears that a crucial prerequisite for successful expansion of HpSCs is to mimic an appropriate microenvironment. When selected on tissue culture plastic tissue, the HpSCs invariably grow as colonies in association with immature mesenchymal cells, identified as angioblasts and hepatic stellate cell precursors (Kubota et al. 2007; Schmelzer et al. 2007; Wang et al. 2010b). Purified HpSCs survive and proliferate in culture only if they are provided with appropriate molecules to replace the paracrine signals normally received from the mesenchymal partners. The stem cells can be expanded for extended periods in Kubota's medium on a substratum of type III collagen or embedded in weakly crosslinked hyaluronic acid hydrogels (McClelland et al. 2008b; Wang et al. 2011c; Wang et al. 2010b). Both type III collagen and hyaluronans are constituents of the liver stem cell niche in bile ductules known as the canals of Hering (see Fig. 5-1) (McClelland et al. 2008a; Wang et al. 2010b; Zhang et al. 2008b). Conversely, other collagen types induce differentiation of the HpSCs toward hepatocytes (type IV collagen) or cholangiocytes (type I collagen) (Wang et al. 2010b).

The hepatic lineage cells also respond to mechanical forces. Initially, it was apparent that HpSCs grew better on flexible mesh (transwells) coated with type III collagen than hard plastic surfaces with the same coating (McClelland et al. 2008b). A systematic study of HpSC behavior in three-dimensional cultures using hyaluronan hydrogels of differing stiffness indicated that rigidity of the microenvironment is an important parameter in regulating maintenance of stemness versus differentiation to more restricted progenitors (Lozoya et al. 2011). This had been studied previously in differentiation of progenitors for bone and other hard tissues but not for internal organs such as the liver. Optimal expansion of the HpSCs for clinical applications likely will be achieved in three-dimensional hydrogels containing type III collagen and possibly additional ECM components or synthetic mimetics.

HpSCs, similar to human ES cells, grow in tight colonies. Dissociating both types of stem cells has proven to be an important practical problem for their efficient expansion ex vivo and for cryopreservation. When treated enzymatically to generate a single cell suspension, both ES cells and HpSCs undergo a high level of cell death. S. Ding's laboratory screened for chemicals that would enable ES cells to survive enzymatic dissociation and remain pluripotent (Xu et al. 2010). They identified two compounds, a 2,4-disubstituted thiazole (Thiazovivin) and a 2,4-disubstituted pyrimidine (Tyrintegin), meeting these criteria. Thiazovivin inhibits Rho-associated kinase (ROCK), a key component of the pathway that controls cytoskeleton remodeling and a likely regulator of cell–ECM and cell–cell interactions. Tyrintegin enhances attachment of dissociated ES cells to ECM and stabilizes E-cadherin. The investigators concluded that ES cell interactions in the normal niche generate signals essential to survival and that small molecules modulating those signals can maintain the viability of dissociated cells. Likewise, we have observed that hyaluronans, a normal component of many stem cell niches, can protect HpSC for dissociation and cryopreservation. This action presumably is mediated through the CD44 hyaluronan receptor, a marker shared by hepatic and many other stem cell populations.

Clinical programs for hepatic stem and progenitor cell therapies are in their early stages but have shown initial promise. A study by the late C.M. Habibullah and colleagues demonstrated potential value of such cells in end-stage liver disease (Khan et al. 2010). They used CD326-selected fetal liver cells, comprising both HpSC and HB. Twenty-five subjects with decompensated liver cirrhosis from various causes received cell infusions into the liver via the hepatic artery. At 6 months of follow-up, multiple diagnostic and biochemical parameters showed clear improvement, and there was a significant ($P < 0.01$) decrease in the mean Mayo End-stage Liver Disease (MELD) score, an accepted metric for clinical severity.

Future efforts to use HpSCs clinically would be facilitated by large-scale manufacturing of the cell population, especially if, from ethical and safety considerations, the choice of donor organs would be postnatal (neonatal or adult) rather than fetal. It may also be desirable to match, to the degree possible, the human leukocyte antigen (HLA; major histocompatibility) types of donor cells and recipients, although Khan et al. (2010) neither attempted such matching nor used immunosuppressive drugs. However, given sufficient expansion, it should be possible to bank expanded populations of stem cells from a modest number of carefully selected donors and achieve a beneficial degree of HLA matching for the large majority of recipients (Taylor et al. 2005).

Differentiation

The pharmacology of stem cell differentiation also must encompass both soluble signals (i.e., conventional biologics or drugs) and ECM components corresponding to cells' three-dimensional microenvironments. Cytokines and other soluble factors necessary for liver development and for the maintenance of differentiated hepatocytes have been known for some time (Kinoshita and Miyajima, 2002; Macdonald et al. 2002). However, the specific and efficient directed differentiation of stem or progenitor cells to fully mature hepatocytes and cholangiocytes ex vivo remained a difficult challenge. This, in fact, is a general problem in much of stem cell biology, whether starting with lineage-restricted adult stem cells or pluripotent ES and iPS cells.

More than 30 years ago, the laboratory of Reid developed a means to provide an environment conducive to maintenance of the differentiated state by presenting cells with ECM components, termed biomatrices, prepared by a high-salt extraction procedure (Rojkind et al. 1980). Frozen sections or pulverized liver biomatrices used as cell culture substrata enabled the long-term survival of highly functional hepatocytes, far beyond what could be achieved on plastic or with simple type I collagen gels. Recently, the Reid laboratory has used comparable extraction approaches to prepare perfused, decellularized organs. These biomatrix scaffolds are tissue specific and potently induce cell differentiation (Wang et al. 2011c). They contain more than 99.5 percent of the collagens and known collagen-bound matrix components, including the proteoglycans, and retain physiological levels of the known cytokines and growth factors found in the tissue. As expected from the original biomatrix studies, mature parenchymal cells plated on the scaffolds in a defined medium remained stable for many weeks and expressed liver-specific functions equivalent to those of freshly isolated cells. When HpSCs were seeded onto the liver biomatrix scaffolds in the same medium, within 1 week, they underwent several rounds of cell division followed by growth arrest and differentiation to mature hepatic parenchymal cells. High levels of specialized hepatocyte and cholangiocyte protein expression and functions could then be maintained for more than 8 weeks (Wang et al. 2011c).

Differentiation of HpSCs to mature parenchymal cells also can be achieved in three-dimensional hydrogels containing defined, purified ECM components (Cardinale et al. 2011; Wang et al. 2010b). Distinct conditions favor the generation of hepatocytes versus cholangiocytes. Ultimately, identification of each of the particular tissue-specific matrix molecules necessary for efficient differentiation will be required for mechanistic understanding. It also may be important for clinical translation. The pharmacology of ECM components and their interactions with cytokines and growth factors, the great majority of which bind to the carbohydrate chains of proteoglycans, is a rich, albeit highly complex area that promises to contribute greatly to regenerative medicine. Understanding of the role of specific carbohydrate sequences in regulating cell differentiation and tissue-specific gene expression is still in its infancy. There is ample opportunity to discover new drugs able to augment or substitute for rare matrix components that may be difficult to manufacture (Fisher et al. 2010).

Multipotent Endodermal Stem Cells

The liver derives from the endoderm, one of the three germ layers that are established at the gastrulation stage of early embryonic development (Zorn and Wells, 2007). Among the other organs of endodermal origin, endogenous adult stem cells have been identified in most, including the small and large intestines (Barker et al. 2008), the stomach (Barker et al. 2010b), and the lungs (Snyder et al. 2009). The situation for the pancreas is less clear cut because lineage-tracing experiments suggested that the postnatal organ lacks stem cells, at least for insulin-producing β cells (Dor et al. 2004; Houbracken and Bouwens, 2010; Xu et al. 2008a).

Recent collaborative work by Reid, Gaudio, Alvaro, and associates revealed previously unknown stem cells throughout the human biliary tree (Cardinale et al. 2011). These cells are located in peribiliary glands, found deep within the intra- and extrahepatic bile ducts (see Fig. 5-1). High numbers are found in the hepatopancreatic common duct, connecting to both the liver and the pancreas. Subpopulations of the biliary tree stem cells resemble the HpSCs in the canals of Hering of the liver (Theise et al. 1999; Zhang et al. 2008b). However, in addition to early endodermal lineage transcription factors, cells of the biliary tree stem cell populations also express moderate levels of certain markers generally associated with pluripotent stem cells, including OCT4, NANOG, SOX2, and KLF4 (Cardinale et al. 2011). Strikingly, some of the biliary tree stem cells also contain high levels of transcription factors specifically required for the development of the entire pancreas (e.g., PDX1) and the endocrine pancreatic islets of Langerhans (e.g., NGN3). Comparable levels of these pancreatic markers are not found in the HpSCs within the liver. Moreover, using appropriate conditions in three-dimensional hydrogels, biliary tree stem cells (a typical colony is shown in Fig. 5-2A) were induced to differentiate toward cholangiocytes (Fig. 5-2B), hepatocytes (Fig. 5-2C), and pancreatic neo-islets (Fig. 5-2D) (Cardinale et al. 2011). Differentiated cells showed characteristic morphology, three-dimensional organization, and lineage-specific patterns of gene expression. Data for representative transcripts are shown in the right-hand panels of Figure 5-2. The stem cell marker CD326/EpCAM is downmodulated under all three differentiation conditions. Conversely, markers of each lineage are upregulated in a cell type–specific manner: cystic fibrosis transmembrane conductance regulator for cholangiocytes; TF for hepatocytes; and proinsulin for pancreatic β cells (>300-fold relative increase).

To our knowledge, no previous study documented in fetal or adult tissue of any mammal a comparable robustly self-renewing, endodermal stem population able to give rise to pancreatic islet–like clusters and glucose-responsive β cells. The neo-islets

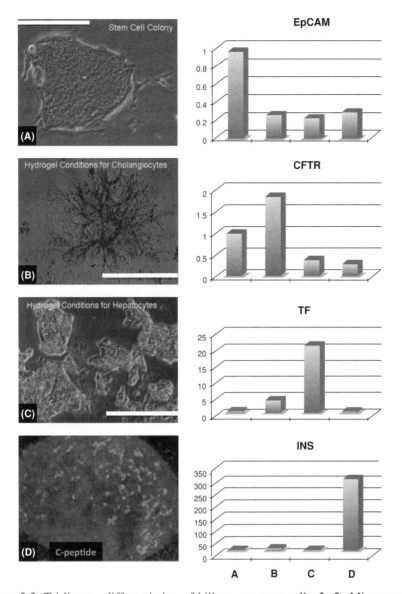

Figure 5-2. Tri-lineage differentiation of biliary tree stem cells. **Left**. Micrographs of (**A**) *undifferentiated biliary tree stem cells* expanded in Kubota's medium on tissue-culture plastic (bar = 0.2 mm) and (**B–D**) differentiation in three-dimensional hydrogels with appropriate growth factors and collagen types for specific fates: (**B**) *cholangiocyte lineage* showing branching ductules (bar = 1.0 mm), (**C**) *hepatocyte lineage* showing large cells with distinct bile canaliculi (bar = 0.2 mm), and (**D**) *endocrine pancreatic lineage* showing an islet-like cell cluster with positive immunofluorescent staining for insulin C-peptide. **Right**. Relative expression of representative lineage-specific transcripts assessed by quantitative polymerase chain reaction. Values are normalized to 1.0 in the undifferentiated stem cells (**A**). Differentiation conditions **B**, **C**, and **D** are as in the micrographs. CFTR = cystic fibrosis transmembrane conductance regulator, a cholangiocyte marker (much greater upregulation is observed with complete tissue-specific matrix in the hydrogel); EpCAM = CD326, expressed in stem cells, downregulated under all three differentiation conditions.; INS = proinsulin, a pancreatic β-cell marker; TR = transferrin, a hepatocyte marker. Many additional lineage markers showed comparably specific expression patterns under these differentiation conditions. (Adapted from Cardinale et al. 2011.) (See color plate 9.)

generated from biliary tree stem cells in vitro contained numerous cells positive for PDX1 and for the pancreatic hormones: glucagon, somatostatin, and, most importantly, insulin (Cardinale et al. 2011). Immunofluorescence staining for human C-peptide confirmed de novo synthesis of proinsulin (see Fig. 5-2D). Secretion of C-peptide was regulated appropriately in response to the level of glucose.

In vivo studies provided further evidence for the multipotency of the human biliary stem cells for hepatic and pancreatic fates. Direct injection of the stem cells into the livers of immune-deficient mice generated hepatocyte-like and cholangiocyte-like cells. To confirm endocrine pancreatic differentiation, pre-induced neo-islet structures were implanted into mouse fat pads, and the animals were treated with a toxin to destroy their own pancreatic β cells. Mice that received the human neo-islets showed significant resistance to hyperglycemia (diabetes) compared with control mice that did not receive cell therapy. The presence of functional β-like cells derived from the biliary tree stem cells could be inferred from circulating human C-peptide, which was regulated appropriately in response to a glucose challenge (Cardinale et al. 2011).

We favor the hypothesis that the extrahepatic biliary tree contains stem cells that are precursors to both HpSCs and pancreatic progenitors, and that these can migrate to the liver and pancreas throughout life as part of normal maturational lineages or in response to injury or disease. This implicates ongoing organogenesis for liver and pancreas, with the biliary tree serving as a stem cell reservoir. The practical utility of such multipotent endodermal stem cells will be enhanced as the tools of regenerative pharmacology are used to drive their expansion and directed differentiation in culture or in vivo (Furth and Christ, 2009).

Mesenchymal Stem Cells for Bone

Two decades ago Caplan proposed that a common mesenchymal stem cell (MSC) exists and gives rise to multiple specialized cell types, including those of bone (osteoblasts), cartilage (chondrocytes), fat (adipocytes), tendon (tenocytes), ligament, dermis, bone marrow stroma, and muscle (Caplan, 1991). Experiments in his and many other laboratories have substantially validated Caplan's hypothesis, and MSCs are now a mainstay of regenerative medicine. Although initially isolated from bone marrow (Lennon et al. 1996), MSCs have been identified throughout the body, with adipose tissue being a particularly rich source (Gimble et al. 2007). MSCs often are defined operationally as adherent cells able to expand for several passages in serum-containing medium and to give rise to various mesenchymal lineages (e.g., osteogenic, chondrogenic, adipogenic). Such bulk populations more properly are called mesenchymal *stromal* cells, reserving the designation "stem cell" for situations in which clonal self-renewal and differentiation potential have been verified (Horwitz et al. 2005). The exact phenotype and frequency within typical MSC cultures of multipotent stem cells actually capable of extensive self-renewal remains incompletely defined (Lee et al. 2010a). Cell sorting analyses indicate that MSCs expanded in culture derive from perivascular cells that surround blood vessels, especially capillaries and microvessels (Crisan et al. 2011; Crisan et al. 2008). In addition to serving as precursors of differentiated mesenchymal cell types, MSCs promote regeneration via secretion of multiple trophic factors and modulation of inflammatory responses (Bernardo et al. 2009; Caplan, 2009; Newman et al. 2009; Parekkadan and Milwid, 2010). Although MSCs have numerous applications in regenerative medicine, we will focus here on pharmacological agents that influence their activity in fracture healing and bone tissue engineering.

Bone Morphogenetic Proteins

The discovery that decalcified bone contained factors able to promote bone regeneration led to the eventual identification of 19 related "bone morphogenetic proteins" (BMPs), all cystine-knot cytokines that share a protein fold characteristic of the transforming growth factor-β (TGF-β) superfamily (Bessa et al. 2008b; Bragdon et al. 2011; Rider and Mulloy, 2010). (Nomenclature of the BMPs is complex, and the family overlaps with the "growth and differentiation factors" [GDFs]; moreover, multiple BMP–GDF homodimers and heterodimers exist and interact with specific receptors to activate competing signal transduction pathways and transcription factors [Bragdon et al. 2011; Miyazono et al. 2010; Rider and Mulloy, 2010; Zeng et al. 2010].) Some of the BMPs stimulate both bone and cartilage formation, and others favor one of these fates. Still others (e.g., BMP-3) are negative regulators of bone morphogenesis. Unrelated antagonists also have been identified, such as the protein Noggin (Krause et al. 2011; Reddi, 2001). A number of the BMPs have important developmental roles unrelated to skeletal morphogenesis. Because of the wide range of cell types potentially responsive to BMPs, clinical development has focused on local application at sites where bone repair or growth is desired.

Two family members, BMP-7 (also known as osteogenic protein-1 [OP-1] or eptotermin alfa) and BMP-2, manufactured as recombinant human proteins, have received regulatory approval in the United States and Europe for specific orthopedic applications. These cytokines are *osteoinductive* – that is, they stimulate the proliferation and differentiation of bone precursor cells, generally assumed to be some type of MSC. BMP-7, delivered locally in a type I collagen carrier, showed comparable efficacy in the treatment of tibial fractures that had failed to heal (non-unions) as grafts of autologous living bone (Friedlaender et al. 2001). The U.S. FDA issued a Humanitarian Device Exemption (HDE) for use of the BMP-7 implant to treat recalcitrant long bone non-unions that could not be autografted. The FDA also approved use under an HDE of a BMP-7–collagen–carboxymethylcellulose putty for revision spinal fusions. BMP-2, likewise, is delivered locally after absorption in a collagen sponge. The FDA has approved this product (INFUSE Bone Graft, Medtronic Spinal and Biologics, Memphis, TN) as a combination biologic device for certain classes of interbody spine fusions, severe long bone fractures, and oral maxillofacial bone grafting procedures (Burkus et al. 2002a; Burkus et al. 2002b; Govender et al. 2002; McKay et al. 2007; Swiontkowski et al. 2006). Currently, the most frequent clinical application of BMPs is for spine fusions (Ong et al. 2010). The total market for BMP devices now approaches $1 billion in the United States (Burks and Nair, 2010; Lysaght et al. 2008), and the large majority (~85 percent) of the procedures are off-label (i.e., they are prescribed by physicians but fall outside the narrow boundaries of indications approved by the FDA) (Lad et al. 2011).

With increasingly wide use of BMPs, serious questions have arisen regarding their efficacy and safety in certain procedures, both those officially sanctioned by the FDA and the off-label applications (Carragee et al. 2011; Lissenberg-Thunnissen et al. 2011; Mirza, 2011). Specific concerns include ectopic bone formation, implant displacement, back and leg pain, infection, and urogenital events. Peer-reviewed articles on company-sponsored BMP clinical trials initially reported excellent efficacy and safety. However, it now seems apparent that the studies suffered from systematic design bias because they did not test for significant improvement in efficacy over conventional procedures (Aro et al. 2011). Moreover, the publications gave the false impression that the BMP products were associated with essentially no adverse events. A much more critical view has now emerged (Carragee et al. 2011; Mirza, 2011). Reanalysis of data on BMPs in spine fusion revealed that the actual incidence of adverse events fell in the range of 10 to 50 percent, depending on the surgical approach. For anterior cervical fusions use of BMP-2 elevated the risk of early postoperative adverse events by about 40 percent, and some of these were life threatening (Carragee et al. 2011). The further possibility exists that, as in the case of EPO, off-target activity of BMPs on non-bone cells bearing functional receptors may promote the growth of cancers (Buijs et al. 2010; Carragee et al. 2011; Singh and Morris, 2010; Thawani et al. 2010).

New Approaches for Bone Regeneration

What future developments might enable more precisely targeted bone regeneration from stem and progenitor cells or decrease the risks of off-target activities and adverse events? One area for potential improvement centers on the materials and mechanics used in the delivery systems for BMPs and other cytokines (Bessa et al. 2008a). It should be possible to replace collagen sponges, which can easily be overloaded and leak excess BMP, with "smart" biomaterials (Furth et al. 2007) that are permissive for bone development (osteoconductive) and may permit significant reductions of cytokine dosage. For example, investigators recently screened a combinatorial library of 120 photo-crosslinked, biodegradable poly(β-amino ester)s and identified a novel scaffold material highly conducive to bone growth when loaded with BMP-2 (Brey et al. 2010).

Other osteoinductive substances may replace a BMP or strongly potentiate its activity, thereby lowering the amount used and the risks of spread from the site of application. The protein NEL-like molecule-1 (NELL1), a novel growth factor believed to target osteochondral lineage progenitors, promotes bone regeneration in several stringent animal models (Aghaloo et al. 2010; Xue et al. 2011). At low doses NELL-1 synergizes with BMP-2. Various additional growth factors and presentation strategies, including genetic delivery of a BMP gene to MSC for sustained local expression, are under active development (Bessa et al. 2008a; Kimelman-Bleich et al. 2011; Nauth et al. 2010).

Conserved Stem Cell Pathways: Wnt and Hedgehog Agonists

Widely used signaling mechanisms common to many stem cells, such as the canonical Wnt pathway (Nusse, 2008), may be specifically targeted to improve bone regeneration. Potentiation of Wnt signaling through genetic manipulation was known to stimulate the proliferation of skeletal stem/progenitor cells, located on the endosteal surfaces of bone, and to enhance their osteogenic differentiation (Bennett et al. 2007; Krishnan et al. 2006). In mice homozygous for a knockout of *Axin2*, a negative feedback regulator of Wnt signaling, the skeleton developed normally. However, these animals showed accelerated bone healing after injury (Minear et al. 2010). Furthermore, delivery of recombinant Wnt3a to the site of a bone injury substantially accelerated tissue regeneration, yielding a 3.5-fold increase in new bone 3 days after a single application compared with a placebo control (Minear et al. 2010). Because Wnt3a is lipid modified and strongly hydrophobic (Willert et al. 2003), a key element in this study was packaging of the purified protein in lipid vesicles that were delivered directly to the site of injury (Minear et al. 2010; Morrell et al. 2008). BMP-2 induces formation of both cartilage and new bone, even after short-term exposure, and can cause excessive bone formation at inappropriate (ectopic) sites (Noel et al. 2004). By contrast, the delivery of Wnt3a in vivo induced a bone-specific pattern of regeneration and did not cause ectopic bone formation. The data appeared consistent with prolongation and enhancement of the endogenous Wnt-mediated healing response in some subset(s) of stem and progenitor cells that migrate to the injured periosteum and bone marrow cavity (Minear et al. 2010). Therefore, lipsomally delivered Wnt3a appears a strong candidate for clinical testing in bone repair. A recent report describes a small molecule agonist of the Wnt pathway that also promotes osteogenic differentiation (Gwak et al. 2011).

The Hh pathway also regulates the behavior of many stem and progenitor cells during development and in adult tissues (Ingham and McMahon, 2001; Parisi and Lin, 1998). A small molecule capable of promoting osteogenic differentiation emerged from a screen of about 50,000 heterocyclics and was identified as an Hh agonist (Wu et al. 2002). This compound, a 2,6,9-trisubstituted purine named purmorphamine, strongly induced the expression of the osteoblast-specific enzyme alkaline phosphatase and other markers of bone differentiation in an MSC-like mouse cell line. The compound also enhanced the osteogenic differentiation of human MSCs (Beloti et al. 2005a; Beloti et al. 2005b). Transcriptional arrays from purmorphamine-treated cells revealed a gene expression profile consistent with Hh signaling; antagonists of the Hh pathway blocked these expression changes (Wu et al. 2004). Purmorphamine targets the seven-transmembrane protein Smoothened (Smo) (Sinha and Chen, 2006). Activation of Smo leads to the release of Gli family transcription factors from an inhibitory binding protein (Suppressor of Fused), allowing Hh-responsive genes to turn on. Normally, Smo activity is repressed by Patched (Ptch1), the cell surface receptor for Hh ligands. Hh binding to Ptch1 releases Smo to initiate the signaling cascade (Aanstad et al. 2009). Thus, by activating Smo directly, purmorphamine bypasses the requirement for an Hh protein to turn up the osteogenic program of gene expression. The importance of the Hh pathway, particularly the role of Smo in promoting bone formation, was confirmed using an MSC population isolated from mouse periosteum healing after a segmental bone autograft. In this system genetic deletion of Smo reduced both osteogenic differentiation of the MSCs in culture and healing of the graft in vivo (Wang et al. 2010a). Whether a small molecule such as purmorphamine could be used clinically to enhance human bone repair remains to be determined. As with BMPs and Wnt proteins, it would appear essential to deliver an Hh agonist locally to avoid significant off-target effects on other normal or cancer stem cells (Dodge and Lum, 2011).

The search for small molecules capable of modulating osteogenesis from bone stem and progenitor cells continues. A recent report describes decalpenic acid, a novel fermentation product from a *Penicillium* species, able to induce MSC to express early markers of the osteoblast lineage (Sakamoto et al. 2010). However, the molecular target of this compound has not yet been reported.

Regenerative Pluripotent Stem Cells

Pluripotent ES and iPS cells provide the greatest potential flexibility to generate many classes of specialized cells. Production of iPS cells has become routine in many research centers. Lines can be made by reprogramming of cells obtained from skin biopsies, blood samples, hair shafts, and even urine (Aasen et al. 2008; Brown et al. 2010; Chou et al. 2011; Kunisato et al. 2010; Staerk et al. 2010).

Efforts to direct pluripotent stem cells to differentiate toward specific fates began with the development of mouse teratocarcinoma cell lines (Martin and Evans, 1975), and intensified with the isolation of mouse and then human ES cells from normal embryos (Evans and Kaufman, 1981; Martin, 1981; Odorico et al. 2001). The emergence of reprogramming and iPS cell technology galvanized the field of regenerative medicine because of the potential to create patient-specific therapeutics, perfectly matched at the HLA loci and so theoretically not susceptible to immune rejection

(Csete, 2010; Nishikawa et al. 2008). It also should be possible to correct a genetic defect in patient-derived iPS cells; generate appropriate stem cells for the lineage(s) critically affected by the mutation; and return them to the individual to effect a long-lasting, possibly permanent cure (Howden et al. 2011; Kazuki et al. 2010; Liu et al. 2011). Finally, the iPS technology offers a possible resolution to ethical debates about the use of cell lines derived from human embryos (Lee et al. 2009; Meyer, 2008).

However, iPS cells should not be viewed as a panacea (Okita and Yamanaka, 2011). Similar to human ES cells, they raise major challenges for large-scale expansion and manufacturing of differentiated derivatives under conditions compliant with regulatory standards for clinical use (Rodriguez-Piza et al. 2010; Skottman et al. 2007; Unger et al. 2008). They also bear potential risks of tumorigenicity because of the teratoma formation intrinsic to pluripotent stem cells and the possibility of oncogene activation. Furthermore, important cautions have been raised concerning the genomic integrity of iPS cells, both genetic and epigenetic (Gore et al. 2011; Hussein et al. 2011; Lister et al. 2011). Moreover, transplantation experiments in syngeneic mice showed unexpected immunogenicity; thus, it cannot be assumed that tissue grafts derived from a patient's own iPS cells necessarily will be accepted as "self" by the immune system (Zhao et al. 2011).

Nevertheless, despite the limitations of current iPS cell technology, this field is developing at breakneck speed. Problems that appear daunting today are likely to be solved in the near future, while unanticipated difficulties may yet emerge. A key focus for regenerative pharmacology will be to discover safer, more robust ways to reprogram somatic cells either to a pluripotent state or to a desired specialized lineage. The reverse of the coin will be to discover small molecules that induce lineage-specific differentiation from pluripotent stem cells. This will both improve mechanistic understanding and facilitate the translation from academic bench to industrial and clinical scale research and development. Advances on both sides are coming fast and furious.

Pharmacology of Reprogramming

Detailed comparisons of gene expression patterns between iPS and ES cells have revealed systematic differences, indicating that reprogramming may be incomplete (Wang et al. 2011a). Similarly, assessments of DNA methylation show that iPS cells retain some epigenetic memory of the particular cells from which they derive (Kim et al. 2010; Stadtfeld et al. 2010). Cells reprogrammed by somatic cell nuclear transfer (SCNT) show more complete resetting to an ES cell-like ground state (Kim et al. 2010). This approach enables the reprogramming even of fully differentiated, postmitotic cells, such as olfactory neurons (Eggan et al. 2004). By contrast, it is easier to generate iPS cells from adult stem and progenitor cells than from more mature cells (Chou et al. 2011; Kim et al. 2008; Moon et al. 2011; Tat et al. 2010). One possible goal for regenerative pharmacology will be to identify molecules that facilitate complete erasure of the epigenetic signature of starting cells in order to produce iPS cells that more closely resemble native ES cells.

Chemistry and pharmacology already are contributing strongly to the production of iPS cells that should be better suited for clinical applications. The first iterations of iPS technology used integrating vectors for four genes (*OCT4–SOX2–KLF4–c-MYC* or *OCT4–SOX2–NANOG–LIN28*), including known oncogenes. Use of self-inactivating or deletable viral vectors, or transient expression of the reprogramming genes via non-integrating plasmid vectors increases safety (Chang et al. 2009; Okita et al. 2008; Yu et al. 2009). Many laboratories are now focused on next-generation iPS technologies, especially the development of DNA-free methods to generate pluripotent cells. Approaches include the use of recombinant transcription factors (Cho et al. 2010; Pan et al. 2010) or synthetic modified mRNA encoding these proteins (Warren et al. 2010) rather than the corresponding genes. In addition, chemical screens have identified small molecules able to enhance the efficiency of reprogramming or to replace some of the genetic factors required to reset cells to the pluripotent state (Desponts and Ding, 2010; Ichida et al. 2009; Li and Ding, 2010; Lyssiotis et al. 2009; Shi et al. 2008; Wang et al. 2011b). Most recently, two groups have reported iPS cell generation using a single genetic factor, either NANOG (Theunissen et al. 2011) or OCT4 (Yuan et al. 2011b), in combination with small molecules. NANOG and OCT4 are the key transcription factors long known to be essential for the pluripotency of ES cells. Whether reprogramming can be accomplished using small molecules alone remains to be seen.

The recognition that somatic cells can be reverted to a pluripotent ground state raises the question whether "transdifferentiation" between unrelated specialized cell lineages can be accomplished by similar means. Indeed, several groups have now reported the direct reprogramming of fibroblasts to functional neurons (Vierbuchen et al. 2010) and to cardiomyocytes (Efe et al. 2011; Ieda et al. 2010). Another potential tactic to produce patient-specific differentiated cells will be to reprogram readily obtained cells, such as fibroblasts or blood cells, to adult stem cells of a desired lineage, such as hepatic or cardiac stem cells, that otherwise could be harvested only through a more invasive biopsy. These stem cells might then be expanded and induced to differentiate more efficiently than would be the case for iPS cells and with less risk of tumorigenicity. The strategies of directed differentiation and reprogramming and transdifferentiation can be viewed as complementary approaches to solve the general problem of providing specialized cells for regenerative medicine (Cohen and Melton, 2011).

Cell Differentiation from Pluripotent Stem Cells

The generation of specialized cell types from pluripotent stem cells has become a global enterprise. It seems safe to predict that at varying efficiencies, cells of virtually any lineage could be generated ex vivo (Darr and Benvenisty, 2006; Trounson, 2006). A review of this burgeoning literature would fill its own book. A few examples include differentiation to neural crest cells (Lee et al. 2010b), various types of functional neurons (Carpenter et al. 2001; Karumbayaram et al. 2009; Lee et al. 2000; Perrier et al. 2004; Salli et al. 2004; Soundararajan et al. 2006), MSC-like mesenchymal precursor cells (Barberi et al. 2005; Boyd et al. 2009; Gruenloh et al. 2011), red and white blood cells (Chicha et al. 2011; Choi et al. 2011; Dias et al. 2011; Kouskoff et al. 2005; Lengerke et al. 2009; Lu et al. 2010; Matsumoto et al. 2009; Niwa et al. 2009; Timmermans et al. 2009; Vodyanik et al. 2005), and hepatic lineage cells (Funakoshi et al. 2011; Hamazaki et al. 2001; Lavon et al. 2004; Loya et al. 2009; Schwartz et al. 2005; Sullivan et al. 2010; Zhao et al. 2009).

Most protocols to obtain specific cell fates have been developed empirically. A powerful general strategy evolved by taking lessons from embryology (Murry and Keller, 2008). Stepwise differentiation through known developmental stages, beginning with the first segregation of the three germ layers, offers a rational framework to reach desired target cell types. Most such efforts have concentrated on the selection of growth factors and cytokines to advance through a lineage series. One example is the generation from human ES or iPS cells of insulin-producing cells akin to pancreatic β cells (D'Amour et al. 2006; Jiang et al. 2007a; Jiang et al. 2007b; Mayhew and Wells, 2010; Van Hoof et al. 2009). The process begins with the induction of the endoderm lineage, generally using activin A, an analog of the embryonic regulatory factor Nodal in the TGF-β family (D'Amour et al. 2005; Kubo et al. 2004). Sequential steps then restrict the cells to stages corresponding to gut tube; posterior foregut; pancreatic endoderm and endocrine precursors; and, finally, hormone-expressing endocrine cells. Initially, the reported yield of insulin-producing cells was low, and their final phenotype resembled that of immature fetal rather than adult pancreatic cells, unless allowed to mature in vivo for several months (Kroon et al. 2008). Even with significant optimization, the highest yield of insulin-positive cells from human ES cells reported to date was about 25 percent (Zhang et al. 2009a).

The problem of achieving fully *adult* cell characteristics in differentiation from ES and iPS cells appears far more daunting than has been generally appreciated. A case in point is the production of hepatocyte-like cells from human ES cells (Funakoshi et al. 2011). Comparison of the differentiated progeny of ES cells with those of adult liver progenitors showed striking differences. Investigators concluded that the ES-derived cells, after 3 weeks of differentiation in culture, remained immature, resembling human fetal hepatocytes at less than 20 weeks of gestation. More broadly, W. Lowry and colleagues carried out a detailed assessment by expression profiling of various differentiated progeny generated from human pluripotent stem cells. They focused on fates representative of the three germ layers, namely, neural (ectoderm), hepatic (endoderm), and mesenchymal (mesoderm) lineages (Patterson et al. 2011). The good news was that the differentiated cells derived from iPS cells were nearly identical to those derived from ES cells, and there was no evidence for reactivation of the exogenous reprogramming genes used to make the iPS cells. However, the progeny from neither ES cells nor iPS cells were identical to mature tissue-derived cells. In all cases the differentiated cells continued to express a subset of genes associated with early embryonic development, such as *LIN28A*, *LIN28B*, and *DPPA4*. The investigators concluded that the phenotypes of the specialized progeny of pluripotent stem cells resembled those of cells present within the first 6 weeks of human development. This finding reinforces the utility of ES and iPS cells as tools to understand human embryology. However, to model human diseases and to produce safe cells for regenerative medicine applications, it may be essential to find efficient methods for induction of further maturation toward later fetal and adult phenotypes. One specific concern will be whether cells that persistently express early embryonic genes are more prone than their adult counterparts to proliferate excessively or even to form frank tumors after implantation in human patients.

Considerable effort is being expended in many laboratories to make differentiation protocols more robust and cost effective, to understand variability among different human ES and iPS cell lines, and to scale up the production of specific cell types for clinical studies and high-throughput screening. As noted in the discussion earlier of adult hepatic and biliary tree stem cells, the use of three-dimensional culture systems and tissue-specific biomatrix scaffolds or defined ECM components to drive differentiation will likely offer substantial advantages in speed, efficiency, and the final degree of maturation achieved (Wang et al. 2011c).

Pharmacology of Pluripotent Stem Cell Differentiation

Small molecules to promote differentiation also are emerging as valuable mechanistic probes and practical tools. High-content screening can use fluorescence imaging to identify and enumerate viable cells and to monitor such drug-induced changes as downregulation of pluripotency markers, induction of lineage-specific differentiation markers or reporters controlled by lineage-specific promoters, or physiological activities of electrically excitable cells such as neurons or cardiomyocytes (Barbaric et al. 2010). The technical feasibility of screening on human ES cells has been established convincingly (Desbordes et al. 2008). Several review articles have catalogued "hits" from phenotypic screens for small molecules that influence stem cell self-renewal or modulate, positively or negatively, the differentiation of various pluripotent and lineage-restricted stem cells (Burton et al. 2010; Eglen et al. 2008; Fang et al. 2007; Li and Ding, 2010; Martinez-Fernandez et al. 2011; Zhang, 2010; Zhou and Ding, 2010). The identification of the molecular targets of small molecules that generate specific phenotypes establishes a "chemical genetics" to elucidate the underlying pathways (Sachinidis et al. 2008).

Ding, Schultz, and colleagues pioneered the use of small molecules to improve the propagation of pluripotent stem cells and to facilitate the production of desired differentiated cell types from them (Ding and Schultz, 2004; Yuan et al. 2011a). For example, in an early proof-of-concept study a high-throughput phenotypic cell-based screen and combinatorial libraries directed at protein kinase targets were used to identify a compound (TWS119, a 4,6-disubstituted pyrrolopyrimidine) that efficiently induced neural cell differentiation from mouse teratocarcinoma and ES cells (Ding et al. 2003). TWS119 targets glycogen synthase kinase-3β (GSK-3β), a serine-threonine kinase that serves as a pivotal enzyme in the Wnt, Hh, and Notch signaling pathways and profoundly influences cell proliferation, differentiation, and apoptosis. GSK-3β previously had been implicated in controlling the proliferation of progenitors of cerebellar neurons (Cui et al. 1998). The neurogenic action of TWS119 may result from the activation of Wnt pathway signaling through the inhibition of phosphorylation-induced degradation of β-catenin, which then migrates to the cell nucleus and upregulates expression of genes under control of the transcription factor TCF/LEF.

Efficient neural differentiation of human ES and iPS cells can be achieved by manipulating other distinct pathways. For example, a near-total blockade of TGF-β family signaling gave robust neural induction. This was achieved via simultaneous inhibition of receptors for TGF-β and Nodal (ALK4, ALK5, ALK7) with a compound (SB431542) that inhibits receptor phosphorylation, and of BMP action with Dorsomorphin (6-[4-(2-piperidin-1-yl-ethyoxy)phenyl]-3-pyridin-4-yl-pyrazolo[1,5-a]pyrimidine), a compound that inhibits a related family of receptors (ALK2, ALK3, and ALK6). The resulting neural lineage progenitor cells were able to differentiate further to yield dopaminergic neurons (Morizane et al. 2011).

More recently, Ding's group extended the manipulation of neural differentiation of human ES cells by devising a way to generate a self-renewing population of primitive neural stem cells. They used a GSK-3 inhibitor (CHIR99021) known to activate canonical Wnt signaling, together with the above-mentioned TGF-β/Nodal pathway inhibitor (SB431542). Finally, they added a Notch signaling pathway blocker, a γ-secretase inhibitor they refer to as Compound E. Normally, binding of a ligand to Notch, a transmembrane receptor, induces proteolytic cleavage and allows the intracellular domain of the receptor to translocate to the nucleus where it activates transcription of Notch-responsive genes. The γ-secretase inhibitors prevent Notch signaling by blocking receptor cleavage. Within 1 week the three-compound cocktail synergistically induced the quantitative conversion of the ES cells to a phenotype corresponding to primitive neuroepithelium, an early precursor of neural lineages (Li et al. 2011). These cells lost expression of the characteristic ES cell transcription factors OCT4 and NANOG but maintained high levels of SOX2, which is expressed in both pluripotent and neural lineage stem cells. The neuroepithelial cells continued to proliferate in culture (i.e., were capable of extended self-renewal) in the presence of the GSK-3 and TGF-β/Nodal inhibitors and a cytokine, leukemia inhibitory factor (LIF). The cells could be described as stable, early stage ("pre-rosette") neural stem cells and were capable of differentiation to a number of subtype-specific neurons in response to appropriate morphogens.

Yet another example of small molecules with utility in controlling differentiation comes from Melton and colleagues, who focused on the pathway from ES cells toward an endocrine pancreatic fate, outlined earlier (Melton, 2011). One screen targeted the initial step of endoderm specification from pluripotent stem cells (Borowiak et al. 2009). Two small molecules with the desired activity, low toxicity, and the ability to enter cells were identified from a set of 4,000 compounds. The investigators designated these compounds "inducers of definitive endoderm" (IDE1: 2-[(6-carboxy-hexanoyl)-hydrazonomethyl]-benzoic acid, and IDE2: 7-[2-cyclopentylidenehydrazino]-7-oxoheptanoic acid). The screening assay used to find IDE1 and IDE2 was based on induction of the endodermal transcription factor SOX17 using a fluorescent reporter under control of that gene's promoter. The two compounds have related structures and display comparable potency (EC_{50} 125 nM and 223 nM, respectively) and will be referred to collectively as IDE1/2. They induced expression of SOX17 and another essential endodermal transcription factor, FOXA2, in 70 to 80 percent of mouse ES cells compared with only about 45 percent induction by Activin A. Similar results were obtained for induction of definitive endoderm from human ES cells. By contrast, similar to Activin A, IDE1/2 failed to induce definitive endoderm markers in stem cells resembling primitive MSCs obtained from umbilical cord blood (Filby et al. 2011). Although IDE1/2 came from a library of putative HDAC inhibitors, the molecular target has not yet been reported. However, the compounds appear to act through the same signaling pathway as the physiological inducer of definitive endoderm formation, Nodal, and its analog Activin A (Borowiak et al. 2009). Similar to other TGF-β family members, these two growth factors activate SMAD transcription factors, as detected by increases in phosphorylated SMAD2. Similarly, ES cells treated with IDE1/2 showed strongly enhanced SMAD2 phosphorylation, and this effect was blocked by SB431542, the inhibitor of the ALK4, ALK5, and ALK7 TGF-β family receptors. Finally, similar to definitive endoderm generated in the presence of Nodal or Activin A, cells that turned on endoderm markers in response to IDE1/2 were fully competent to continue along the differentiation path to gut tube endoderm and pancreatic progenitors.

A search for small molecules able to promote the subsequent step(s) in differentiation, downstream from definitive endoderm, also proved fruitful (Chen et al. 2009). High content screening was carried out on human ES cells that had been pre-induced with Activin A to identify compounds able to act on endodermal precursor cells and turn on expression of the transcription factor PDX1, a master regulator of pancreatic development expressed by pancreatic progenitors. The best hit found in a library of 5,000 compounds was (−)-indolactam V (ILV). Detailed analysis confirmed that ILV acts specifically on definitive endoderm cells and induces differentiation to pancreatic progenitors. These respond normally to factors that stimulate proliferation (e.g., FGF10) and can differentiate further to endocrine-restricted progenitors. ILV promoted robust differentiation to pancreatic progenitors from definitive endoderm, regardless of whether commitment from ES cells to endoderm was induced with Activin A or with the small molecules IE1/2. It appears that ILV achieves this function through activation of protein kinase C (PKC) signaling, although the specific isoform the compound targets among the 11 known members of the PKC family remains to be identified.

Taken together, these examples and numerous additional studies give compelling motivation to seek small molecules that influence stem cell differentiation. These compounds provide excellent probes to better understand underlying mechanisms of cell signaling and commitment to lineage pathways. They are easier to produce and in many instances more efficacious than growth factors and cytokines. Eventually, they should prove well suited to cost-effective scale up of cells for human therapy.

Clinical Trials of Embryonic Stem Cell–Derived Products

One of the ultimate goals of directed differentiation of pluripotent stem cells is the generation of cells and tissue-based medicines to treat injuries and degenerative diseases. Within the past year the first FDA-approved clinical trials of cell therapy products derived from human ES cells have begun to enroll subjects, marking a major milestone toward medical translation of stem cell technology. One trial sponsored by Geron Corporation uses oligodendrocyte progenitor cells (GRNOPC1) to treat spinal cord injury (Bretzner et al. 2011; Strauss, 2010). Two further trials sponsored by Advanced Cell Technology will test retinal pigment epithelial (RPE) cells (Ma09-hRPE Cellular Therapy) with the goal of slowing or reversing related disorders of the retina, dry age-related macular degeneration, and Stargardt's macular dystrophy (Klimanskaya et al. 2004; Rowland et al. 2011; Uygun et al. 2009). Although primarily designed to assess safety, especially to address concerns that even small numbers of residual undifferentiated ES cells could form teratoma tumors, these first-in-human studies will be followed closely for evidence of efficacy as well.

The current clinical trials with ES cells are designed for "off-the-shelf" therapy with a single cellular product. If iPS cells can be generated, expanded, and differentiated efficiently, and assuming that regulations for safety testing do not make them cost prohibitive, then future therapies could be customized for individual patients. Clearly, the importance of this approach depends largely on the degree to which personalized cell therapy actually would obviate requirements for immune suppression to prevent graft rejection.

Disease Models from Patient-Specific Pluripotent Stem Cells

Beyond personalized medicines, the production of disease-specific iPS cells promises to impact profoundly the creation of new in vitro models for human disease – pithily described by the phrase "disease in a dish" (Gage, 2010; Walker, 2010). The notion is that by capturing in pluripotent stem cells the genotypes of individuals who have a disease, it should be possible to produce cell types in which there will be a phenotypic readout reflecting the underlying genetic susceptibility. The affected cells can be used to develop screens for molecules that overcome the phenotypic abnormality. These, in turn, will potentially correct the disease in individuals with the corresponding genotype.

The logic of the disease-in-a-dish strategy is most compelling for disorders with a straightforward genetic cause, especially those that display simple Mendelian inheritance (i.e., result from mutations in a single gene). The underlying basis of most human disease is far more complex, with contributions from multiple genetic polymorphisms and even more substantial contributions from environmental variables. However, it should be remembered that lessons learned about drug targets based on rare mutant individuals sometimes can be extrapolated to populations at large. The seminal work by Goldstein and Brown on the low-density lipoprotein (LDL) receptor offers a dramatic example. They focused initially on familial hypercholesterolemia (FH), an inborn error of metabolism causing extreme elevation of blood cholesterol and early heart attacks. They found that the disease results from genetic defects in the LDL receptor, disrupting the normal regulation of cholesterol metabolism. The severe form of FH affects only one individual per 1 million in the population. However, understanding gained from studying this small group led to the elucidation of several major concepts in the biology of receptors and to the widespread introduction of statins to prevent heart disease (Goldstein and Brown, 2009).

A powerful initial demonstration that patient-specific iPS cells could be differentiated to an appropriate cell type to model a degenerative disease phenotype ex vivo came from human spinal muscular atrophy (SMA) (Ebert et al. 2009). In this autosomal recessive disorder, mutations that reduce levels of the widely expressed protein survival motor neuron 1 (SMN1) cause selective degeneration of lower α-motor neurons. Although the biochemistry of the disease had been studied in patient fibroblasts, no system was available previously to study the specific effects of SMN1 deficiency in the affected cell type, motor neurons. Pluripotent stem cells generated by reprogramming SMA patient fibroblasts enabled the production of neurons with the disease genotype. These showed the expected deficiency in SMN1 protein. After 4 weeks of in vitro differentiation, the overall production and survival of total neurons and motor neurons were comparable between the SMA and control iPS lines. However, over the next 2 weeks, whereas the SMA cells showed a striking fivefold drop in the number in motor neurons and a reduction in their average size, other neurons remained unaffected. This presumably resulted from a specific developmental failure or increased degeneration as a direct consequence of the SMN1 deficiency. Furthermore, treatment of the patient-specific cells with compounds known to boost SMN1 protein levels (valproic acid or tobramycin) induced a two- to threefold increase in the amount of SMN1 in the mutant motor neurons and a corresponding increase in sites of nuclear structures ("gems") containing the protein (Ebert et al. 2009). These observations provide encouraging validation for the use of patient-specific cells in drug screening.

The development of iPS cell lines from individuals with a variety of disorders, both simple Mendelian and complex, was first reported in 2008, particularly from the Daley laboratory, and continues at a hurtling pace (Park et al. 2008). Several excellent current review articles cover in depth the rationale, strategies, and range of diseases for which progress in the preparation of iPS cell lines has been reported (Kiskinis and Eggan, 2010; Unternaehrer and Daley, 2011; Zhu et al. 2011). Some patient-specific iPS cells of direct relevance to regenerative medicine and pharmacology include Parkinson's disease (sporadic) (Park et al. 2008; Soldner et al. 2009), Parkinson's disease (PINK1 mutation with mitochondrial degradation) (Seibler et al. 2011), amyotrophic lateral sclerosis (sporadic) (Dimos et al. 2008), amyotrophic lateral sclerosis (ALS8 autosomal dominant, familial) (Mitne-Neto et al. 2011), gyrate atrophy of the choroid and retina (Howden et al. 2011), retinitis pigmentosa (Jin et al. 2011), type I diabetes (Maehr et al. 2009), Huntington's disease (Park et al. 2008), long QT syndrome (Itzhaki et al. 2011; Matsa et al. 2011; Yazawa et al. 2011), LEOPARD (lentigines, electrocardiographic conduction abnormalities, ocular hypertelorism, pulmonary stenosis, abnormal genitalia, retarded growth, and sensorineural deafness) syndrome (Carvajal-Vergara et al. 2010), and Duchenne and Becker muscular dystrophies (Park et al. 2008).

Duchenne Muscular Dystrophy as a Model for Regenerative Pharmacology

We (Childers, Furth) have begun a program geared to identify compounds able to ameliorate abnormalities in the heart muscle of patients with Duchenne muscular dystrophy (DMD). We present the strategy here as exemplary of a disease-in-a-dish strategy (Fig. 5-3).

Duchenne muscular dystrophy, an X-linked genetic disorder resulting from mutations in the dystrophin gene (DYS), affects one in 3,300 male births, causing devastating skeletal and cardiac muscle weakness. Although efforts to develop treatments have generally focused on the defect in skeletal muscle, early death in DMD patients results from cardiorespiratory failure (Cox and Kunkel, 1997). Cardiomyocytes isolated from dystrophin-deficient animals (mice or dogs) manifest increased susceptibility to damage in vitro, especially in response to mechanical stress. Despite many years of effort, gene therapy has not yet succeeded in correcting either the skeletal or cardiac defects in DMD patients. Moreover, without correction of the deteriorating heart muscle, improvements in skeletal muscle would be unlikely to increase the lifespan of DMD patients and might actually increase the workload on the diseased heart and accelerate cardiomyopathy (Duan, 2006).

We therefore propose to screen specifically for new compounds that protect DMD cardiomyocytes from stress-induced damage. To do this, we are isolating DMD patient-specific iPS cell clones by reprogramming of fibroblasts and blood cells from

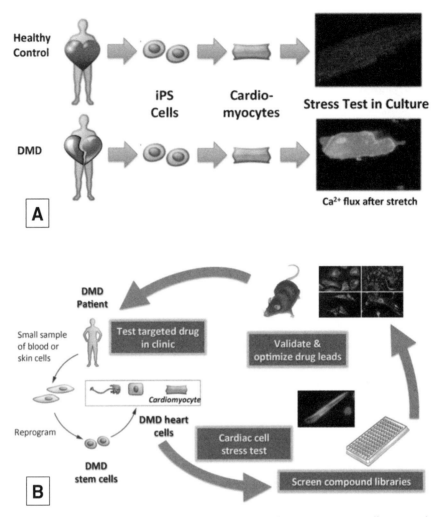

Figure 5-3. Disease-in-a-dish strategy to discover drugs to treat cardiomyopathy associated with Duchenne muscular dystrophy (DMD). (**A**) Screening assays will be developed using cardiomyocytes derived from DMD patient-specific induced pluripotent stem (iPS) cells. Dystrophin deficiency makes membranes of DMD cardiomyocytes more sensitive to mechanical stress. This can be detected using assays discussed in text, such as potentiation of Ca^{2+} flux, illustrated here. "Healthy control" will be syngeneic iPS cells in which the DMD mutation is corrected by introduction of a functional mini-dystrophin transgene. (**B**) Schematic of pathway from generation of DMD patient-specific iPS cells through drug discovery and preclinical development to clinical testing in DMD subjects. (See color plate 10.)

individuals with common mutations in the *DYS* gene, similar to a line previously reported (Park et al. 2008). We are inducing differentiation of the DMD mutant stem cells to cardiomyocytes and comparing responses to cardiomyocytes derived from patient-specific iPS cells in which the dystrophin deficiency has been corrected genetically by introduction of a mini-dystrophin gene (Li et al. 2006). This approach of using syngeneic cells is designed to eliminate perturbations caused by background genetic variation that could affect drug metabolism, toxicity, or the cardiac phenotype. Cardiomyocytes derived from other well-characterized human pluripotent (ES, iPS, or both) stem cell lines will serve as reference standards.

To enable high-throughput screening, it is important to generate sufficient numbers of highly enriched iPS cell–derived cardiomyocytes of consistent phenotype. Several methods to induce differentiation of murine and human pluripotent stem cells to cardiomyocytes have been described in the literature. We are using an approach introduced by Field and colleagues in which selection for a drug-resistance gene controlled by a cardiac-specific promoter eliminates cells that have not differentiated to the cardiomyocyte lineage (Zandstra et al. 2003). Kamp, a collaborator in this work, has developed methods to standardize cardiac differentiation and functionally characterize the cells produced from human ES and iPS cells by electrophysiology (Mohr et al. 2010; Zhang et al. 2009b).

We have devised several phenotypic screens that are designed to discriminate between normal and dystrophin-deficient cardiomyocytes. All rely on a generally accepted finding that physiological levels of mechanical stress cause abnormal leakiness of the membrane of dystrophin-deficient muscle cells, whether of cardiomyocytes or striated muscle. We will confirm that dystrophin deficiency results in abnormal response to mechanical stress by first testing available mutant murine cardiomyocytes. One approach to phenotypic screening rests on the use of a sensitive assay for changes in cardiomyocyte behavior encompassing morphology, beating, metabolism, signal transduction, or viability. Time-dependent cell response profiling (TCRP), using microelectrode arrays embedded in multi-well dishes to determine impedance, robustly measures such changes without the need for cell labeling (Xi et al. 2008). The TCRP assay is ideally suited for moderate to high-throughput screening without bias regarding the mechanism by which a molecule induces a desired phenotypic change. This will enable us to cast a wide net to find diverse hits within a library of druglike molecules. We will then focus on the specific effects of these compounds on electrophysiology, calcium trafficking, and other cellular parameters that we confirm are perturbed in DMD mutant cardiomyocytes. These secondary assays will identify lead compounds suitable for further optimization. We also are exploring high-content screening (Zock, 2009) focused primarily on assessment of Ca^{2+} ion fluxes, detected using a reporter dye (Fluo-4). We anticipate that compared with normal (dystrophin-corrected) control cardiomyocytes, the DMD cardiomyocytes will manifest significantly greater calcium entry, membrane microruptures, and susceptibility to cell death after physiologically relevant membrane stretching.

Our initial screening plan is geared for a library of about 5,000 compounds with the goal of identifying hits that normalize the phenotype of DMD cardiomyocytes. We anticipate then carrying out lead optimization and, if needed, scaling up to screen a library that is larger by one to two orders of magnitude.

A key element of regenerative pharmacology envisioned in our approach will be to use lead compounds to enable working backward from phenotypic observations at the cellular level to identify specific molecular targets. As we have seen in other examples in this chapter, in some instances, this happens by chance because an existing drug with a known target induces the desired phenotypic effect. In other cases, the tools of chemical genomics are required to identify targets. In either case the gist of the strategy is to develop assays sufficiently faithful to the human disease so that compounds active in an ex vivo model derived from patient-specific stem cells will accurately predict useful pharmaceutical activity.

References

Aanstad, P., N. Santos, K.C. Corbit, P.J. Scherz, L.A. Trinh, W. Salvenmoser, J. Huisken, J.F. Reiter, and D.Y. Stainier. 2009. The extracellular domain of Smoothened regulates ciliary localization and is required for high-level Hh signaling. *Curr Biol.* 19:1034–1039.

Aasen, T., A. Raya, M.J. Barrero, E. Garreta, A. Consiglio, F. Gonzalez, R. Vassena, J. Bilic, V. Pekarik, G. Tiscornia, M. Edel, S. Boue, and J.C. Belmonte. 2008. Efficient and rapid generation of induced pluripotent stem cells from human keratinocytes. *Nat Biotechnol.* 26:1276–1284.

Aghaloo, T., C.M. Cowan, X. Zhang, E. Freymiller, C. Soo, B. Wu, K. Ting, and Z. Zhang. 2010. The effect of NELL1 and bone morphogenetic protein-2 on calvarial bone regeneration. *J Oral Maxillofac Surg.* 68:300–308.

Alison, M.R., and S. Islam. 2009. Attributes of adult stem cells. *J Pathol.* 217:144–160.

Andersson, K.E., and G.J. Christ. 2007. Regenerative pharmacology: the future is now. *Mol Interv.* 7:79–86.

Antman, K.H. 1990. G-CSF and GM-CSF in clinical trials. *Yale J Biol Med.* 63:387–410.

Anversa, P., J. Kajstura, A. Leri, and R. Bolli. 2006. Life and death of cardiac stem cells: a paradigm shift in cardiac biology. *Circulation.* 113:1451–1463.

Araki, H., N. Mahmud, M. Milhem, R. Nunez, M. Xu, C.A. Beam, and R. Hoffman. 2006. Expansion of human umbilical cord blood SCID-repopulating cells using chromatin-modifying agents. *Exp Hematol.* 34:140–149.

Aro, H.T., S. Govender, A.D. Patel, P. Hernigou, A. Perera de Gregorio, G.I. Popescu, J.D. Golden, J. Christensen, and A. Valentin. 2011. Recombinant human bone morphogenetic protein-2: a randomized trial in open tibial fractures treated with reamed nail fixation. *J Bone Joint Surg.* 93:801–808.

Baptista, P.M., M.M. Siddiqui, G. Lozier, S.R. Rodriguez, A. Atala, and S. Soker. 2011. The use of whole organ decellularization for the generation of a vascularized liver organoid. *Hepatology.* 53:604–617.

Barbaric, I., P.J. Gokhale, and P.W. Andrews. 2010. High-content screening of small compounds on human embryonic stem cells. *Biochem Soc Trans.* 38:1046–1050.

Barberi, T., L.M. Willis, N.D. Socci, and L. Studer. 2005. Derivation of multipotent mesenchymal precursors from human embryonic stem cells. *PLoS Med.* 2:e161.

Barker, N., S. Bartfeld, and H. Clevers. 2010a. Tissue-resident adult stem cell populations of rapidly self-renewing organs. *Cell Stem Cell.* 7:656–670.

Barker, N., M. Huch, P. Kujala, M. van de Wetering, H.J. Snippert, J.H. van Es, T. Sato, D.E. Stange, H. Begthel, M. van den Born, E. Danenberg, S. van den Brink, J. Korving, A. Abo, P.J. Peters, N. Wright, R. Poulsom, and H. Clevers. 2010b. Lgr5(+ve) stem cells drive self-renewal in the stomach and build long-lived gastric units in vitro. *Cell Stem Cell.* 6:25–36.

Barker, N., M. van de Wetering, and H. Clevers. 2008. The intestinal stem cell. *Genes Dev.* 22:1856–1864.

Beier, J.I., G.E. Arteel, and C.J. McClain. 2011. Advances in alcoholic liver disease. *Curr Gastroenterol Rep.* 13:56–64.

Beloti, M.M., L.S. Bellesini, and A.L. Rosa. 2005a. The effect of purmorphamine on osteoblast phenotype expression of human bone marrow mesenchymal cells cultured on titanium. *Biomaterials.* 26:4245–4248.

Beloti, M.M., L.S. Bellesini, and A.L. Rosa. 2005b. Purmorphamine enhances osteogenic activity of human osteoblasts derived from bone marrow mesenchymal cells. *Cell Biol Int.* 29:537–541.

Bennett, C.N., H. Ouyang, Y.L. Ma, Q. Zeng, I. Gerin, K.M. Sousa, T.F. Lane, V. Krishnan, K.D. Hankenson, and O.A. MacDougald. 2007. Wnt10b increases postnatal bone formation by enhancing osteoblast differentiation. *J Bone Miner Res.* 22:1924–1932.

Bernardo, M.E., F. Locatelli, and W.E. Fibbe. 2009. Mesenchymal stromal cells. *Ann N Y Acad Sci.* 1176:101–117.

Bessa, P.C., M. Casal, and R.L. Reis. 2008a. Bone morphogenetic proteins in tissue engineering: the road from laboratory to clinic, part II (BMP delivery). *J Tissue Eng Regen Med.* 2:81–96.

Bessa, P.C., M. Casal, and R.L. Reis. 2008b. Bone morphogenetic proteins in tissue engineering: the road from the laboratory to the clinic, part I (basic concepts). *J Tissue Eng Regen Med.* 2:1–13.

Blau, C.A. 2007. Erythropoietin in cancer: presumption of innocence? *Stem Cells.* 25:2094–2097.

Boitano, A.E., J. Wang, R. Romeo, L.C. Bouchez, A.E. Parker, S.E. Sutton, J.R. Walker, C.A. Flaveny, G.H. Perdew, M.S. Denison, P.G. Schultz, and M.P. Cooke. 2010. Aryl hydrocarbon receptor antagonists promote the expansion of human hematopoietic stem cells. *Science.* 329:1345–1348.

Bonnefoix, T., and M. Callanan. 2010. Accurate hematopoietic stem cell frequency estimates by fitting multicell Poisson models substituting to the single-hit Poisson model in limiting dilution transplantation assays. *Blood.* 116:2472–2475.

Borowiak, M., R. Maehr, S. Chen, A.E. Chen, W. Tang, J.L. Fox, S.L. Schreiber, and D.A. Melton. 2009. Small molecules efficiently direct endodermal differentiation of mouse and human embryonic stem cells. *Cell Stem Cell.* 4:348–358.

Boyd, N.L., K.R. Robbins, S.K. Dhara, F.D. West, and S.L. Stice. 2009. Human embryonic stem cell-derived mesoderm-like epithelium transitions to mesenchymal progenitor cells. *Tissue Eng Part A.* 15:1897–1907.

Bragdon, B., O. Moseychuk, S. Saldanha, D. King, J. Julian, and A. Nohe. 2011. Bone morphogenetic proteins: a critical review. *Cell Signal.* 23:609–620.

Brave, M., A. Farrell, S. Ching Lin, T. Ocheltree, S. Pope Miksinski, S.L. Lee, H. Saber, J. Fourie, C. Tornoe, B. Booth, W. Yuan, K. He, R. Justice, and R. Pazdur. 2010. FDA review summary: Mozobil in combination with granulocyte colony-stimulating factor to mobilize hematopoietic stem cells to the peripheral blood for collection and subsequent autologous transplantation. *Oncology.* 78:282–288.

Bretzner, F., F. Gilbert, F. Baylis, and R.M. Brownstone. 2011. Target populations for first-in-human embryonic stem cell research in spinal cord injury. *Cell Stem Cell.* 8:468–475.

Brey, D.M., C. Chung, K.D. Hankenson, J.P. Garino, and J.A. Burdick. 2010. Identification of osteoconductive and biodegradable polymers from a combinatorial polymer library. *J Biomed Mater Res A.* 93:807–816.

Brown, M.E., E. Rondon, D. Rajesh, A. Mack, R. Lewis, X. Feng, L.J. Zitur, R.D. Learish, and E.F. Nuwaysir. 2010. Derivation of induced pluripotent stem cells from human peripheral blood T lymphocytes. *PLoS One.* 5:e11373.

Bruder, S.P., N. Jaiswal, and S.E. Haynesworth. 1997. Growth kinetics, self-renewal, and the osteogenic potential of purified human mesenchymal stem cells during extensive subcultivation and following cryopreservation. *J Cell Biochem.* 64:278–294.

Bryder, D., D.J. Rossi, and I.L. Weissman. 2006. Hematopoietic stem cells: the paradigmatic tissue-specific stem cell. *Am J Pathol.* 169:338–346.

Buijs, J.T., M. Petersen, G. van der Horst, and G. van der Pluijm. 2010. Bone morphogenetic proteins and its receptors; therapeutic targets in cancer progression and bone metastasis? *Curr Pharm Des.* 16:1291–1300.

Burks, M.V., and L. Nair. 2010. Long-term effects of bone morphogenetic protein-based treatments in humans. *J Long Term Eff Med Implants.* 20:277–293.

Burkus, J.K., M.F. Gornet, C.A. Dickman, and T.A. Zdeblick. 2002a. Anterior lumbar interbody fusion using rhBMP-2 with tapered interbody cages. *J Spinal Disord Tech.* 15:337–349.

Burkus, J.K., E.E. Transfeldt, S.H. Kitchel, R.G. Watkins, and R.A. Balderston. 2002b. Clinical and radiographic outcomes of anterior lumbar interbody fusion using recombinant human bone morphogenetic protein-2. *Spine.* 27:2396–2408.

Burton, P., D.R. Adams, A. Abraham, R.W. Allcock, Z. Jiang, A. McCahill, J. Gilmour, J. McAbney, N.M. Kane, G.S. Baillie, F.R. McKenzie, A.H. Baker, M.D. Houslay, J.C. Mountford, and G. Milligan. 2010. Identification and characterization of small-molecule ligands that maintain pluripotency of human embryonic stem cells. *Biochem Soc Trans.* 38:1058–1061.

Cao, Y., J.D. Lathia, C.E. Eyler, Q. Wu, Z. Li, H. Wang, R.E. McLendon, A.B. Hjelmeland, and J.N. Rich. 2010. Erythropoietin receptor signaling through STAT3 Is required for glioma stem cell maintenance. *Genes Cancer.* 1:50–61.

Cao, Y.A., A.J. Wagers, A. Beilhack, J. Dusich, M.H. Bachmann, R.S. Negrin, I.L. Weissman, and C.H. Contag. 2004. Shifting foci of hematopoiesis during reconstitution from single stem cells. *Proc Natl Acad Sci U S A.* 101:221–226.

Caplan, A.I. 1991. Mesenchymal stem cells. *J Orthop Res.* 9:641–650.

Caplan, A.I. 2009. Why are MSC therapeutic? New data: new insight. *J Pathol.* 217:318–324.

Cardinale, V., Y. Wang, G. Carpino, C.B. Cui, M. Gatto, M. Rossi, P.B. Berloco, A. Cantafora, E. Wauthier, M.E. Furth, L. Inverardi, J. Dominguez-Bendala, C. Ricordi, D. Gerber, E. Gaudio, D. Alvaro, and L. Reid. 2011. Multipotent stem/progenitor cells in human biliary tree give rise to hepatocytes, cholangiocytes and pancreatic islets. *Hepatology* 54:2159–2172.

Carpenter, M.K., M.S. Inokuma, J. Denham, T. Mujtaba, C.P. Chiu, and M.S. Rao. 2001. Enrichment of neurons and neural precursors from human embryonic stem cells. *Exp Neurol.* 172:383–397.

Carragee, E.J., E.L. Hurwitz, and B.K. Weiner. 2011. A critical review of recombinant human bone morphogenetic protein-2 trials in spinal surgery: emerging safety concerns and lessons learned. *Spine J.* 11:471–491.

Carvajal-Vergara, X., A. Sevilla, S.L. D'Souza, Y.S. Ang, C. Schaniel, D.F. Lee, L. Yang, A.D. Kaplan, E.D. Adler, Y. Rozov, Y. Ge, N. Cohen, L.J. Edelmann, B. Chang, A. Waghray, J. Su, S. Pardo, K.D. Lichtenbelt, M. Tartaglia, B.D. Gelb, and I.R. Lemischka. 2010. Patient-specific induced pluripotent stem-cell-derived models of LEOPARD syndrome. *Nature.* 465:808–812.

Cerdan, C., and M. Bhatia. 2010. Novel roles for Notch, Wnt and Hedgehog in hematopoesis derived from human pluripotent stem cells. *Int J Dev Biol.* 54:955–963.

Chang, C.W., Y.S. Lai, K.M. Pawlik, K. Liu, C.W. Sun, C. Li, T.R. Schoeb, and T.M. Townes. 2009. Polycistronic lentiviral vector for "hit and run" reprogramming of adult skin fibroblasts to induced pluripotent stem cells. *Stem Cells.* 27:1042–1049.

Chen, S., M. Borowiak, J.L. Fox, R. Maehr, K. Osafune, L. Davidow, K. Lam, L.F. Peng, S.L. Schreiber, L.L. Rubin, and D. Melton. 2009. A small molecule that directs differentiation of human ESCs into the pancreatic lineage. *Nat Chem Biol*. 5:258–265.

Chen, Z.Y., P. Asavaritikrai, J.T. Prchal, and C.T. Noguchi. 2007. Endogenous erythropoietin signaling is required for normal neural progenitor cell proliferation. *J Biol Chem*. 282:25875–25883.

Chicha, L., A. Feki, A. Boni, O. Irion, O. Hovatta, and M. Jaconi. 2011. Human pluripotent stem cells differentiated in fully defined medium generate hematopoietic CD34$^-$ and CD34$^+$ progenitors with distinct characteristics. *PLoS One*. 6:e14733.

Chitu, V., and E.R. Stanley. 2006. Colony-stimulating factor-1 in immunity and inflammation. *Curr Opin Immunol*. 18:39–48.

Cho, H.J., C.S. Lee, Y.W. Kwon, J.S. Paek, S.H. Lee, J. Hur, E.J. Lee, T.Y. Roh, I.S. Chu, S.H. Leem, Y. Kim, H.J. Kang, Y.B. Park, and H.S. Kim. 2010. Induction of pluripotent stem cells from adult somatic cells by protein-based reprogramming without genetic manipulation. *Blood*. 116(3):386–395.

Choi, K.D., M. Vodyanik, and Slukvin, II. 2011. Hematopoietic differentiation and production of mature myeloid cells from human pluripotent stem cells. *Nat Protoc*. 6:296–313.

Chou, B.K., P. Mali, X. Huang, Z. Ye, S.N. Dowey, L.M. Resar, C. Zou, Y.A. Zhang, J. Tong, and L. Cheng. 2011. Efficient human iPS cell derivation by a non-integrating plasmid from blood cells with unique epigenetic and gene expression signatures. *Cell Res*. 21:518–529.

Chow, D.C., L.A. Wenning, W.M. Miller, and E.T. Papoutsakis. 2001. Modeling pO(2) distributions in the bone marrow hematopoietic compartment. II. Modified Kroghian models. *Biophys J*. 81:685–696.

Cohen, D.E., and D. Melton. 2011. Turning straw into gold: directing cell fate for regenerative medicine. *Nat Rev Genet*. 12:243–252.

Cohen, J.C., J.D. Horton, and H.H. Hobbs. 2011. Human fatty liver disease: old questions and new insights. *Science*. 332:1519–1523.

Congdon, K.L., C. Voermans, E.C. Ferguson, L.N. DiMascio, M. Uqoezwa, C. Zhao, and T. Reya. 2008. Activation of Wnt signaling in hematopoietic regeneration. *Stem Cells*. 26:1202–1210.

Cox, G.F., and L.M. Kunkel. 1997. Dystrophies and heart disease. *Curr Opin Cardiol*. 12:329–343.

Crisan, M., M. Corselli, C.W. Chen, and B. Peault. 2011. Multilineage stem cells in the adult: a perivascular legacy? *Organogenesis*. 7:101–104.

Crisan, M., S. Yap, L. Casteilla, C.W. Chen, M. Corselli, T.S. Park, G. Andriolo, B. Sun, B. Zheng, L. Zhang, C. Norotte, P.N. Teng, J. Traas, R. Schugar, B.M. Deasy, S. Badylak, H.J. Buhring, J.P. Giacobino, L. Lazzari, J. Huard, and B. Peault. 2008. A perivascular origin for mesenchymal stem cells in multiple human organs. *Cell Stem Cell*. 3:301–313.

Csete, M. 2005. Oxygen in the cultivation of stem cells. *Ann N Y Acad Sci*. 1049:1–8.

Csete, M. 2010. Translational prospects for human induced pluripotent stem cells. *Regen Med*. 5:509–519.

Cui, H., Y. Meng, and R.F. Bulleit. 1998. Inhibition of glycogen synthase kinase 3beta activity regulates proliferation of cultured cerebellar granule cells. *Brain Res Dev Brain Res*. 111:177–188.

D'Amour, K.A., A.D. Agulnick, S. Eliazer, O.G. Kelly, E. Kroon, and E.E. Baetge. 2005. Efficient differentiation of human embryonic stem cells to definitive endoderm. *Nat Biotechnol*. 23:1534–1541.

D'Amour, K.A., A.G. Bang, S. Eliazer, O.G. Kelly, A.D. Agulnick, N.G. Smart, M.A. Moorman, E. Kroon, M.K. Carpenter, and E.E. Baetge. 2006. Production of pancreatic hormone-expressing endocrine cells from human embryonic stem cells. *Nat Biotechnol.* 24:1392–1401.

D'Ippolito, G., S. Diabira, G.A. Howard, P. Menei, B.A. Roos, and P.C. Schiller. 2004. Marrow-isolated adult multilineage inducible (MIAMI) cells, a unique population of postnatal young and old human cells with extensive expansion and differentiation potential. *J Cell Sci.* 117:2971–2981.

Damon, L.E. 2009. Mobilization of hematopoietic stem cells into the peripheral blood. *Expert Rev Hematol.* 2:717–733.

Darr, H., and N. Benvenisty. 2006. Human embryonic stem cells: the battle between self-renewal and differentiation. *Regen Med.* 1:317–325.

De Coppi, P., G. Bartsch, M.M. Siddiqui, T. Xu, C.C. Santos, L. Perin, G. Mostoslavsky, A.C. Serre, E.Y. Snyder, J.J. Yoo, M.E. Furth, S. Soker, and A. Atala. 2007. Isolation of amniotic stem cell lines with potential for therapy. *Nat Biotechnol.* 25:100–106.

Demetri, G.D., and K.H. Antman. 1992. Granulocyte-macrophage colony-stimulating factor (GM-CSF): preclinical and clinical investigations. *Semin Oncol.* 19:362–385.

Desbordes, S.C., D.G. Placantonakis, A. Ciro, N.D. Socci, G. Lee, H. Djaballah, and L. Studer. 2008. High-throughput screening assay for the identification of compounds regulating self-renewal and differentiation in human embryonic stem cells. *Cell Stem Cell.* 2:602–612.

Desponts, C., and S. Ding. 2010. Using small molecules to improve generation of induced pluripotent stem cells from somatic cells. *Methods Mol Biol.* 636:207–218.

Deuel, T.F., N. Zhang, H.J. Yeh, I. Silos-Santiago, and Z.Y. Wang. 2002. Pleiotrophin: a cytokine with diverse functions and a novel signaling pathway. *Arch Biochem Biophys.* 397:162–171.

Dias, J., M. Gumenyuk, H. Kang, M. Vodyanik, J. Yu, J. Thomson, and I. Slukvin. 2011. Generation of red blood cells from human induced pluripotent stem cells. *Stem Cells Dev.* 200(9):1639–1647.

Dicato, M., and L. Plawny. 2010. Erythropoietin in cancer patients: pros and cons. *Curr Opin Oncol.* 22:307–311.

Dimos, J.T., K.T. Rodolfa, K.K. Niakan, L.M. Weisenthal, H. Mitsumoto, W. Chung, G.F. Croft, G. Saphier, R. Leibel, R. Goland, H. Wichterle, C.E. Henderson, and K. Eggan. 2008. Induced pluripotent stem cells generated from patients with ALS can be differentiated into motor neurons. *Science.* 321:1218–1221.

Ding, S., and P.G. Schultz. 2004. A role for chemistry in stem cell biology. *Nat Biotechnol.* 22:833–840.

Ding, S., T.Y. Wu, A. Brinker, E.C. Peters, W. Hur, N.S. Gray, and P.G. Schultz. 2003. Synthetic small molecules that control stem cell fate. *Proc Natl Acad Sci U S A.* 100:7632–7637.

Dodge, M.E., and L. Lum. 2011. Drugging the cancer stem cell compartment: lessons learned from the hedgehog and Wnt signal transduction pathways. *Ann Rev Pharmacol Toxicol.* 51:289–310.

Dor, Y., J. Brown, O.I. Martinez, and D.A. Melton. 2004. Adult pancreatic beta-cells are formed by self-duplication rather than stem-cell differentiation. *Nature.* 429:41–46.

Drake, A.C., M. Khoury, I. Leskov, B.P. Iliopoulou, M. Fragoso, H. Lodish, and J. Chen. 2011. Human CD34$^+$ CD133$^+$ hematopoietic stem cells cultured with growth factors including Angptl5 efficiently engraft adult NOD-SCID Il2rgamma$^{-/-}$ (NSG) mice. *PLoS One.* 6:e18382.

Duan, D. 2006. Challenges and opportunities in dystrophin-deficient cardiomyopathy gene therapy. *Hum Mol Genet.* 15(Spec No 2):R253–R261.

Duncan, A.W., C. Dorrell, and M. Grompe. 2009. Stem cells and liver regeneration. *Gastroenterology.* 137:466–481.

Duncan, A.W., F.M. Rattis, L.N. DiMascio, K.L. Congdon, G. Pazianos, C. Zhao, K. Yoon, J.M. Cook, K. Willert, N. Gaiano, and T. Reya. 2005. Integration of Notch and Wnt signaling in hematopoietic stem cell maintenance. *Nat Immunol.* 6:314–322.

Ebert, A.D., J. Yu, F.F. Rose, Jr., V.B. Mattis, C.L. Lorson, J.A. Thomson, and C.N. Svendsen. 2009. Induced pluripotent stem cells from a spinal muscular atrophy patient. *Nature.* 457:277–280.

Eder, M., G. Geissler, and A. Ganser. 1997. IL-3 in the clinic. *Stem Cells.* 15:327–333.

Efe, J.A., S. Hilcove, J. Kim, H. Zhou, K. Ouyang, G. Wang, J. Chen, and S. Ding. 2011. Conversion of mouse fibroblasts into cardiomyocytes using a direct reprogramming strategy. *Nat Cell Biol.* 13:215–222.

Eggan, K., K. Baldwin, M. Tackett, J. Osborne, J. Gogos, A. Chess, R. Axel, and R. Jaenisch. 2004. Mice cloned from olfactory sensory neurons. *Nature.* 428:44–49.

Eglen, R.M., A. Gilchrist, and T. Reisine. 2008. An overview of drug screening using primary and embryonic stem cells. *Comb Chem High Throughput Screen.* 11:566–572.

Evans, M.J., and M.H. Kaufman. 1981. Establishment in culture of pluripotential cells from mouse embryos. *Nature.* 292:154–156.

Fandrey, J., and M. Dicato. 2009. Examining the involvement of erythropoiesis-stimulating agents in tumor proliferation (erythropoietin receptors, receptor binding, signal transduction), angiogenesis, and venous thromboembolic events. *Oncologist.* 14 Suppl 1:34–42.

Fang, Y.Q., W.Q. Wong, Y.W. Yap, and B.P. Orner. 2007. Stem cells and combinatorial science. *Comb Chem High Throughput Screen.* 10:635–651.

Fatrai, S., A.T. Wierenga, S.M. Daenen, E. Vellenga, and J.J. Schuringa. 2011. Identification of HIF2alpha as an important STAT5 target gene in human hematopoietic stem cells. *Blood.* 117:3320–3330.

Faulds, D., and E.M. Sorkin. 1989. Epoetin (recombinant human erythropoietin). A review of its pharmacodynamic and pharmacokinetic properties and therapeutic potential in anaemia and the stimulation of erythropoiesis. *Drugs.* 38:863–899.

Fennelly, D., L. Vahdat, J. Schneider, L. Reich, N. Hamilton, T. Hakes, G. Raptis, C. Wasserheit, A. Kritz, S. Gulati, and et al. 1994. High-intensity chemotherapy with peripheral blood progenitor cell support. *Semin Oncol.* 21:21–25; quiz 26, 58.

Filby, C.E., R. Williamson, P. van Kooy, A. Pebay, M. Dottori, N.J. Elwood, and F. Zaibak. 2011. Stimulation of Activin A/Nodal signaling is insufficient to induce definitive endoderm formation of cord blood-derived unrestricted somatic stem cells. *Stem Cell Res Ther.* 2:16.

Fisher, O.Z., A. Khademhosseini, R. Langer, and N.A. Peppas. 2010. Bioinspired materials for controlling stem cell fate. *Accounts of Chemical Research.* 43:419–428.

Forristal, C.E., K.L. Wright, N.A. Hanley, R.O. Oreffo, and F.D. Houghton. 2010. Hypoxia inducible factors regulate pluripotency and proliferation in human embryonic stem cells cultured at reduced oxygen tensions. *Reproduction.* 139:85–97.

Frampton, J.E., C.R. Lee, and D. Faulds. 1994. Filgrastim. A review of its pharmacological properties and therapeutic efficacy in neutropenia. *Drugs.* 48:731–760.

Fried, W. 2009. Erythropoietin and erythropoiesis. *Exp Hematol.* 37:1007–1015.

Friedlaender, G.E., C.R. Perry, J.D. Cole, S.D. Cook, G. Cierny, G.F. Muschler, G.A. Zych, J.H. Calhoun, A.J. LaForte, and S. Yin. 2001. Osteogenic protein-1 (bone morphogenetic protein-7) in the treatment of tibial nonunions. *J Bone Joint Surg.* 83-A Suppl 1:S151–158.

Fukumitsu, K., H. Yagi, and A. Soto-Gutierrez. 2011. Bioengineering in organ transplantation: targeting the liver. *Transplant Proc.* 43:2137–2138.

Funakoshi, N., C. Duret, J.M. Pascussi, P. Blanc, P. Maurel, M. Daujat-Chavanieu, and S. Gerbal-Chaloin. 2011. Comparison of hepatic-like cell production from human embryonic stem cells and adult liver progenitor cells: CAR transduction activates a battery of detoxification genes. *Stem Cell Rev.* 7:518–531.

Furth, M.E., A. Atala, and M.E. Van Dyke. 2007. Smart biomaterials design for tissue engineering and regenerative medicine. *Biomaterials.* 28:5068–5073.

Furth, M.E., and G.J. Christ. 2009. Regenerative pharmacology for diabetes mellitus. *Mol Interv.* 9:171–174.

Gage, F. 2010. The promise and the challenge of modelling human disease in a dish. *EMBO Mol Med.* 2:77–78.

Gage, F.H. 2000. Mammalian neural stem cells. *Science.* 287:1433–1438.

Gazit, R., I.L. Weissman, and D.J. Rossi. 2008. Hematopoietic stem cells and the aging hematopoietic system. *Semin Hematol.* 45:218–224.

Gertz, M.A. 2010. Current status of stem cell mobilization. *Br J Haematol.* 150:647–662.

Giese, A.K., J. Frahm, R. Hubner, J. Luo, A. Wree, M.J. Frech, A. Rolfs, and S. Ortinau. 2010. Erythropoietin and the effect of oxygen during proliferation and differentiation of human neural progenitor cells. *BMC Cell Biol.* 11:94.

Gimble, J.M., A.J. Katz, and B.A. Bunnell. 2007. Adipose-derived stem cells for regenerative medicine. *Circ Res.* 100:1249–1260.

Glaspy, J.A. 2009. Erythropoietin in cancer patients. *Annu Rev Med.* 60:181–192.

Goldstein, J.L., and M.S. Brown. 2009. The LDL receptor. *Arterioscler Thromb Vasc Biol.* 29:431–438.

Gore, A., Z. Li, H.L. Fung, J.E. Young, S. Agarwal, J. Antosiewicz-Bourget, I. Canto, A. Giorgetti, M.A. Israel, E. Kiskinis, J.H. Lee, Y.H. Loh, P.D. Manos, N. Montserrat, A.D. Panopoulos, S. Ruiz, M.L. Wilbert, J. Yu, E.F. Kirkness, J.C. Izpisua Belmonte, D.J. Rossi, J.A. Thomson, K. Eggan, G.Q. Daley, L.S. Goldstein, and K. Zhang. 2011. Somatic coding mutations in human induced pluripotent stem cells. *Nature.* 471:63–67.

Govender, S., C. Csimma, H.K. Genant, A. Valentin-Opran, Y. Amit, R. Arbel, H. Aro, D. Atar, M. Bishay, M.G. Borner, P. Chiron, P. Choong, J. Cinats, B. Courtenay, R. Feibel, B. Geulette, C. Gravel, N. Haas, M. Raschke, E. Hammacher, D. van der Velde, P. Hardy, M. Holt, C. Josten, R.L. Ketterl, B. Lindeque, G. Lob, H. Mathevon, G. McCoy, D. Marsh, R. Miller, E. Munting, S. Oevre, L. Nordsletten, A. Patel, A. Pohl, W. Rennie, P. Reynders, P.M. Rommens, J. Rondia, W.C. Rossouw, P.J. Daneel, S. Ruff, A. Ruter, S. Santavirta, T.A. Schildhauer, C. Gekle, R. Schnettler, D. Segal, H. Seiler, R.B. Snowdowne, J. Stapert, G. Taglang, R. Verdonk, L. Vogels, A. Weckbach, A. Wentzensen, and T. Wisniewski. 2002. Recombinant human bone morphogenetic protein-2 for treatment of open tibial fractures: a prospective, controlled, randomized study of four hundred and fifty patients. *J Bone Joint Surg.* 84:2123–2134.

Grant, S.M., and R.C. Heel. 1992. Recombinant granulocyte-macrophage colony-stimulating factor (rGM-CSF). A review of its pharmacological properties and prospective role in the management of myelosuppression. *Drugs.* 43:516–560.

Gruenloh, W., A. Kambal, C. Sondergaard, J. McGee, C. Nacey, S. Kalomoiris, K. Pepper, S. Olson, F. Fierro, and J.A. Nolta. 2011. Characterization and in vivo testing of mesenchymal stem cells derived from human embryonic stem cells. *Tissue Eng Part A.* 17:1517–1525.

Gu, Y.Z., J.B. Hogenesch, and C.A. Bradfield. 2000. The PAS superfamily: sensors of environmental and developmental signals. *Ann Rev Pharmacol Toxicol.* 40:519–561.

Gupta, S., C. Verfaillie, D. Chmielewski, S. Kren, K. Eidman, J. Connaire, Y. Heremans, T. Lund, M. Blackstad, Y. Jiang, A. Luttun, and M.E. Rosenberg. 2006. Isolation and characterization of kidney-derived stem cells. *J Am Soc Nephrol.* 17:3028–3040.

Gwak, J., S.G. Hwang, H.S. Park, S.R. Choi, S.H. Park, H. Kim, N.C. Ha, S.J. Bae, J.K. Han, D.E. Kim, J.W. Cho, and S. Oh. 2011. Small molecule-based disruption of the

Axin/beta-catenin protein complex regulates mesenchymal stem cell differentiation. *Cell Res.* 22(1):237–247.

Hamazaki, T., Y. Iiboshi, M. Oka, P.J. Papst, A.M. Meacham, L.I. Zon, and N. Terada. 2001. Hepatic maturation in differentiating embryonic stem cells in vitro. *FEBS Lett.* 497:15–19.

Hidaka, T., S. Akada, A. Teranishi, H. Morikawa, S. Sato, Y. Yoshida, A. Yajima, N. Yaegashi, K. Okamura, and S. Saito. 2003. Mirimostim (macrophage colony-stimulating factor; M-CSF) improves chemotherapy-induced impaired natural killer cell activity, Th1/Th2 balance, and granulocyte function. *Cancer Sci.* 94:814–820.

Himburg, H.A., G.G. Muramoto, P. Daher, S.K. Meadows, J.L. Russell, P. Doan, J.T. Chi, A.B. Salter, W.E. Lento, T. Reya, N.J. Chao, and J.P. Chute. 2010. Pleiotrophin regulates the expansion and regeneration of hematopoietic stem cells. *Nat Med.* 16:475–482.

Hoggatt, J., and L.M. Pelus. 2011. Many mechanisms mediating mobilization: an alliterative review. *Curr Opin Hematol.* 18(4):231–238.

Horwitz, E.M., K. Le Blanc, M. Dominici, I. Mueller, I. Slaper-Cortenbach, F.C. Marini, R.J. Deans, D.S. Krause, and A. Keating. 2005. Clarification of the nomenclature for MSC: the International Society for Cellular Therapy position statement. *Cytotherapy.* 7:393–395.

Hosokawa, K., F. Arai, H. Yoshihara, Y. Nakamura, Y. Gomei, H. Iwasaki, K. Miyamoto, H. Shima, K. Ito, and T. Suda. 2007. Function of oxidative stress in the regulation of hematopoietic stem cell-niche interaction. *Biochem Biophys Res Commun.* 363:578–583.

Houbracken, I., and L. Bouwens. 2010. The quest for tissue stem cells in the pancreas and other organs, and their application in beta-cell replacement. *Rev Diabet Stud.* 7:112–123.

Howden, S.E., A. Gore, Z. Li, H.L. Fung, B.S. Nisler, J. Nie, G. Chen, B.E. McIntosh, D.R. Gulbranson, N.R. Diol, S.M. Taapken, D.T. Vereide, K.D. Montgomery, K. Zhang, D.M. Gamm, and J.A. Thomson. 2011. Genetic correction and analysis of induced pluripotent stem cells from a patient with gyrate atrophy. *Proc Natl Acad Sci U S A.* 108:6537–6542.

Hussein, S.M., N.N. Batada, S. Vuoristo, R.W. Ching, R. Autio, E. Narva, S. Ng, M. Sourour, R. Hamalainen, C. Olsson, K. Lundin, M. Mikkola, R. Trokovic, M. Peitz, O. Brustle, D.P. Bazett-Jones, K. Alitalo, R. Lahesmaa, A. Nagy, and T. Otonkoski. 2011. Copy number variation and selection during reprogramming to pluripotency. *Nature.* 471:58–62.

Ichida, J.K., J. Blanchard, K. Lam, E.Y. Son, J.E. Chung, D. Egli, K.M. Loh, A.C. Carter, F.P. Di Giorgio, K. Koszka, D. Huangfu, H. Akutsu, D.R. Liu, L.L. Rubin, and K. Eggan. 2009. A small-molecule inhibitor of TGF-Beta signaling replaces Sox2 in reprogramming by inducing Nanog. *Cell Stem Cell.* 5:491–503.

Ieda, M., J.D. Fu, P. Delgado-Olguin, V. Vedantham, Y. Hayashi, B.G. Bruneau, and D. Srivastava. 2010. Direct reprogramming of fibroblasts into functional cardiomyocytes by defined factors. *Cell.* 142:375–386.

Ihle, J.N. 1992. Interleukin-3 and hematopoiesis. *Chem Immunol.* 51:65–106.

Ingham, P.W., and A.P. McMahon. 2001. Hedgehog signaling in animal development: paradigms and principles. *Genes Dev.* 15:3059–3087.

Istvanffy, R., M. Kroger, C. Eckl, S. Gitzelmann, B. Vilne, F. Bock, S. Graf, M. Schiemann, U.B. Keller, C. Peschel, and R.A. Oostendorp. 2011. Stromal pleiotrophin regulates repopulation behavior of hematopoietic stem cells. *Blood.* 118(10):2712–2722.

Itzhaki, I., L. Maizels, I. Huber, L. Zwi-Dantsis, O. Caspi, A. Winterstern, O. Feldman, A. Gepstein, G. Arbel, H. Hammerman, M. Boulos, and L. Gepstein. 2011. Modelling the long QT syndrome with induced pluripotent stem cells. *Nature.* 471:225–229.

Ivanovic, Z. 2004. Interleukin-3 and ex vivo maintenance of hematopoietic stem cells: facts and controversies. *Euro Cytokine Netw.* 15:6–13.

Jiang, J., M. Au, K. Lu, A. Eshpeter, G. Korbutt, G. Fisk, and A.S. Majumdar. 2007a. Generation of insulin-producing islet-like clusters from human embryonic stem cells. *Stem Cells.* 25:1940–1953.

Jiang, W., Y. Shi, D. Zhao, S. Chen, J. Yong, J. Zhang, T. Qing, X. Sun, P. Zhang, M. Ding, D. Li, and H. Deng. 2007b. In vitro derivation of functional insulin-producing cells from human embryonic stem cells. *Cell Res.* 17:333–344.

Jiang, Y., B. Vaessen, T. Lenvik, M. Blackstad, M. Reyes, and C.M. Verfaillie. 2002. Multipotent progenitor cells can be isolated from postnatal murine bone marrow, muscle, and brain. *Exp Hematol.* 30:896–904.

Jin, Z.B., S. Okamoto, F. Osakada, K. Homma, J. Assawachananont, Y. Hirami, T. Iwata, and M. Takahashi. 2011. Modeling retinal degeneration using patient-specific induced pluripotent stem cells. *PLoS One.* 6:e17084.

Karumbayaram, S., B.G. Novitch, M. Patterson, J.A. Umbach, L. Richter, A. Lindgren, A.E. Conway, A.T. Clark, S.A. Goldman, K. Plath, M. Wiedau-Pazos, H.I. Kornblum, and W.E. Lowry. 2009. Directed differentiation of human-induced pluripotent stem cells generates active motor neurons. *Stem Cells.* 27:806–811.

Katsumoto, K., N. Shiraki, R. Miki, and S. Kume. 2010. Embryonic and adult stem cell systems in mammals: ontology and regulation. *Dev Growth Differ.* 52:115–129.

Kazuki, Y., M. Hiratsuka, M. Takiguchi, M. Osaki, N. Kajitani, H. Hoshiya, K. Hiramatsu, T. Yoshino, K. Kazuki, C. Ishihara, S. Takehara, K. Higaki, M. Nakagawa, K. Takahashi, S. Yamanaka, and M. Oshimura. 2010. Complete genetic correction of iPS cells from Duchenne muscular dystrophy. *Mol Ther.* 18:386–393.

Kent, D., M. Copley, C. Benz, B. Dykstra, M. Bowie, and C. Eaves. 2008. Regulation of hematopoietic stem cells by the steel factor/KIT signaling pathway. *Clin Cancer Res.* 14:1926–1930.

Khan, A.A., M.V. Shaik, N. Parveen, A. Rajendraprasad, M.A. Aleem, M.A. Habeeb, G. Srinivas, T.A. Raj, S.K. Tiwari, K. Kumaresan, J. Venkateswarlu, G. Pande, and C.M. Habibullah. 2010. Human fetal liver-derived stem cell transplantation as supportive modality in the management of end-stage decompensated liver cirrhosis. *Cell Transplant.* 19:409–418.

Khoury, M., A. Drake, Q. Chen, D. Dong, I. Leskov, M.F. Fragoso, Y. Li, B.P. Iliopoulou, W. Hwang, H.F. Lodish, and J. Chen. 2011. Mesenchymal stem cells secreting angiopoietin-like-5 support efficient expansion of human hematopoietic stem cells without compromising their repopulating potential. *Stem Cells Dev.* 20(8):1371–1381.

Kim, J.B., H. Zaehres, G. Wu, L. Gentile, K. Ko, V. Sebastiano, M.J. Arauzo-Bravo, D. Ruau, D.W. Han, M. Zenke, and H.R. Scholer. 2008. Pluripotent stem cells induced from adult neural stem cells by reprogramming with two factors. *Nature.* 454:646–650.

Kim, K., A. Doi, B. Wen, K. Ng, R. Zhao, P. Cahan, J. Kim, M.J. Aryee, H. Ji, L.I. Ehrlich, A. Yabuuchi, A. Takeuchi, K.C. Cunniff, H. Hongguang, S. McKinney-Freeman, O. Naveiras, T.J. Yoon, R.A. Irizarry, N. Jung, J. Seita, J. Hanna, P. Murakami, R. Jaenisch, R. Weissleder, S.H. Orkin, I.L. Weissman, A.P. Feinberg, and G.Q. Daley. 2010. Epigenetic memory in induced pluripotent stem cells. *Nature.* 467:285–290.

Kimelman-Bleich, N., G. Pelled, Y. Zilberman, I. Kallai, O. Mizrahi, W. Tawackoli, Z. Gazit, and D. Gazit. 2011. Targeted gene-and-host progenitor cell therapy for nonunion bone fracture repair. *Mol Ther.* 19:53–59.

Kinoshita, T., and A. Miyajima. 2002. Cytokine regulation of liver development. *Biochim Biophys Acta.* 1592:303–312.

Kiskinis, E., and K. Eggan. 2010. Progress toward the clinical application of patient-specific pluripotent stem cells. *J Clin Invest.* 120:51–59.

Klimanskaya, I., J. Hipp, K.A. Rezai, M. West, A. Atala, and R. Lanza. 2004. Derivation and comparative assessment of retinal pigment epithelium from human embryonic stem cells using transcriptomics. *Cloning Stem Cells*. 6:217–245.

Kouskoff, V., G. Lacaud, S. Schwantz, H.J. Fehling, and G. Keller. 2005. Sequential development of hematopoietic and cardiac mesoderm during embryonic stem cell differentiation. *Proc Natl Acad Sci U S A*. 102:13170–13175.

Krause, C., A. Guzman, and P. Knaus. 2011. Noggin. *Int J Biochem Cell Biol*. 43:478–481.

Krishnan, V., H.U. Bryant, and O.A. Macdougald. 2006. Regulation of bone mass by Wnt signaling. *J Clin Invest*. 116:1202–1209.

Kroon, E., L.A. Martinson, K. Kadoya, A.G. Bang, O.G. Kelly, S. Eliazer, H. Young, M. Richardson, N.G. Smart, J. Cunningham, A.D. Agulnick, K.A. D'Amour, M.K. Carpenter, and E.E. Baetge. 2008. Pancreatic endoderm derived from human embryonic stem cells generates glucose-responsive insulin-secreting cells in vivo. *Nat Biotechnol*. 26:443–452.

Kubo, A., K. Shinozaki, J.M. Shannon, V. Kouskoff, M. Kennedy, S. Woo, H.J. Fehling, and G. Keller. 2004. Development of definitive endoderm from embryonic stem cells in culture. *Development*. 131:1651–1662.

Kubota, H., and L.M. Reid. 2000. Clonogenic hepatoblasts, common precursors for hepatocytic and biliary lineages, are lacking classical major histocompatibility complex class I antigen. *Proc Natl Acad Sci U S A*. 97:12132–12137.

Kubota, H., H.L. Yao, and L.M. Reid. 2007. Identification and characterization of vitamin A-storing cells in fetal liver: implications for functional importance of hepatic stellate cells in liver development and hematopoiesis. *Stem Cells*. 25:2339–2349.

Kunisato, A., M. Wakatsuki, H. Shinba, T. Ota, I. Ishida, and K. Nagao. 2010. Direct generation of induced pluripotent stem cells from human non-mobilized blood. *Stem Cells Dev*.

Kuster, O., P. Simon, M. Mittelbronn, G. Tabatabai, C. Hermann, H. Strik, K. Dietz, F. Roser, R. Meyermann, and J. Schittenhelm. 2009. Erythropoietin receptor is expressed in meningiomas and lower levels are associated with tumour recurrence. *Neuropathol Appl Neurobio*. 35:555–565.

Lad, S.P., J.K. Nathan, and M. Boakye. 2011. Trends in the use of bone morphogenetic protein as a substitute to autologous iliac crest bone grafting for spinal fusion procedures in the United States. *Spine*. 36:E274–281.

Lavon, N., O. Yanuka, and N. Benvenisty. 2004. Differentiation and isolation of hepatic-like cells from human embryonic stem cells. *Differentiation*. 72:230–238.

Lee, C.C., J.E. Christensen, M.C. Yoder, and A.F. Tarantal. 2010a. Clonal analysis and hierarchy of human bone marrow mesenchymal stem and progenitor cells. *Exp Hematol*. 38:46–54.

Lee, G., S.M. Chambers, M.J. Tomishima, and L. Studer. 2010b. Derivation of neural crest cells from human pluripotent stem cells. *Nat Protoc*. 5:688–701.

Lee, H., J. Park, B.G. Forget, and P. Gaines. 2009. Induced pluripotent stem cells in regenerative medicine: an argument for continued research on human embryonic stem cells. *Regen Med*. 4:759–769.

Lee, S.H., N. Lumelsky, L. Studer, J.M. Auerbach, and R.D. McKay. 2000. Efficient generation of midbrain and hindbrain neurons from mouse embryonic stem cells. *Nat Biotechnol*. 18:675–679.

Lei, Y., S. Gojgini, J. Lam, and T. Segura. 2011. The spreading, migration and proliferation of mouse mesenchymal stem cells cultured inside hyaluronic acid hydrogels. *Biomaterials*. 32:39–47.

Lengerke, C., M. Grauer, N.I. Niebuhr, T. Riedt, L. Kanz, I.H. Park, and G.Q. Daley. 2009. Hematopoietic development from human induced pluripotent stem cells. *Ann N Y Acad Sci*. 1176:219–227.

Lennon, D.P., S.E. Haynesworth, S.P. Bruder, N. Jaiswal, and A.I. Caplan. 1996. Human and animal mesenchymal progenitor cells from bone marrow: identification of serum for optimal selection and proliferation. *In Vitro Cell Dev Biol Anim.* 32:602–611.

Li, L., and H. Clevers. 2010. Coexistence of quiescent and active adult stem cells in mammals. *Science.* 327:542–545.

Li, L., and T. Xie. 2005. Stem cell niche: structure and function. *Annu Rev Cell Dev Biol.* 21:605–631.

Li, S., E. Kimura, R. Ng, B.M. Fall, L. Meuse, M. Reyes, J.A. Faulkner, and J.S. Chamberlain. 2006. A highly functional mini-dystrophin/GFP fusion gene for cell and gene therapy studies of Duchenne muscular dystrophy. *Hum Mol Genet.* 15:1610–1622.

Li, W., and S. Ding. 2010. Small molecules that modulate embryonic stem cell fate and somatic cell reprogramming. *Trends Pharmacol Sci.* 31:36–45.

Li, W., W. Sun, Y. Zhang, W. Wei, R. Ambasudhan, P. Xia, M. Talantova, T. Lin, J. Kim, X. Wang, W.R. Kim, S.A. Lipton, K. Zhang, and S. Ding. 2011. Rapid induction and long-term self-renewal of primitive neural precursors from human embryonic stem cells by small molecule inhibitors. *Proc Natl Acad Sci U S A.* 108:8299–8304.

Lindemann, A., and R. Mertelsmann. 1995. Interleukin-3 and its receptor. *Cancer Treat Res.* 80:107–142.

Lissenberg-Thunnissen, S.N., D.J. de Gorter, C.F. Sier, and I.B. Schipper. 2011. Use and efficacy of bone morphogenetic proteins in fracture healing. *Int Orthop.* 35:1271–1280.

Lister, R., M. Pelizzola, Y.S. Kida, R.D. Hawkins, J.R. Nery, G. Hon, J. Antosiewicz-Bourget, R. O'Malley, R. Castanon, S. Klugman, M. Downes, R. Yu, R. Stewart, B. Ren, J.A. Thomson, R.M. Evans, and J.R. Ecker. 2011. Hotspots of aberrant epigenomic reprogramming in human induced pluripotent stem cells. *Nature.* 471:68–73.

Liu, G.H., K. Suzuki, J. Qu, I. Sancho-Martinez, F. Yi, M. Li, S. Kumar, E. Nivet, J. Kim, R.D. Soligalla, I. Dubova, A. Goebl, N. Plongthongkum, H.L. Fung, K. Zhang, J.F. Loring, L.C. Laurent, and J.C. Izpisua Belmonte. 2011. Targeted gene correction of laminopathy-associated LMNA mutations in patient-specific iPSCs. *Cell Stem Cell.* 8:688–694.

Loo, D., C. Beltejar, J. Hooley, and X. Xu. 2008. Primary and multipassage culture of human fetal kidney epithelial progenitor cells. *Methods Cell Biol.* 86:241–255.

Loya, K., R. Eggenschwiler, K. Ko, M. Sgodda, F. Andre, M. Bleidissel, H.R. Scholer, and T. Cantz. 2009. Hepatic differentiation of pluripotent stem cells. *Biol Chem.* 390:1047–1055.

Lozoya, O.A., E. Wauthier, R.A. Turner, C. Barbier, G.D. Prestwich, F. Guilak, R. Superfine, S.R. Lubkin, and L.M. Reid. 2011. Regulation of hepatic stem/progenitor phenotype by microenvironment stiffness in hydrogel models of the human liver stem cell niche. *Biomaterials.* 32:7389–7402.

Lu, S.J., Q. Feng, J.S. Park, and R. Lanza. 2010. Directed differentiation of red blood cells from human embryonic stem cells. *Methods Mol Biol.* 636:105–121.

Lyman, S.D., and S.E. Jacobsen. 1998. c-kit ligand and Flt3 ligand: stem/progenitor cell factors with overlapping yet distinct activities. *Blood.* 91:1101–1134.

Lysaght, M.J., A. Jaklenec, and E. Deweerd. 2008. Great expectations: private sector activity in tissue engineering, regenerative medicine, and stem cell therapeutics. *Tissue Eng Part A.* 14:305–315.

Lyssiotis, C.A., R.K. Foreman, J. Staerk, M. Garcia, D. Mathur, S. Markoulaki, J. Hanna, L.L. Lairson, B.D. Charette, L.C. Bouchez, M. Bollong, C. Kunick, A. Brinker, C.Y. Cho, P.G. Schultz, and R. Jaenisch. 2009. Reprogramming of murine fibroblasts to induced pluripotent stem cells with chemical complementation of Klf4. *Proc Natl Acad Sci U S A.* 106:8912–8917.

Macdonald, J.M., A. Xu, H. Kubota, E. LeCluyse, G. Hamilton, H. Liu, Y. Rong, N. Moss, C. Lodestro, T. Luntz, S.P. Wolfe, and L.M. Reid. 2002. Liver cell culture and lineage biology. In *Methods of Tissue Engineering*. A. Atala and R.P. Lanza, editors. Academic Press, San Diego. 151–202.

Maehr, R., S. Chen, M. Snitow, T. Ludwig, L. Yagasaki, R. Goland, R.L. Leibel, and D.A. Melton. 2009. Generation of pluripotent stem cells from patients with type 1 diabetes. *Proc Natl Acad Sci U S A*. 106:15768–15773.

Maitra, A., D.E. Arking, N. Shivapurkar, M. Ikeda, V. Stastny, K. Kassauei, G. Sui, D.J. Cutler, Y. Liu, S.N. Brimble, K. Noaksson, J. Hyllner, T.C. Schulz, X. Zeng, W.J. Freed, J. Crook, S. Abraham, A. Colman, P. Sartipy, S. Matsui, M. Carpenter, A.F. Gazdar, M. Rao, and A. Chakravarti. 2005. Genomic alterations in cultured human embryonic stem cells. *Nat Genet*. 37:1099–1103.

Martin, G.R. 1981. Isolation of a pluripotent cell line from early mouse embryos cultured in medium conditioned by teratocarcinoma stem cells. *Proc Natl Acad Sci U S A*. 78:7634–7638.

Martin, G.R., and M.J. Evans. 1975. Differentiation of clonal lines of teratocarcinoma cells: formation of embryoid bodies in vitro. *Proc Natl Acad Sci U S A*. 72:1441–1445.

Martinez-Fernandez, A., T.J. Nelson, and A. Terzic. 2011. Nuclear reprogramming strategy modulates differentiation potential of induced pluripotent stem cells. *J Cardiovasc Transl Res*. 4:131–137.

Masarone, M., and M. Persico. 2011. Antiviral therapy: why does it fail in HCV-related chronic hepatitis? *Exp Rev Anti-infect Ther*. 9:535–543.

Matsa, E., D. Rajamohan, E. Dick, L. Young, I. Mellor, A. Staniforth, and C. Denning. 2011. Drug evaluation in cardiomyocytes derived from human induced pluripotent stem cells carrying a long QT syndrome type 2 mutation. *Eur Heart J*. 32(8):952–962.

Matsumoto, K., T. Isagawa, T. Nishimura, T. Ogaeri, K. Eto, S. Miyazaki, J. Miyazaki, H. Aburatani, H. Nakauchi, and H. Ema. 2009. Stepwise development of hematopoietic stem cells from embryonic stem cells. *PLoS One*. 4:e4820.

Maurer, M.H., W.R. Schabitz, and A. Schneider. 2008. Old friends in new constellations–the hematopoetic growth factors G-CSF, GM-CSF, and EPO for the treatment of neurological diseases. *Curr Med Chem*. 15:1407–1411.

Mayhew, C.N., and J.M. Wells. 2010. Converting human pluripotent stem cells into beta-cells: recent advances and future challenges. *Curr Opin Organ Transplant*. 15:54–60.

McClelland, R., E. Wauthier, J. Uronis, and L. Reid. 2008a. Gradients in the liver's extracellular matrix chemistry from periportal to pericentral zones: influence on human hepatic progenitors. *Tissue Eng Part A*. 14:59–70.

McClelland, R., E. Wauthier, L. Zhang, A. Melhem, E. Schmelzer, C. Barbier, and L.M. Reid. 2008b. Ex vivo conditions for self-replication of human hepatic stem cells. *Tissue Eng Part C Methods*. 14:341–351.

McKay, W.F., S.M. Peckham, and J.M. Badura. 2007. A comprehensive clinical review of recombinant human bone morphogenetic protein-2 (INFUSE Bone Graft). *Int Orthop*. 31:729–734.

Melton, D.A. 2011. Using stem cells to study and possibly treat type 1 diabetes. *Philos Trans R Soc Lond B Biol Sci*. 366:2307–2311.

Mendez-Ferrer, S., D. Lucas, M. Battista, and P.S. Frenette. 2008. Haematopoietic stem cell release is regulated by circadian oscillations. *Nature*. 452:442–447.

Metcalf, D. 2008. Hematopoietic cytokines. *Blood*. 111:485–491.

Meyer, J.R. 2008. The significance of induced pluripotent stem cells for basic research and clinical therapy. *J Med Ethics*. 34:849–851.

Michalopoulos, G.K. 2011. Liver regeneration: alternative epithelial pathways. *Int J Biochem Cell Biol*. 43:173–179.

Michalopoulos, G.K., and M. DeFrances. 2005. Liver regeneration. *Adv Biochem Eng Biotechnol.* 93:101–134.

Minear, S., P. Leucht, J. Jiang, B. Liu, A. Zeng, C. Fuerer, R. Nusse, and J.A. Helms. 2010. Wnt proteins promote bone regeneration. *Sci Transl Med.* 2:29ra30.

Mirza, S.K. 2011. Commentary: folly of FDA-approval studies for bone morphogenetic protein. *Spine J.* 11:495–499.

Mitchell, K.E., M.L. Weiss, B.M. Mitchell, P. Martin, D. Davis, L. Morales, B. Helwig, M. Beerenstrauch, K. Abou-Easa, T. Hildreth, D. Troyer, and S. Medicetty. 2003. Matrix cells from Wharton's jelly form neurons and glia. *Stem Cells.* 21:50–60.

Mitne-Neto, M., M. Machado-Costa, M.C. Marchetto, M.H. Bengtson, C.A. Joazeiro, H. Tsuda, H.J. Bellen, H.C. Silva, A.S. Oliveira, M. Lazar, A.R. Muotri, and M. Zatz. 2011. Downregulation of VAPB expression in motor neurons derived from induced pluripotent stem cells of ALS8 patients. *Hum Mol Genet.* 20(18):3642–3652.

Miyazono, K., Y. Kamiya, and M. Morikawa. 2010. Bone morphogenetic protein receptors and signal transduction. *J Biochem.* 147:35–51.

Mohr, J.C., J. Zhang, S.M. Azarin, A.G. Soerens, J.J. de Pablo, J.A. Thomson, G.E. Lyons, S.P. Palecek, and T.J. Kamp. 2010. The microwell control of embryoid body size in order to regulate cardiac differentiation of human embryonic stem cells. *Biomaterials.* 31:1885–1893.

Moon, J.H., J.S. Heo, J.S. Kim, E.K. Jun, J.H. Lee, A. Kim, J. Kim, K.Y. Whang, Y.K. Kang, S. Yeo, H.J. Lim, D.W. Han, D.W. Kim, S. Oh, B.S. Yoon, H.R. Scholer, and S. You. 2011. Reprogramming fibroblasts into induced pluripotent stem cells with Bmi1. *Cell Res.* 21(9):1305–1315.

Morizane, A., D. Doi, T. Kikuchi, K. Nishimura, and J. Takahashi. 2011. Small-molecule inhibitors of bone morphogenic protein and activin/nodal signals promote highly efficient neural induction from human pluripotent stem cells. *J Neurosci Res.* 89:117–126.

Morrell, N.T., P. Leucht, L. Zhao, J.B. Kim, D. ten Berge, K. Ponnusamy, A.L. Carre, H. Dudek, M. Zachlederova, M. McElhaney, S. Brunton, J. Gunzner, M. Callow, P. Polakis, M. Costa, X.M. Zhang, J.A. Helms, and R. Nusse. 2008. Liposomal packaging generates Wnt protein with in vivo biological activity. *PLoS One.* 3:e2930.

Morrison, S.J., and J. Kimble. 2006. Asymmetric and symmetric stem-cell divisions in development and cancer. *Nature.* 441:1068–1074.

Muraca, M. 2011. Evolving concepts in cell therapy of liver disease and current clinical perspectives. *Dig Liver Dis.* 43:180–187.

Murry, C.E., and G. Keller. 2008. Differentiation of embryonic stem cells to clinically relevant populations: lessons from embryonic development. *Cell.* 132:661–680.

Nauth, A., P.V. Giannoudis, T.A. Einhorn, K.D. Hankenson, G.E. Friedlaender, R. Li, and E.H. Schemitsch. 2010. Growth factors: beyond bone morphogenetic proteins. *J Orthop Trauma.* 24:543–546.

Nemeth, M.J., and D.M. Bodine. 2007. Regulation of hematopoiesis and the hematopoietic stem cell niche by Wnt signaling pathways. *Cell Res.* 17:746–758.

Newman, R.E., D. Yoo, M.A. LeRoux, and A. Danilkovitch-Miagkova. 2009. Treatment of inflammatory diseases with mesenchymal stem cells. *Inflamm Allergy Drug Targets.* 8:110–123.

Ninos, J.M., L.C. Jefferies, C.R. Cogle, and W.G. Kerr. 2006. The thrombopoietin receptor, c-Mpl, is a selective surface marker for human hematopoietic stem cells. *J Transl Med.* 4:9.

Nishikawa, S., R.A. Goldstein, and C.R. Nierras. 2008. The promise of human induced pluripotent stem cells for research and therapy. *Nat Rev Mol Cell Biol.* 9:725–729.

Niwa, A., K. Umeda, H. Chang, M. Saito, K. Okita, K. Takahashi, M. Nakagawa, S. Yamanaka, T. Nakahata, and T. Heike. 2009. Orderly hematopoietic development of induced pluripotent stem cells via Flk-1(+) hemoangiogenic progenitors. *J Cell Physiol*. 221:367–377.

Noel, D., D. Gazit, C. Bouquet, F. Apparailly, C. Bony, P. Plence, V. Millet, G. Turgeman, M. Perricaudet, J. Sany, and C. Jorgensen. 2004. Short-term BMP-2 expression is sufficient for in vivo osteochondral differentiation of mesenchymal stem cells. *Stem Cells*. 22:74–85.

Notta, F., S. Doulatov, E. Laurenti, A. Poeppl, I. Jurisica, and J.E. Dick. 2011. Isolation of single human hematopoietic stem cells capable of long-term multilineage engraftment. *Science*. 333:218–221.

Nusse, R. 2008. Wnt signaling and stem cell control. *Cell Res*. 18:523–527.

Odorico, J.S., D.S. Kaufman, and J.A. Thomson. 2001. Multilineage differentiation from human embryonic stem cell lines. *Stem Cells*. 19:193–204.

Okita, K., M. Nakagawa, H. Hyenjong, T. Ichisaka, and S. Yamanaka. 2008. Generation of mouse induced pluripotent stem cells without viral vectors. *Science*. 322:949–953.

Okita, K., and S. Yamanaka. 2011. Induced pluripotent stem cells: opportunities and challenges. *Philos Trans R Soc Lond B Biol Sci*. 366:2198–2207.

Ong, K.L., M.L. Villarraga, E. Lau, L.Y. Carreon, S.M. Kurtz, and S.D. Glassman. 2010. Off-label use of bone morphogenetic proteins in the United States using administrative data. *Spine*. 35:1794–1800.

Osawa, M., K. Hanada, H. Hamada, and H. Nakauchi. 1996. Long-term lymphohematopoietic reconstitution by a single CD34-low/negative hematopoietic stem cell. *Science*. 273:242–245.

Pan, C., B. Lu, H. Chen, and C.E. Bishop. 2010. Reprogramming human fibroblasts using HIV-1 TAT recombinant proteins OCT4, SOX2, KLF4 and c-MYC. *Mol Biol Rep*. 37:2117–2124.

Papini, S., D. Cecchetti, D. Campani, W. Fitzgerald, J.C. Grivel, S. Chen, L. Margolis, and R.P. Revoltella. 2003. Isolation and clonal analysis of human epidermal keratinocyte stem cells in long-term culture. *Stem Cells*. 21:481–494.

Parekkadan, B., and J.M. Milwid. 2010. Mesenchymal stem cells as therapeutics. *Annu Rev Biomed Eng*. 12:87–117.

Parisi, M.J., and H. Lin. 1998. The role of the hedgehog/patched signaling pathway in epithelial stem cell proliferation: from fly to human. *Cell Res*. 8:15–21.

Park, I.H., N. Arora, H. Huo, N. Maherali, T. Ahfeldt, A. Shimamura, M.W. Lensch, C. Cowan, K. Hochedlinger, and G.Q. Daley. 2008. Disease-specific induced pluripotent stem cells. *Cell*. 134:877–886.

Parmar, K., P. Mauch, J.A. Vergilio, R. Sackstein, and J.D. Down. 2007. Distribution of hematopoietic stem cells in the bone marrow according to regional hypoxia. *Proc Natl Acad Sci U S A*. 104:5431–5436.

Patterson, M., D.N. Chan, I. Ha, D. Case, Y. Cui, B.V. Handel, H.K. Mikkola, and W.E. Lowry. 2011. Defining the nature of human pluripotent stem cell progeny. *Cell Res*. 22(1):178–193.

Perrier, A.L., V. Tabar, T. Barberi, M.E. Rubio, J. Bruses, N. Topf, N.L. Harrison, and L. Studer. 2004. Derivation of midbrain dopamine neurons from human embryonic stem cells. *Proc Natl Acad Sci U S A*. 101:12543–12548.

Perry, D. 2000. Patients' voices: the powerful sound in the stem cell debate. *Science*. 287:1423.

Pusic, I., and J.F. DiPersio. 2008. The use of growth factors in hematopoietic stem cell transplantation. *Curr Pharm Des*. 14:1950–1961.

Pusic, I., and J.F. DiPersio. 2010. Update on clinical experience with AMD3100, an SDF-1/CXCL12-CXCR4 inhibitor, in mobilization of hematopoietic stem and progenitor cells. *Curr Opin Hematol.* 17:319–326.

Reddi, A.H. 2001. Interplay between bone morphogenetic proteins and cognate binding proteins in bone and cartilage development: noggin, chordin and DAN. *Arthritis Res.* 3:1–5.

Rider, C.C., and B. Mulloy. 2010. Bone morphogenetic protein and growth differentiation factor cytokine families and their protein antagonists. *Biochem J.* 429:1–12.

Rodriguez, A.M., D. Pisani, C.A. Dechesne, C. Turc-Carel, J.Y. Kurzenne, B. Wdziekonski, A. Villageois, C. Bagnis, J.P. Breittmayer, H. Groux, G. Ailhaud, and C. Dani. 2005. Transplantation of a multipotent cell population from human adipose tissue induces dystrophin expression in the immunocompetent mdx mouse. *J Exp Med.* 201:1397–1405.

Rodriguez-Piza, I., Y. Richaud-Patin, R. Vassena, F. Gonzalez, M.J. Barrero, A. Veiga, A. Raya, and J.C. Belmonte. 2010. Reprogramming of human fibroblasts to induced pluripotent stem cells under xeno-free conditions. *Stem Cells.* 28:36–44.

Rojkind, M., Z. Gatmaitan, S. Mackensen, M.A. Giambrone, P. Ponce, and L.M. Reid. 1980. Connective tissue biomatrix: its isolation and utilization for long-term cultures of normal rat hepatocytes. *J Cell Biol.* 87:255–263.

Rowland, T.J., D.E. Buchholz, and D.O. Clegg. 2011. Pluripotent human stem cells for the treatment of retinal disease. *J Cell Physiol.* 227(2)455–466.

Russo, F.P., and M. Parola. 2011. Stem and progenitor cells in liver regeneration and repair. *Cytotherapy.* 13:135–144.

Sachinidis, A., I. Sotiriadou, B. Seelig, A. Berkessel, and J. Hescheler. 2008. A chemical genetics approach for specific differentiation of stem cells to somatic cells: a new promising therapeutical approach. *Comb Chem High Throughput Screen.* 11:70–82.

Saha, K., and R. Jaenisch. 2009. Technical challenges in using human induced pluripotent stem cells to model disease. *Cell Stem Cell.* 5:584–595.

Said, Z.N. 2011. An overview of occult hepatitis B virus infection. *World J Gastroenterol.* 17:1927–1938.

Sakamoto, S., F. Kojima, M. Igarashi, R. Sawa, M. Umekita, Y. Kubota, K. Nakae, S. Yamaguchi, H. Adachi, Y. Nishimura, and Y. Akamatsu. 2010. Decalpenic acid, a novel small molecule from Penicillium verruculosum CR37010, induces early osteoblastic markers in pluripotent mesenchymal cells. *J Antibiot (Tokyo).* 63:703–708.

Salli, U., A.P. Reddy, N. Salli, N.Z. Lu, H.C. Kuo, F.K. Pau, D.P. Wolf, and C.L. Bethea. 2004. Serotonin neurons derived from rhesus monkey embryonic stem cells: similarities to CNS serotonin neurons. *Exp Neurol.* 188:351–364.

Scadden, D.T. 2006. The stem-cell niche as an entity of action. *Nature.* 441:1075–1079.

Schepers, A.G., R. Vries, M. van den Born, M. van de Wetering, and H. Clevers. 2011. Lgr5 intestinal stem cells have high telomerase activity and randomly segregate their chromosomes. *EMBO J.* 30(6):1104–1109.

Schmelzer, E., and L.M. Reid. 2009. Human telomerase activity, telomerase and telomeric template expression in hepatic stem cells and in livers from fetal and postnatal donors. *Eur J Gastroenterol Hepatol.* 21:1191–1198.

Schmelzer, E., L. Zhang, A. Bruce, E. Wauthier, J. Ludlow, H.L. Yao, N. Moss, A. Melhem, R. McClelland, W. Turner, M. Kulik, S. Sherwood, T. Tallheden, N. Cheng, M.E. Furth, and L.M. Reid. 2007. Human hepatic stem cells from fetal and postnatal donors. *J Exp Med.* 204:1973–1987.

Schwartz, R.E., J.L. Linehan, M.S. Painschab, W.S. Hu, C.M. Verfaillie, and D.S. Kaufman. 2005. Defined conditions for development of functional hepatic cells from human embryonic stem cells. *Stem Cells Dev.* 14:643–655.

Seibler, P., J. Graziotto, H. Jeong, F. Simunovic, C. Klein, and D. Krainc. 2011. Mitochondrial Parkin recruitment is impaired in neurons derived from mutant PINK1 induced pluripotent stem cells. *J Neurosci.* 31:5970–5976.

Seita, J., and I.L. Weissman. 2010. Hematopoietic stem cell: self-renewal versus differentiation. *Wiley Interdiscip Rev Syst Biol Med.* 2:640–653.

Sell, S. 2004. Stem cell origin of cancer and differentiation therapy. *Crit Rev Oncol Hematol.* 51:1–28.

Shamblott, M.J., J. Axelman, S. Wang, E.M. Bugg, J.W. Littlefield, P.J. Donovan, P.D. Blumenthal, G.R. Huggins, and J.D. Gearhart. 1998. Derivation of pluripotent stem cells from cultured human primordial germ cells. *Proc Natl Acad Sci U S A.* 95:13726–13731.

Shi, Y., C. Desponts, J.T. Do, H.S. Hahm, H.R. Scholer, and S. Ding. 2008. Induction of pluripotent stem cells from mouse embryonic fibroblasts by Oct4 and Klf4 with small-molecule compounds. *Cell Stem Cell.* 3:568–574.

Shupe, T., and B.E. Petersen. 2011. Potential applications for cell regulatory factors in liver progenitor cell therapy. *Int J Biochem Cell Biol.* 43:214–221.

Sicklick, J.K., Y.X. Li, A. Melhem, E. Schmelzer, M. Zdanowicz, J. Huang, M. Caballero, J.H. Fair, J.W. Ludlow, R.E. McClelland, L.M. Reid, and A.M. Diehl. 2006. Hedgehog signaling maintains resident hepatic progenitors throughout life. *Am J Physiol Gastrointest Liver Physiol.* 290:859–870.

Simons, B.D., and H. Clevers. 2011. Strategies for homeostatic stem cell self-renewal in adult tissues. *Cell.* 145:851–862.

Simsek, T., F. Kocabas, J. Zheng, R.J. Deberardinis, A.I. Mahmoud, E.N. Olson, J.W. Schneider, C.C. Zhang, and H.A. Sadek. 2010. The distinct metabolic profile of hematopoietic stem cells reflects their location in a hypoxic niche. *Cell Stem Cell.* 7:380–390.

Singh, A., and R.J. Morris. 2010. The Yin and Yang of bone morphogenetic proteins in cancer. *Cytokine Growth Factor Rev.* 21:299–313.

Sinha, S., and J.K. Chen. 2006. Purmorphamine activates the Hedgehog pathway by targeting Smoothened. *Nat Chem Biol.* 2:29–30.

Sizonenko, S.V., N. Bednarek, and P. Gressens. 2007. Growth factors and plasticity. *Semin Fetal Neonatal Med.* 12:241–249.

Skottman, H., S. Narkilahti, and O. Hovatta. 2007. Challenges and approaches to the culture of pluripotent human embryonic stem cells. *Regen Med.* 2:265–273.

Smith, M.A., E.L. Court, and J.G. Smith. 2001. Stem cell factor: laboratory and clinical aspects. *Blood Rev.* 15:191–197.

Snyder, J.C., R.M. Teisanu, and B.R. Stripp. 2009. Endogenous lung stem cells and contribution to disease. *J Pathol.* 217:254–264.

Soldner, F., D. Hockemeyer, C. Beard, Q. Gao, G.W. Bell, E.G. Cook, G. Hargus, A. Blak, O. Cooper, M. Mitalipova, O. Isacson, and R. Jaenisch. 2009. Parkinson's disease patient-derived induced pluripotent stem cells free of viral reprogramming factors. *Cell.* 136:964–977.

Solter, D. 2006. From teratocarcinomas to embryonic stem cells and beyond: a history of embryonic stem cell research. *Nat Rev Genet.* 7:319–327.

Soundararajan, P., G.B. Miles, L.L. Rubin, R.M. Brownstone, and V.F. Rafuse. 2006. Motoneurons derived from embryonic stem cells express transcription factors and develop phenotypes characteristic of medial motor column neurons. *J Neurosci.* 26:3256–3268.

Spalding, K.L., R.D. Bhardwaj, B.A. Buchholz, H. Druid, and J. Frisen. 2005. Retrospective birth dating of cells in humans. *Cell.* 122:133–143.

Stachelscheid, H., T. Urbaniak, A. Ring, B. Spengler, J.C. Gerlach, and K. Zeilinger. 2009. Isolation and characterization of adult human liver progenitors from ischemic liver tissue derived from therapeutic hepatectomies. *Tissue Eng Part A*. 15:1633–1643.

Stadtfeld, M., E. Apostolou, H. Akutsu, A. Fukuda, P. Follett, S. Natesan, T. Kono, T. Shioda, and K. Hochedlinger. 2010. Aberrant silencing of imprinted genes on chromosome 12qF1 in mouse induced pluripotent stem cells. *Nature*. 465:175–181.

Staerk, J., M.M. Dawlaty, Q. Gao, D. Maetzel, J. Hanna, C.A. Sommer, G. Mostoslavsky, and R. Jaenisch. 2010. Reprogramming of human peripheral blood cells to induced pluripotent stem cells. *Cell Stem Cell*. 7:20–24.

Strauss, S. 2010. Geron trial resumes, but standards for stem cell trials remain elusive. *Nat Biotechnol*. 28:989–990.

Studer, L., M. Csete, S.H. Lee, N. Kabbani, J. Walikonis, B. Wold, and R. McKay. 2000. Enhanced proliferation, survival, and dopaminergic differentiation of CNS precursors in lowered oxygen. *J Neurosci*. 20:7377–7383.

Sullivan, G.J., D.C. Hay, I.H. Park, J. Fletcher, Z. Hannoun, C.M. Payne, D. Dalgetty, J.R. Black, J.A. Ross, K. Samuel, G. Wang, G.Q. Daley, J.H. Lee, G.M. Church, S.J. Forbes, J.P. Iredale, and I. Wilmut. 2010. Generation of functional human hepatic endoderm from human induced pluripotent stem cells. *Hepatology*. 51:329–335.

Suzuki, T., Y. Yokoyama, K. Kumano, M. Takanashi, S. Kozuma, T. Takato, T. Nakahata, M. Nishikawa, S. Sakano, M. Kurokawa, S. Ogawa, and S. Chiba. 2006. Highly efficient ex vivo expansion of human hematopoietic stem cells using Delta1-Fc chimeric protein. *Stem Cells*. 24:2456–2465.

Swiontkowski, M.F., H.T. Aro, S. Donell, J.L. Esterhai, J. Goulet, A. Jones, P.J. Kregor, L. Nordsletten, G. Paiement, and A. Patel. 2006. Recombinant human bone morphogenetic protein-2 in open tibial fractures. A subgroup analysis of data combined from two prospective randomized studies. *J Bone Joint Surg*. 88:1258–1265.

Takahashi, K., and S. Yamanaka. 2006. Induction of pluripotent stem cells from mouse embryonic and adult fibroblast cultures by defined factors. *Cell*. 126:663–676.

Takubo, K., N. Goda, W. Yamada, H. Iriuchishima, E. Ikeda, Y. Kubota, H. Shima, R.S. Johnson, A. Hirao, M. Suematsu, and T. Suda. 2010. Regulation of the HIF-1alpha level is essential for hematopoietic stem cells. *Cell Stem Cell*. 7:391–402.

Tanaka, M., T. Itoh, N. Tanimizu, and A. Miyajima. 2011. Liver stem/progenitor cells: their characteristics and regulatory mechanisms. *J Biochem*. 149:231–239.

Tat, P.A., H. Sumer, K.L. Jones, K. Upton, and P.J. Verma. 2010. The efficient generation of induced pluripotent stem (iPS) cells from adult mouse adipose tissue-derived and neural stem cells. *Cell Transplant*. 19:525–536.

Taylor, B.L., and I.B. Zhulin. 1999. PAS domains: internal sensors of oxygen, redox potential, and light. *Microbiol Mol Biol Rev*. 63:479–506.

Taylor, C.J., E.M. Bolton, S. Pocock, L.D. Sharples, R.A. Pedersen, and J.A. Bradley. 2005. Banking on human embryonic stem cells: estimating the number of donor cell lines needed for HLA matching. *Lancet*. 366:2019–2025.

Thawani, J.P., A.C. Wang, K.D. Than, C.Y. Lin, F. La Marca, and P. Park. 2010. Bone morphogenetic proteins and cancer: review of the literature. *Neurosurgery*. 66:233–246; discussion 246.

Theise, N.D., R. Saxena, B.C. Portmann, S.N. Thung, H. Yee, L. Chiriboga, A. Kumar, and J.M. Crawford. 1999. The canals of Hering and hepatic stem cells in humans. *Hepatology*. 30:1425–1433.

Theunissen, T.W., A.L. van Oosten, G. Castelo-Branco, J. Hall, A. Smith, and J.C. Silva. 2011. Nanog overcomes reprogramming barriers and induces pluripotency in minimal conditions. *Curr Biol*. 21:65–71.

Thomas, E., R. Storb, R.A. Clift, A. Fefer, F.L. Johnson, P.E. Neiman, K.G. Lerner, H. Glucksberg, and C.D. Buckner. 1975a. Bone-marrow transplantation (first of two parts). *N Engl J Med*. 292:832–843.

Thomas, E.D., R. Storb, R.A. Clift, A. Fefer, L. Johnson, P.E. Neiman, K.G. Lerner, H. Glucksberg, and C.D. Buckner. 1975b. Bone-marrow transplantation (second of two parts). *N Engl J Med*. 292:895–902.

Thomson, J.A., J. Itskovitz-Eldor, S.S. Shapiro, M.A. Waknitz, J.J. Swiergiel, V.S. Marshall, and J.M. Jones. 1998. Embryonic stem cell lines derived from human blastocysts. *Science*. 282:1145–1147.

Timmermans, F., I. Velghe, L. Vanwalleghem, M. De Smedt, S. Van Coppernolle, T. Taghon, H.D. Moore, G. Leclercq, A.W. Langerak, T. Kerre, J. Plum, and B. Vandekerckhove. 2009. Generation of T cells from human embryonic stem cell-derived hematopoietic zones. *J Immunol*. 182:6879–6888.

Tovari, J., R. Pirker, J. Timar, G. Ostoros, G. Kovacs, and B. Dome. 2008. Erythropoietin in cancer: an update. *Curr Mol Med*. 8:481–491.

Trounson, A. 2006. The production and directed differentiation of human embryonic stem cells. *Endocr Rev*. 27:208–219.

Tsai, P.T., J.J. Ohab, N. Kertesz, M. Groszer, C. Matter, J. Gao, X. Liu, H. Wu, and S.T. Carmichael. 2006. A critical role of erythropoietin receptor in neurogenesis and post-stroke recovery. *J Neurosci*. 26:1269–1274.

Turner, R., O. Lozoya, Y. Wang, V. Cardinale, E. Gaudio, G. Alpini, G. Mendel, E. Wauthier, C. Barbier, D. Alvaro, and L.M. Reid. 2011. Human hepatic stem cell and maturational liver lineage biology. *Hepatology*. 53:1035–1045.

Unger, C., H. Skottman, P. Blomberg, M.S. Dilber, and O. Hovatta. 2008. Good manufacturing practice and clinical-grade human embryonic stem cell lines. *Hum Mol Genet*. 17:R48–53.

Untergasser, G., R. Koeck, D. Wolf, H. Rumpold, H. Ott, P. Debbage, C. Koppelstaetter, and E. Gunsilius. 2006. CD34+/CD133- circulating endothelial precursor cells (CEP): characterization, senescence and in vivo application. *Exp Gerontol*. 41:600–608.

Unternaehrer, J.J., and G.Q. Daley. 2011. Induced pluripotent stem cells for modelling human diseases. *Philos Trans R Soc Lond B Biol Sci*. 366:2274–2285.

Uygun, B.E., N. Sharma, and M. Yarmush. 2009. Retinal pigment epithelium differentiation of stem cells: current status and challenges. *Crit Rev Biomed Eng*. 37:355–375.

Vadhan-Raj, S. 1994. PIXY321 (GM-CSF/IL-3 fusion protein): biology and early clinical development. *Stem Cells*. 12:253–261.

Van Hoof, D., K.A. D'Amour, and M.S. German. 2009. Derivation of insulin-producing cells from human embryonic stem cells. *Stem Cell Res*. 3:73–87.

Veiby, O.P., A.A. Mikhail, and H.R. Snodgrass. 1997. Growth factors and hematopoietic stem cells. *Hematology/oncology clinics of North America*. 11:1173-1184.

Verstappen, J., C. Katsaros, R. Torensma, and J.W. Von den Hoff. 2009. A functional model for adult stem cells in epithelial tissues. *Wound Repair Regen*. 17:296–305.

Vierbuchen, T., A. Ostermeier, Z.P. Pang, Y. Kokubu, T.C. Sudhof, and M. Wernig. 2010. Direct conversion of fibroblasts to functional neurons by defined factors. *Nature*. 463:1035–1041.

Vitellaro-Zuccarello, L., S. Mazzetti, L. Madaschi, P. Bosisio, A. Gorio, and S. De Biasi. 2007. Erythropoietin-mediated preservation of the white matter in rat spinal cord injury. *Neuroscience*. 144:865–877.

Vodyanik, M.A., J.A. Bork, J.A. Thomson, and I.I. Slukvin. 2005. Human embryonic stem cell-derived CD34+ cells: efficient production in the coculture with OP9 stromal cells and analysis of lymphohematopoietic potential. *Blood*. 105:617–626.

Volkers, N. 1999. Colony-stimulating factors stimulate some treatments, continue to evolve. *J Natl Cancer Inst*. 91:210–212.

Wagner, J.E., C. Brunstein, W. Tse, and M. Laughlin. 2009. Umbilical cord blood transplantation. *Cancer Treat Res*. 144:233–255.

Walker, J. 2010. Disease in a dish: a new approach to drug discovery. *Regen Med.* 5:505–507.

Wang, A., K. Huang, Y. Shen, Z. Xue, C. Cai, S. Horvath, and G. Fan. 2011a. Functional modules distinguish human induced pluripotent stem cells from embryonic stem cells. *Stem Cells Dev.* 20:1937–1950.

Wang, Q., C. Huang, F. Zeng, M. Xue, and X. Zhang. 2010a. Activation of the Hh pathway in periosteum-derived mesenchymal stem cells induces bone formation in vivo: implication for postnatal bone repair. *Am J Pathol.* 177:3100–3111.

Wang, Q., X. Xu, J. Li, J. Liu, H. Gu, R. Zhang, J. Chen, Y. Kuang, J. Fei, C. Jiang, P. Wang, D. Pei, S. Ding, and X. Xie. 2011b. Lithium, an anti-psychotic drug, greatly enhances the generation of induced pluripotent stem cells. *Cell Res.* 21:1424–1435.

Wang, Y., C.B. Cui, M. Yamauchi, P. Miguez, M. Roach, R. Malavarca, M.J. Costello, V. Cardinale, E. Wauthier, C. Barbier, D.A. Gerber, D. Alvaro, and L.M. Reid. 2011c. Lineage restriction of human hepatic stem cells to mature fates is made efficient by tissue-specific biomatrix scaffolds. *Hepatology.* 53:293–305.

Wang, Y., J. Kellner, L. Liu, and D. Zhou. 2011d. Inhibition of p38 mitogen-activated protein kinase promotes ex vivo hematopoietic stem cell expansion. *Stem Cells Dev.* 20:1143–1152.

Wang, Y., H.-L. Yao, E. Wauthier, C. Barbier, M. Costello, N. Moss, M. Yamauchi, M. Sricholpech, C.-B. Cui, D. Gerber, E. Loboa, and L. Reid. 2010b. Paracrine signals from mesenchymal cell populations govern the expansion and differentiation of human hepatic stem cells to adult liver fates. *Hepatology.* 52:1443–1454.

Wang, Y., M. Yao, C. Zhou, D. Dong, Y. Jiang, G. Wei, and X. Cui. 2010c. Erythropoietin promotes spinal cord-derived neural progenitor cell proliferation by regulating cell cycle. *Neuroscience.* 167:750–757.

Warren, L., P.D. Manos, T. Ahfeldt, Y.H. Loh, H. Li, F. Lau, W. Ebina, P.K. Mandal, Z.D. Smith, A. Meissner, G.Q. Daley, A.S. Brack, J.J. Collins, C. Cowan, T.M. Schlaeger, and D.J. Rossi. 2010. Highly efficient reprogramming to pluripotency and directed differentiation of human cells with synthetic modified mRNA. *Cell Stem Cell.* 7:618–630.

Wauthier, E., E. Schmelzer, W. Turner, L. Zhang, E. LeCluyse, J. Ruiz, R. Turner, M.E. Furth, H. Kubota, O. Lozoya, C. Barbier, R. McClelland, H.L. Yao, N. Moss, A. Bruce, J. Ludlow, and L.M. Reid. 2008. Hepatic stem cells and hepatoblasts: identification, isolation, and ex vivo maintenance. *Methods Cell Biol.* 86:137–225.

Weissman, I.L., D.J. Anderson, and F. Gage. 2001. Stem and progenitor cells: origins, phenotypes, lineage commitments, and transdifferentiations. *Annu Rev Cell Dev Biol.* 17:387–403.

Willert, K., J.D. Brown, E. Danenberg, A.W. Duncan, I.L. Weissman, T. Reya, J.R. Yates, 3rd, and R. Nusse. 2003. Wnt proteins are lipid-modified and can act as stem cell growth factors. *Nature.* 423:448–452.

Wu, X., S. Ding, Q. Ding, N.S. Gray, and P.G. Schultz. 2002. A small molecule with osteogenesis-inducing activity in multipotent mesenchymal progenitor cells. *J Am Chem Soc.* 124:14520–14521.

Wu, X., J. Walker, J. Zhang, S. Ding, and P.G. Schultz. 2004. Purmorphamine induces osteogenesis by activation of the hedgehog signaling pathway. *Chem Biol.* 11:1229–1238.

Xi, B., N. Yu, X. Wang, X. Xu, and Y.A. Abassi. 2008. The application of cell-based label-free technology in drug discovery. *Biotechnol J.* 3:484–495.

Xu, X., J. D'Hoker, G. Stange, S. Bonne, N. De Leu, X. Xiao, M. Van de Casteele, G. Mellitzer, Z. Ling, D. Pipeleers, L. Bouwens, R. Scharfmann, G. Gradwohl, and H. Heimberg. 2008a. Beta cells can be generated from endogenous progenitors in injured adult mouse pancreas. *Cell.* 132:197–207.

Xu, Y., Y. Shi, and S. Ding. 2008b. A chemical approach to stem-cell biology and regenerative medicine. *Nature*. 453:338–344.

Xu, Y., X. Zhu, H.S. Hahm, W. Wei, E. Hao, A. Hayek, and S. Ding. 2010. Revealing a core signaling regulatory mechanism for pluripotent stem cell survival and self-renewal by small molecules. *Proc Natl Acad Sci USA* 107:8129–8134.

Xue, J., J. Peng, M. Yuan, A. Wang, L. Zhang, S. Liu, M. Fan, Y. Wang, W. Xu, K. Ting, X. Zhang, and S. Lu. 2011. NELL1 promotes high-quality bone regeneration in rat femoral distraction osteogenesis model. *Bone*. 48:485–495.

Yamazaki, S., and H. Nakauchi. 2009. Insights into signaling and function of hematopoietic stem cells at the single-cell level. *Curr Opin Hematol*. 16:255–258.

Yazawa, M., B. Hsueh, X. Jia, A.M. Pasca, J.A. Bernstein, J. Hallmayer, and R.E. Dolmetsch. 2011. Using induced pluripotent stem cells to investigate cardiac phenotypes in Timothy syndrome. *Nature*. 471:230–234.

Yu, J., K. Hu, K. Smuga-Otto, S. Tian, R. Stewart, I.I. Slukvin, and J.A. Thomson. 2009. Human induced pluripotent stem cells free of vector and transgene sequences. *Science*. 324:797–801.

Yu, J., M.A. Vodyanik, K. Smuga-Otto, J. Antosiewicz-Bourget, J.L. Frane, S. Tian, J. Nie, G.A. Jonsdottir, V. Ruotti, R. Stewart, I.I. Slukvin, and J.A. Thomson. 2007. Induced pluripotent stem cell lines derived from human somatic cells. *Science*. 318:1917–1920.

Yuan, X., W. Li, and S. Ding. 2011a. Small molecules in cellular reprogramming and differentiation. *Prog Drug Res*. 67:253–266.

Yuan, X., H. Wan, X. Zhao, S. Zhu, Q. Zhou, and S. Ding. 2011b. Combined chemical treatment enables Oct4-induced reprogramming from mouse embryonic fibroblasts. *Stem Cells*. 29:549–553.

Zandstra, P.W., C. Bauwens, T. Yin, Q. Liu, H. Schiller, R. Zweigerdt, K.B. Pasumarthi, and L.J. Field. 2003. Scalable production of embryonic stem cell-derived cardiomyocytes. *Tissue Eng*. 9:767–778.

Zeng, S., J. Chen, and H. Shen. 2010. Controlling of bone morphogenetic protein signaling. *Cell Signal*. 22:888–893.

Zhang, C.C., M. Kaba, S. Iizuka, H. Huynh, and H.F. Lodish. 2008a. Angiopoietin-like 5 and IGFBP2 stimulate ex vivo expansion of human cord blood hematopoietic stem cells as assayed by NOD/SCID transplantation. *Blood*. 111:3415–3423.

Zhang, C.C., and H.F. Lodish. 2008. Cytokines regulating hematopoietic stem cell function. *Curr Opin Hematol*. 15:307–311.

Zhang, D., W. Jiang, M. Liu, X. Sui, X. Yin, S. Chen, Y. Shi, and H. Deng. 2009a. Highly efficient differentiation of human ES cells and iPS cells into mature pancreatic insulin-producing cells. *Cell Res*. 19:429–438.

Zhang, J., G.F. Wilson, A.G. Soerens, C.H. Koonce, J. Yu, S.P. Palecek, J.A. Thomson, and T.J. Kamp. 2009b. Functional cardiomyocytes derived from human induced pluripotent stem cells. *Circ Res*. 104:e30–41.

Zhang, L., N. Theise, M. Chua, and L.M. Reid. 2008b. The stem cell niche of human livers: symmetry between development and regeneration. *Hepatology*. 48:1598–1607.

Zhang, X.Z. 2010. Modulation of embryonic stem cell fate and somatic cell reprogramming by small molecules. *Reprod Biomed Online*. 21:26–36.

Zhao, D., S. Chen, J. Cai, Y. Guo, Z. Song, J. Che, C. Liu, C. Wu, M. Ding, and H. Deng. 2009. Derivation and characterization of hepatic progenitor cells from human embryonic stem cells. *PLoS One*. 4:e6468.

Zhao, T., Z.N. Zhang, Z. Rong, and Y. Xu. 2011. Immunogenicity of induced pluripotent stem cells. *Nature*. 474:212–215.

Zhou, H., and S. Ding. 2010. Evolution of induced pluripotent stem cell technology. *Curr Opin Hematol*. 17:276–280.

Zhu, H., M.W. Lensch, P. Cahan, and G.Q. Daley. 2011. Investigating monogenic and complex diseases with pluripotent stem cells. *Nat Rev Genet.* 12:266–275.

Zock, J.M. 2009. Applications of high content screening in life science research. *Comb Chem High Throughput Screen.* 12:870–876.

Zorn, A.M., and J.M. Wells. 2007. Molecular basis of vertebrate endoderm development. *Int Rev Cytol.* 259:49–111.

6

Micro- and Nanoscale Delivery of Therapeutic Agents for Regenerative Therapy

JUSTIN M. SAUL AND BENJAMIN S. HARRISON

Micro- and nanotechnology are heavily studied for applications ranging from renewable energy to textiles to the petrochemical industry. Within the context of regenerative medicine, micro- and nanotechnology have received attention primarily as a means to achieve the delivery or release of therapeutic agents. Micro- and nano-delivery systems provide the opportunity to regulate the dose, timing, and location of delivery. Furthermore, such systems can be used in combination with imaging modalities such as quantum dots and other nanoscale technologies to allow real-time monitoring of physiological responses to release compounds or other regenerative processes. This ability to monitor physiological responses through imaging or other noninvasive modalities will be essential as these technologies are translated from preclinical animal models to human clinical patients in whom histologic analysis cannot be used. Throughout this chapter, the term "nano" carriers is used to refer to carriers with diameters of less than 200 nm. Although the term "nano" typically refers to substances of 100 nm or smaller, the size of 200 nm is useful for these discussions because of important physiological capabilities of these sized carriers such as the ability to leave the vasculature or to be internalized by cells. "Microcarriers" is used to refer to carriers larger than 1 μm in diameter, and a gray area between 200 nm and 1 μm will be assumed in which some of the generalizations about nano- and microcarriers may not fully apply. In this chapter, we consider the applications of micro- and nanotechnology within regenerative medicine, describing the principles governing their behavior and application as well as ongoing challenges.

Need for Controlled Release Systems in Regenerative Medicine

The use of controlled-release technology has several clinical, scientific, and industrial advantages. From the clinical perspective, patient compliance with drug dosing regimens is a major challenge. This can impact both safety and efficacy of drugs because maintaining plasma levels within the therapeutic window is problematic.

127

Scientifically, controlled release systems offer the potential to alter biodistribution and pharmacokinetic profiles to improve the safety and efficacy of the drugs. From an industrial perspective, these improvements can provide market leverage for a particular compound. Furthermore, interest in controlled-release systems has taken on increased importance in the era of long drug development pipelines as a means to extend the patent lifetimes of novel compounds [1].

Although similar in nature to delivery of classical pharmaceutical drug compounds, the application of controlled-release systems to regenerative medicine applications faces several hurdles, some of which are unique to this field. The primary compounds to be delivered for most regenerative applications are biologic molecules such as peptides, growth factors and other proteins, glycoproteins, and nucleic acids. Delivered systemically, the rates of clearance of these molecules are typically rapid and the biodistribution unfavorable. For example, growth factors are considerably larger in size than traditional pharmaceutics and are typically cleared from the body on the order of minutes, often through the liver [2,3]. In addition, biologically active therapeutic molecules are susceptible to degradative processes such as hydrolysis and enzymatic digestion. This combination of rapid clearance and degradation leads to poor bioactivity when delivered intravenously because of a lack of rapid localization to a site of action. Delivery of nucleic acids is even more complicated because these molecules have to be delivered not only to the cells of interest (e.g., damaged, injured, or diseased cells) but also to the nucleus – the subcellular site of action. Short half-lives and effective delivery to the site of action are significant challenges because of the high production costs associated with the manufacture of growth factors and nucleic acids. Because of these challenges of systemic delivery, current clinical and preclinical examples seeking delivery of therapeutic agents for regenerative purposes rely on release of the agent from local delivery through means such as implantable biomaterial scaffolds. After release from the local implant or delivery to the cell, however, subcellular aspects of delivery remain the same as for systemically delivered agents.

An understanding of the principles guiding delivery of therapeutic agents as well as knowledge of the capabilities of this technology is important for understanding their potential to impact the field. Although both rapid and slow release of therapeutics are possible with current delivery systems, in this chapter, we focus on the ability to achieve sustained release of drugs in the case of local delivery systems and in achieving the localization of agents to their sites of action when delivered systemically.

The vast majority of controlled release delivery systems are polymer or lipid based and typically self-assemble into structures at the nano- and micro-scales. These will therefore be focused upon here. These systems play important roles in (1) protecting the molecules from rapid degradation and clearance; (2) promoting increased uptake at the tissue, cellular, and subcellular site(s) of action; and (3) altering the biodistribution of molecules therapeutics to improve efficacy and minimize systemic side effects. Systemic delivery is clinically useful because it allows repeated administration of a therapeutic at the discretion of the physician. However, polymer and lipid-based encapsulation of therapeutics are also important concepts for local delivery, whether by direct injection or as part of an implantable scaffold. The use of micro- and nano-delivery systems provides the ability to achieve prolonged release of biologic compounds at the site of action in doses that promote functional utility of the molecule. We consider challenges to both systemic and local delivery in more depth below.

Systemic Delivery Systems

The concept of using particulate delivery systems might be traced to the concept of Ehrlich's "magic bullet" postulate more than 100 years ago [4,5], suggesting that drugs could go directly to an intended cellular target. Although Ehrlich conceived of chemotherapy drugs that specifically killed tumor cells, modifications to particulate delivery systems have the capability of achieving high levels of selectivity for cells, thereby eliciting a similar effect. As mentioned earlier, the application of systemic delivery of therapeutic agents is a challenge in the field of regenerative medicine because of the unique nature of engineered tissues including irregular vasculature and lymph drainage. To date, the vast majority of research for the application of systemic particulate carriers is related to delivery of chemical and biologic agents for the treatment of diseases such as cancer. Table 6-1 highlights a select few broad categories of particulate carrier systems that are important for systemic delivery applications.

Polymeric modifications to peptides and drug molecules have proven effective in enhancing circulation time and efficacy of these therapeutics [6]. For example, the covalent attachment of polyethylene glycol (PEG) to therapeutic polypeptides such as adenosine deaminase, asparaginase, and interferon-alpha derived from bovine or bacterial sources provides improved pharmacokinetic profiles of these compounds without loss of bioactivity, providing modalities for the clinical treatment of severe combined immunodeficiency disease, leukemia, and chronic hepatitis C infection, respectively [7–9]. Although the principles of polymer technology such as PEG are important for improving circulation half-lives, the focus of this section is on particulate delivery systems that can entrap *multiple* therapeutic molecules (small drugs, polypeptides, or nucleic acids) for the delivery of a larger "payload" to the site of action. As described later, the incorporation of PEG or similar polymeric agents is also applicable and, in fact, very important to delivery of particulate delivery systems for several reasons as well.

Figure 6-1 schematically highlights the hurdles that agents must overcome when delivered systemically with particulate carrier systems. First, they must be transported to the tissue of interest via the vasculature and then extravasate at this location. They must then diffuse through the tissue to, ideally, reach all of the cells requiring the therapeutic agent. These therapeutic agents may require delivery to specific cells, intracellular delivery, and even delivery to subcellular organelles (e.g., the nucleus in the case of DNA delivery). Thus, micro- and nanoscale carriers require vascular, tissue, cellular, and subcellular levels of localization to achieve physiological effect.

Table 6-1. *Description of select particulate micro- and nanocarrier systems*

Type	Description	Applications	References
Liposomes	Self-assembling lipid bilayer vesicles with aqueous core. ~50–200 nm diameter. Common components include phosphocholine (for bilayer) and cholesterol (for bilayer stability).	Chemotherapy, antibiotic and antifungal delivery, and protein delivery	[10–12]
Cationic lipid vectors (e.g., cationic liposomes)	Similar to liposomes, but containing cationic lipids (e.g., DOTAP) or other cationic molecules (e.g., protamine). May not consist of inner aqueous core and may form complex structures with anionic molecules such as DNA.	Nucleic acid delivery	[13–16]
Lipid micelles	Lipid-based systems similar to liposomes but typically with a high density of hydrophilic surface groups leading to a hydrophobic core rather than an aqueous core. Diameters ~10–50 nm.	Chemotherapy, nucleic acid delivery, and protein delivery	[17,18]
Dendrimers	Branched or hyperbranched polymer systems. Size (hydrodynamic diameter) depends on the number of generations but is in the range of several nanometers to about 25 nm.	Chemotherapy, nucleic acid delivery, and imaging	[19–22]
Polymeric micelles	Polymers often in a diblock configuration that allows for self-assembly often with a hydrophobic core and hydrophilic corona, allowing encapsulation of hydrophilic therapeutics. Size (hydrodynamic diameter) varies greatly depending on polymers used but is typically ~30–200 nm.	Chemotherapy, nucleic acid delivery, and protein delivery	[23–26]

Type	Description	Applications	References
Polyplexes	Cationic polymers (e.g., polyethylenimine) complexed with anionic agents such as DNA. Diameter ~50–200 nm.	Nucleic acid and protein and vaccine delivery	[27–29]
Polymersomes	Vesicles formed from diblock polymers that consist of an aqueous core. Diameters are variable from ~tens of nanometers to 1 micron or larger diameter.	Protein delivery, nucleic acid delivery, imaging	[30–33]
Quantum dots	Not typically used as a delivery system but an increasingly useful system for imaging that may be compatible with delivery of therapeutics. Semiconductor crystal fluorophores with tunable emission spectra. Emission spectra depends in part on particle diameter, but diameters of several nanometers to tens of nanometers are common.	Imaging, cell tracking, and subcellular localization imaging	[34–37]
Polymeric microparticles	Single or co-polymer systems formed by numerous techniques. Particle diameters may be anywhere from several microns to several hundred microns depending on polymers and preparation methods.	Small molecule drugs, nucleic acid, and protein and growth factor delivery	[38–40]
Microbubbles	Lipid-based vesicles containing a gaseous core useful for ultrasonic imaging. Diameters are typically on the order of tens of microns.	Imaging and chemotherapy	[41–43]

DOTAP = N-[1-(2,3-dioleoyloxy)-propyl]-N,N,N-trimethylammonium methyl sulfate.

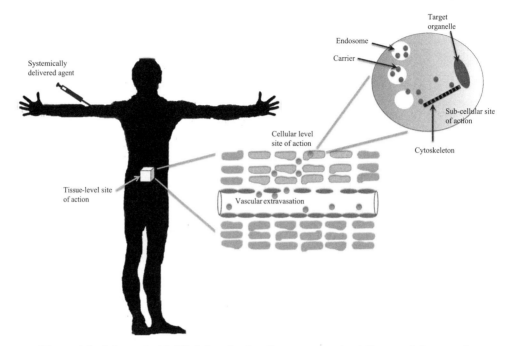

Figure 6-1. Schematic highlighting the hurdles to systemic delivery of therapeutic agents with micro- or nano-scale particulate carriers. These carriers are often delivered intravenously. They reach all areas of the body, including the intended tissue-level site of action, via the bloodstream. To reach the tissue, the carriers must extravasate from the vasculature. In tumors, this occurs by the enhanced permeation retention effect or "leaky vasculature." Vascular disruption may be required to allow extravasation to occur, and nanocarriers much more readily extravasate than microcarriers. Ideally, the carriers will localize to specific cells to which the therapeutic is being delivered (*gray cells*) while sparing off-target cells (*green cells*). Several mechanisms exist to achieve cellular uptake, including the use of targeting ligands. After cellular uptake, the carriers or their payload (or both) must reach the subcellular site of action. This often requires achieving escape from the endosome, after which the carrier may traffic to the target organelle (e.g., the nucleus) via actin or other cytoskeletal components. (See color plate 11.)

Although a challenge for regenerative medicine, much has been learned about the ability to overcome these hurdles for the treatment of solid tumors. Furthermore, these underlying principles present design criteria for delivery in regenerative applications. In the following sections, the current strategies and challenges to delivery of therapeutics are discussed. The four areas that are addressed are:

- vascular-level delivery
- tissue-level delivery
- cellular-level delivery
- sub-cellular localization

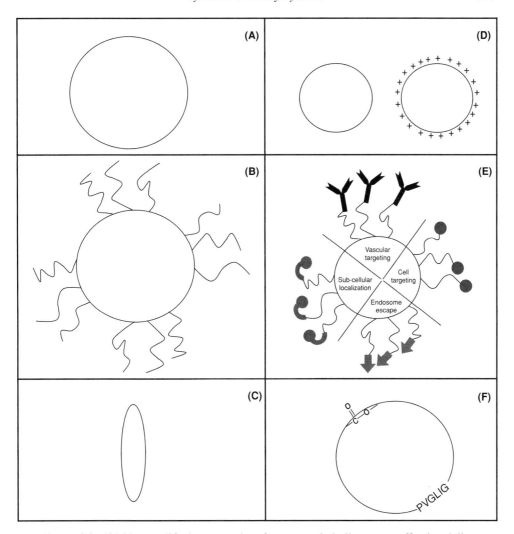

Figure 6-2. (**A**) Nonmodified nanocarriers face several challenges to effective delivery, including rapid clearance, low diffusion, poor cellular entry, and lack of subcellular localization. Strategies to improve the characteristics of nanocarriers include the following: (**B**) Incorporation of hydrophilic molecules such as polyethylene glycol to improve circulation time. (**C**) Modification of the particle shape to improve extravasation or cellular uptake. (**D**) Alteration of surface charge to alter extravasation or cellular uptake. (**E**) Incorporation of ligands to achieve vascular binding, cellular uptake through endocytosis, endosomal escape, or subcellular localization. (**F**) Modification with sequences to allow particle degradation by low pH environments or enzymatic degradation.

Figure 6-2 highlights modifications to nanocarrier systems that are being used or investigated as means to overcome these hurdles; these modifications are described in more depth later.

Vascular-Level Delivery

Unlike traditional chemotherapy drugs that can reach their site of action primarily through diffusion, nano- and microcarriers are generally too large to diffuse to a site of action. Microcarriers are, in fact, restricted to the vascular compartment because they are too large to leave the vasculature (extravasate). These systems are cleared rapidly, typically on a first pass through the liver because of size and the adsorption of opsonin proteins of the complement system.

A large number of microcarrier systems are under investigation that are composed of both natural and synthetic polymers, as highlighted in Table 6-2. Not all of these systems are used or suitable for systemic delivery but are provided as a reference because of their utility for local release (see later discussion). Two examples of microparticles under investigation for therapeutic delivery at the systemic level are synthetic polymer microparticles and lipid microbubbles.

Microparticles fabricated in the 10- to 50-μm diameter range are able to mimic the rolling and adhesion behavior of leukocytes. The surfaces of these microparticles can be modified to present ligands that provide a high degree of selectivity to cell surface receptors. Examples include monoclonal antibodies, proteins (e.g., cell adhesion molecules), and carbohydrates. Because of their size, microparticles have sufficient drag and sedimentation characteristics to contact the surface of the endothelium, thereby allowing adhesion events with surface ligands. An important example of this behavior is the modification of these systems with Sialyl Lewis^x and an antibody against intercellular adhesion molecule 1 (ICAM-1), which has been applied to systems including polymersomes and polystyrene microparticles, among others [44,45]. Sialyl Lewis^x interacts with P-selectin to provide a relatively weak binding under rolling conditions, and the ICAM-1 antibody binds with ICAM-1 to provide a tight adhesion. Other ligand–receptor alternatives can be considered, but this approach mimics the behavior of leukocyte binding to activated endothelium and is therefore a viable means to achieve pharmacological delivery to sites of endothelial inflammation and damage.

The use of lipid microbubbles is focused on their use as an imaging modality. The application of ultrasound energy can generate cavitation of the bubble, promoting visualization of the carriers within the bloodstream. Disruption of microbubbles within the vasculature is capable of inducing porosity in the vascular wall sufficient to allow for the extravasation of therapeutic agents delivered at the same time as microbubbles or from the microbubbles themselves. The application of targeting ligands to promote rolling and adhesion can also be applied to these imaging and therapeutic delivery systems [46,47]. The ability to image (diagnose) and deliver therapeutics has been coined "theragnostics," and microbubbles are a good example of this type of system.

Table 6-2. *Examples of materials used for the formation of microparticle delivery systems*

Delivery system	Description and notes	References
Synthetic Polymers		
Poly(lactic acid) (PLA)	Poly (L-lactic acid) is expected to show longer term release than PLGA because of the tacticity of side chains. Near zero-order release over course of 9–11 days in vitro and in vivo for human epidermal growth factor. Particle diameters on order of 50–200 μm. Often used for long-term delivery of small molecule therapeutics.	[83]
Poly(lactide-co-glycolide) (PLGA)	PLGA is typically a mixture of PLA and poly(glycolic acid) (PGA) in the form of blends. Typically, these systems show burst release and then near zero-order release caused by diffusion followed by release because of degradation of the particles. Particle diameters range from several microns to several hundred microns depending on the method of fabrication. Release of 14 days or more is common. Porosity can be incorporated into these particles in ways similar to biomaterial scaffolds as a means to modulate the rate of diffusion-controlled release.	[84,85]
Poly-ε-caprolactone (PCL)	PCL is expected to achieve longer release than PLA, PGA, and PLGA because of a slower rate of degradation provided by the more hydrophobic region of the polymer backbone. Particles of 10–50 μm are reported. Encapsulation efficiencies of 20%–50% and release over the course of 20–50 days.	[75,86,87]
Natural Polymers		
Chitosan	Chitosan is polycationic and therefore often used for delivery of anionic plasmid DNA. This property is also useful for control over the release of negatively charged proteins. Particle diameters of 5–30 μm give release over the course of 8 hours for lactoferrin.	[88]
Gelatin	Gelatin microparticles are based on denatured collagen. Collagen microparticles are commonly described, but those processed through organic solvents are likely denatured. Release from gelatin can occur by diffusion but can be delayed by binding interactions. Gelatin has an isoelectric point less than neutral and therefore releases more basic proteins at a slower rate than acidic proteins. Particle diameters are approximately 10 μm. Release of BMP-2 is nearly zero order for 5 days after an initial 24-hour burst release. Subsequently the burst release is followed by a very slow release of basic FGF. Gelatin can be cross-linked by genepin, glutaraldehyde, and other agents.	[89,90]

(continued)

Table 6-2 *(continued)*

Delivery system	Description and notes	References
Alginate	Alginate is a polysaccharide that is cross-linked in the presence of divalent cations such as calcium. It is widely used for cell encapsulation but has been used for delivery of several growth factors as a microparticle delivery system. Particles of ∼15–70 μm achieved release of VEGF over 1–6 days, with release time modulated by the level of cross-linking. Larger particles (up to several hundred microns) can be fabricated. Loss of bioactivity has been reported with spray-drying technique.	[40,91]
Hyaluronic acid (HA)	HA is a glycosaminoglycan that is often use as a hydrogel and can be formed into microparticles. Particles of approximately 5–10 μm diameter have been fabricated by spray drying methods to achieve release of human growth hormone.	[92,93]
Lipid Systems		
Lipid microrods	Microrods have large aspect ratio with cross-sectional diameters of only several hundred nanometers but longitudinal lengths on the order of tens of microns. Release of therapeutic proteins is diffusion mediated and occurs on the order of several days. These systems can also be incorporated into hydrogels to achieve a two-stage release.	[94]

BMP-2 = bone morphogenetic protein 2; FGF = fibroblast growth factor; VEGF = vascular endothelial growth factor.

Tissue-Level Delivery

Applications of microcarriers within the vasculature are theoretically applicable to nanoscale systems on the order of less than 200 nm. However, the smaller size of the particles requires higher numbers of endothelial targeting ligands or reduced shear forces acting on the particles to achieve stable interactions [48]. Thus, achieving binding to target the vascular endothelium with nanocarriers has been challenging. The greater utility of nanocarrier systems has been in their ability to extravasate from the vascular compartment. One example of this phenomenon is in vascularized tumors by a process known as the enhanced permeation and retention (EPR) effect [49,50]. Enhanced permeation is attributable to poor cell–cell adhesion between endothelial cells of the vascular wall ("leaky vasculature") that occurs because of angiogenesis within the tumor. Depending on the tissue and disease state, the size of the gaps in the endothelium may range from several hundred nanometers (e.g., in the brain) to microns. The retention aspect of this phenomenon is associated with the poor lymphatic drainage within the tumor. This mechanism of uptake in tumors has also been described as "passive" targeting because it results from physiological flow of fluids in tumors with aberrant vasculature without major modifications to the carrier itself.

The accumulation of nanocarriers by this passive targeting, however, benefits from prolonged circulation times. That is, multiple passes through the vasculature increase the probability of extravasation at the site of action (i.e., site of the leaky vasculature). Nanocarriers are typically cleared through opsonization of the carrier and subsequent removal by the resident macrophages of the reticulo-endothelial system (RES) such as Kupffer cells of the liver. Long circulation time can be achieved by the use of so-called "Stealth" technology, which prevents adsorption of opsonin proteins of the complement system to the nanocarrier. This technology is best embodied in PEG. As described briefly earlier, PEG has been demonstrated to increase the circulation time of polypeptides and other therapeutic molecules. The incorporation of PEG onto the surface of nanocarriers is also known to prolong the circulation times of the carriers (see Fig. 6-2B). The precise mechanism by which this occurs remains somewhat unclear, but the general principles are as follows. At a high enough PEG concentration (e.g., 5 percent mol volume in liposomal drug carriers), the PEG takes a brush conformation that prevents protein adsorption through steric hindrance by the PEG chains or through the presence of an aqueous layer around the nanoparticle surface because of interaction between PEG and water. With the lower rate of protein adsorption such as those of the complement system (opsonins), the circulation time of the nanocarrier can be significantly extended because they are not recognized by residence macrophages. The use of PEG to achieve long-circulating formulations of nanocarriers such as liposomes has been critical to achieving clinical success of the systems.

An alternative approach that has been explored to achieve delivery of nanoparticles beyond the vasculature is the use of transcytosis. Transcytosis is a trafficking mechanism used by cells to shuttle macromolecules from one side of a cell to the other [51]. One example in which the delivery of nanoparticles is particularly challenging is in the brain, where the tight packing of endothelial cells known as the blood–brain barrier (BBB) can exclude many nanocarriers based on size and surface charge. In the case of endothelial cells of the BBB, transcytosis would involve the transport from the vessel lumen to the abluminal side. Several approaches have been used that seem to indicate the ability to achieve transcytosis of nanocarriers if their surfaces are appropriately modified. One example is the modification of nanocarrier surface charge (Fig. 6-2D) through the use of cationic albumin coupled to a PEG–poly(lactic acid) nanoparticle [52]. Others have used targeting ligands on the surface of nanoparticles to achieve transcytosis across the BBB [53] (Fig. 6-2E). These approaches are also under investigation to other epithelial barriers [54]. Most nanocarrier systems are currently designed for intravenous injection, but the ability to achieve transcytosis of the gut would open the possibility of oral administration of these carriers.

The mechanisms of transcytosis are well documented, but achieving effective and reproducible levels of transcytosis for delivery of therapeutic agents remains a future challenge.

From a nonmaterials perspective, approaches have been investigated to overcome the challenge of extravasation and diffusion through tissue. One such approach is the use of hyperthermia to enhance the extravasation of nanocarriers to the site of action [55–57]. Increased temperature is believed to improve extravasation by increasing blood flow and the diameters of microvascular pores [55,58]. This approach, however, requires fine control over temperature to avoid cell toxicity and hemorrhage. Approaches to improve movement of carrier systems through the vasculature by material modification or therapeutic intervention are essential to allowing application of these technologies to regenerative medicine needs.

Cell-Level and Subcellular Delivery

The long-circulating nanocarriers described earlier accumulate within a particular tissue such as a tumor. When this occurs, the nanocarriers are effectively lodged in the extracellular region of the tissue, where they slowly release their contents. This approach to delivery significantly alters the biodistribution of drugs within the body by increasing the amount of material in the tissue as well as by altering routes of clearance and localization of free drug to other tissues. One drawback to this approach, however, is that when free drug is released from the nanocarriers at the tissue level, it can diffuse either back to the vascular compartment or to nearby cells that are not being targeted (e.g., nontumor cells in the case of cancer targeting).

An approach to overcome this drawback is to achieve cell-level delivery of the carrier and its payload. As described earlier for microparticles targeting the vascular endothelium, an active area of research is in the presentation of targeting motifs on the surface of both micro and especially nanocarrier systems. PEG used to achieve long circulation times also provides an excellent means of achieving targeting ligand presentation because it can be anchored into nanoparticles through covalent interactions (see Fig. 6-2E). Perhaps more importantly, the PEG chain provides three-dimensional freedom of rotation of the targeting ligand, allowing the ligand to properly interact with its receptor [59,60]. PEG with reactive terminal groups such as carboxyls, amines, and maleimides are commercially available or can be synthesized by relatively straightforward means. By coupling ligands to the terminal ends of these PEG motifs, it is then possible to direct nanocarriers to the cell surface. The presence of multiple ligands on the nanocarrier surface along with the flexibility of the PEG chain allows for a strong interaction to occur at the cell surface if the appropriate receptor for the ligand is present, thereby preventing detachment of the carrier. This type of strong binding affinity through multiple binding events is sometimes referred to as avidity.

Interaction between certain ligand–receptor pairs can, in turn, trigger endocytosis of the carrier upon binding. It is well established, for example, that targeting the folate receptor, transferrin receptor, epidermal growth factor receptor, and others leads to cellular uptake of nanocarriers with diameters of several hundred nanometers or less. Thus, when the carrier has a therapeutic payload, the nanocarrier is using the cell's inherent machinery to achieve delivery – a "Trojan horse" effect. Several mechanisms of endocytosis include clathrin-coated pits, caveolae and lipid rafts, and macropinocytosis. Endocytosis can be achieved through nonspecific means such as the use of a positive surface charge on the nanocarrier. However, the advantage to the use of targeting ligands is the ability to more selectively deliver therapeutic cargo to cells that express a unique receptor or greatly overexpress more common receptors, thereby minimizing delivery to cells not intended for delivery (nontargeted cells). In addition to modification of the nanocarrier surface with ligands to promote cellular uptake, several other key material properties are known to affect these process. These include particle size (see Fig. 6-2D), geometry (see Fig. 6-2C), and surface chemistry (e.g., as surface chemistry relates to surface charge).

Several specific micro- and nanoparticle systems were described earlier. However, many of these systems are formed primarily through self-assembly processes, affording some lack of control over the final properties of the system. Recently, investigations have been conducted exploring the role of parameters such as charge and geometry on cellular uptake through endocytosis (see Fig. 6-2C). In one example, the geometry of particles can be modulated by subjecting the materials to specific forces to stretch the particles into nonspherical shapes [61]. In another approach, lithographic techniques are used to generate particles of known and well-defined size, geometry, and surface chemistry [62]. These approaches provide a means by which to study the effects of each of these parameters. Based on these and similar studies, it appears that more rodlike materials may have advantages in achieving cellular uptake via endocytosis and may also promote more favorable extravasation. Potential drawbacks to these highly technical fabrication approaches include the ability to obtain sufficient quantities for clinical applications and the need for exposure of biologic agents to chemical solvents.

Unless the site of action is the cell surface, it is still necessary to traffic the nanocarrier payload to its subcellular site of action after cellular uptake. The route of cellular uptake is believed to be important in the unpackaging and delivery of the contents of the nanocarrier. For example, delivery via the clathrin-mediated pathway leads to the endosome. The ability to achieve release of therapeutic agents from the endosome is therefore essential to their ability to reach their intracellular target. In the case of chemotherapy agents, the endosome may lead to the degradation of the nanocarrier, allowing the drug to diffuse to the cytoplasm. Alternatively, the nanocarrier may be modified to allow for its rapid and specific degradation upon entering the cell (endosome or otherwise) by incorporating sequences within the carrier that make it susceptible to hydrolytic cleavage (e.g., under the low pH environment of the endosome) or to proteolytic cleavage (e.g., by matrix metalloproteinases), as illustrated in Figure 6-2F.

For delivery of biologic molecules such as DNA and proteins, the therapeutic itself as well as the nanocarrier is too large to simply diffuse from the endosome. For this reason, so-called "smart" agents (polymers and lipids) that are lytic to the endosome have been developed. One example of this type of material is polyethylenimine (PEI), which has been used extensively for the delivery of DNA. PEI is a cationic polymer that complexes with DNA to form self-assembled constructs of approximately 50 to 200 nm in diameter depending on processing conditions such as the molecular weight of the polymer. It does not require the use of targeting ligands to achieve cellular uptake because of its net positive charge, although the use of PEG coatings and targeting motifs have been used to alter pharmacokinetics [63] and cell uptake [64–66], respectively. One theory for the efficacy of PEI for the delivery of DNA is the proton sponge hypothesis. According to this hypothesis, the amine groups of PEI are mostly not protonated at neutral pH. However, in the low-pH environment (pH ~5.5) of the endosome, the amine groups become protonated, leading to an influx of hydrogen ions, chloride counter ions, and water into the endosome. This process ultimately leads to lysis of the endosome and therefore release of the DNA payload. It remains unclear how DNA, after release into the cytoplasm from the endosome, reaches the nucleus. As an alternative approach to nanocarriers that do not inherently achieve spontaneous endosomal escape, it is possible to modify the surface of these carriers with endosomal escape peptides (see Fig. 6-2E and [67]).

The delivery of DNA through nonviral means is an important example of the concept of achieving subcellular localization. Although many growth factors work through cell surface–binding events, many drugs as well as DNA and protein therapies must reach intracellular targets such as the nucleus, mitochondria, or cytoskeletal components. Approaches to shuttle nanocarriers and their payloads to these locations is currently an active area of research that is expected to bring about the next generation of nanocarrier systems. One approach is the modification of carrier surfaces to allow them to harness intracellular machinery in a fashion similar to that used by pathogenic bacteria for intracellular transport. For example, modification of the surface of PEI–DNA complexes with ActA protein (the protein key to intracellular *Listeria monocytogenes* transport) has been demonstrated to promote the propulsion of these complexes in a cytoplasmic media containing actin components [68]. Such approaches may allow intact nanocarriers to overcome intracellular diffusion barriers such as the cytoplasm (Fig. 6-2E shows subcellular targeting).

Achieving subcellular delivery to the nucleus in the case of DNA delivery puts additional design constraints on the nanocarrier if the carrier itself is to deliver the DNA payload. Nuclear pores are on the order of 30 nm, requiring carriers that can cross these pores. Nuclear localization sequences (NLS) have been used to improve delivery of DNA without nanocarriers [69] and have also been used by conjugating to nanocarrier surface to enhance uptake for DNA delivery [70] and gold nanoparticles [71]. Despite the theoretical basis for this approach, however, there are relatively few reports in which NLS have been successfully applied to nanocarriers, indicating that other components to the system, including diameter, geometry, and surface charge, likely play a confounding role.

Taken together, the current state of the art indicates that the combination of ligand sequences that promote cellular uptake, endosomal escape, cellular transport, and subcellular localization provide the paradigm to use human-made carrier systems for effective delivery of therapeutic agents. These human-made carriers offer the promise of allowing for tailored design characteristics and improved safety profiles while acting with efficiencies similar to those of pathogenic agents such as bacteria and viruses.

Local Delivery Systems

Chapter 8 discusses numerous biomaterial systems as they are used to promote tissue regeneration with an emphasis on natural and synthetic polymers. An important aspect of these materials is their ability to modulate cellular behavior through the presentation of immobilized chemical cues in a fashion similar to the native extracellular matrix, thereby promoting cell attachment and adhesion, migration, proliferation, and differentiation. Another useful aspect of these material constructs is their ability to release soluble chemical factors, including growth factors. The specific role of the materials in promoting this release for directing cellular behavior is considered in more detail in Chapter 8. However, it is important to realize that the incorporation of nanoparticles, microparticles, and nanotechnology into these systems is often an important means by which to achieve spatial and temporal control over the rates of drug delivery. In this section, we discuss some of the similarities and differences between systemic and local delivery and describe several local delivery systems that take advantage of micro- and nanoscale technology, often as a modification to or manipulation of a biomaterial system. We also explore several other approaches to the local delivery of therapeutic agents, particularly biomolecules that rely on properties similar to those governing micro- and nanoparticulate delivery, including concepts of self-assembly.

The principles governing local delivery of therapeutic agents are similar to those described earlier for systemic delivery systems and illustrated in Figure 6-1. An important consideration in the development of local delivery platforms is the concept of spatiotemporal control. This refers to the ability of these platforms to control the location of delivery in three-dimensional space (spatial control) and time (temporal control). Numerous approaches can be used to achieve spatiotemporal control of therapeutic delivery for therapeutic agents. Figure 6-3 highlights several of these, which are also discussed further below.

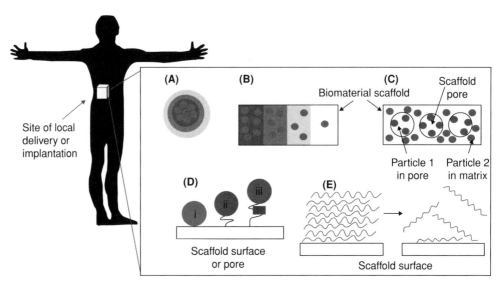

Figure 6-3. Micro- and nanoparticles may be used to achieve spatiotemporal control over delivery of therapeutic agents when delivered locally. (**A**) When delivered alone, the release profile may establish a gradient because of diffusional control over movement of the therapeutic agent. (**B**) When incorporated into a biomaterial scaffold, a similar gradient profile may be established. (**C**) By controlling the spatial location of the particulate carrier, control over the timing of release of single or multiple agents may be controlled. (**D**) Nanoscale carriers may be attached to the surface of biomaterials by adsorption (i) or covalent cross-linking (ii). Enzymatic cleavage sites may also be incorporated into tethers (iii) used to achieve covalent cross-linking to allow cell-mediated release. (**E**) Layer-by-layer release of therapeutic agents allows for temporal control as the layers of the system sequentially degrade, slowly releasing the contents of the subsequent layer. (See color plate 12.)

One advantage to the use of local delivery systems is that molecules with short half-lives in the systemic circulation can be immediately localized to a site of interest without incorporation into micro- or nanocarriers. Clearly, when therapeutic agents are delivered locally either directly within the biomaterial construct or encapsulated in micro- or nanoparticles, they do not need to reach the tissue level via extravasation from the vasculature. However, it is important to note that processes of uptake *into* the vasculature after local delivery can occur. Depending on the potency and systemic half-life of the therapeutic agent being released, this must be considered because of possible systemic side effects.

For systemic delivery of therapeutic agents (especially traditional chemical drug compounds), there is typically a well-defined window within which the blood serum levels should remain to achieve therapeutic effect. For local delivery systems, a challenge is that serum levels cannot be easily monitored to estimate the local effect. This challenge is particularly evident in considering the delivery of biologically active molecules such as growth factors because the effect of these compounds on the local tissue microenvironment can be pronounced. This may be most evident from a nonmaterial example of delivery of vascular endothelial growth factor (VEGF), which showed that the local microenvironmental concentration of VEGF had a pronounced effect on the formation of vascular structures at sites of implants, such as lack of capillary formation or aberrant vasculature [72]. This same principle is applicable to local delivery systems in that relatively small changes at the microenvironmental level can lead to pronounced physiological differences because of the potency of these molecules [73].

One consideration in the design of such systems is the dimensions to use, that is, nano- or micro-scale. The primary advantage of nanoscale systems is they are more diffusible and can be more readily internalized by cells than micro-scale systems. However, micro-scale systems are often used because (1) carriers of these dimensions are more readily prepared, (2) the size does not typically adversely affect cellular growth, and (3) the ratio of volume to surface area scales with the particle diameter. For systems in which diffusion of the compound from the carrier dominates, the flux of the therapeutic from the particle from the carrier depends on the concentration gradient and the surface area. Therefore, because micro-scale systems provide more volume per surface area, they can maintain the concentration gradient more readily, thereby providing sustained release.

Controlled-release systems for local delivery can be used through direct injection or, increasingly, as components of biomaterial scaffolds (Fig. 6-3). Although metal and ceramic delivery systems have been described, polymeric systems are by far the most heavily used controlled release systems at the micro- and nanoscales for regenerative applications. Lipid-based systems at these dimensional ranges are systems are also used [74], although these systems may be thought of as a type of "noncovalent polymer" system because of their self-assembly and higher order structure. When delivered locally, microparticle systems are capable of achieving, in many cases, nearly zero-order release for extended periods of time. These microsphere or microparticle systems can act as a small depot for the release of biologic compounds. When considered as a point source and neglecting uptake into the vascular compartment, these systems can elicit a gradient effect (see Fig. 6-3A). A similar gradient effect may also be achieved when incorporated into biomaterial scaffolds (see Fig. 6-3B) [75,76]. However, it is more common to embed these particulate carrier systems within biomaterial scaffolds as a means to achieve a more sustained release. In this context, the therapeutic agent must first be released from the microparticle and then diffuse out of the scaffold before reaching cells [77].

Alternatively, spatiotemporal control has been achieved by using a biomaterial scaffold and microparticles together to achieve distinct release profiles for multiple therapeutic agents (see Fig. 6-3C [78]). The biologic processes involved in development, healing, and regeneration involve a tight interplay between many signaling molecules. Therefore, this approach of multiple agent delivery is particularly useful for regenerative applications that seek to mimic these processes. Growth factors are the most recognizable of these agents, and to recapitulate these processes with a materials approach (i.e., without cells), spatiotemporal control of the delivery of these molecules is necessary. In one example of this approach, VEGF and platelet-derived growth factor were released in a temporally controlled fashion through modulation of their placement within a biomaterial construct, leading to vasculature within the material construct of a more stable and mature nature [78]. Increasingly complex systems are being used to sequentially deliver growth factors [79–81]. Other systems that rely on specific cellular or enzymatic processes afford even more control over the temporal delivery of growth factors [82].

Some specific challenges related to the use of particulate carriers for growth factor delivery are discussed later. Several additional approaches to deliver micro- or nanoparticles or systems taking advantage of nanotechnology for local delivery include electrospinning, surface-mediated delivery (see Fig. 6-3D), layer-by-layer (LBL) delivery (see Fig. 6-3E), and stimulus-responsive systems.

Polymeric Microparticles

The number of microparticle systems is too numerous to describe each in detail. Table 6-2 highlights examples of microparticle systems fabricated from commonly used biomaterials and investigated for regenerative applications. When possible, Table 6-2 cites references in which the polymer carrier was not a mixture, blend, or composite and was used to achieve release of polypeptides such as growth factors with applications to regenerative medicine. Because different polypeptides are used for the various studies, differences in the duration and profile of release are affected. Several additional parameters to these materials must be considered in regard to their release profiles. The molecular weights of the polymers affect their degradation and rate of release. The tacticity of the side groups as it related to the crystalline nature of the polymer also impacts its rate of degradation and rate of release. The method of formation may consist of emulsions, spray drying, freeze drying, and others. These processing methods can greatly impact the size of the carriers and the bioactivity of the therapeutic. Finally, although in vitro release conditions can be standardized, the conditions for a specific in vivo application may vary, adding an additional challenge when trying to compare different microparticle systems. Therefore, the descriptions in Table 6-2 should be thought of as "case examples" rather than definitive descriptions encompassing all aspects of the delivery system. Stated differently, the appropriate polymer to use and expected release profiles must often be tested for a specific application.

The most commonly used microparticle systems are based on poly(lactide-co-glycolide) (PLGA). PLGA is widely used in regenerative medicine applications because it is used in numerous products that have been approved by the Food and Drug Administration, has sufficient mechanical integrity to withstand normal physiology forces, and can be tailored to achieve sustained release from several days to several months depending on the ratio of lactic acid to glycol acid. PLGA and most other synthetic microparticle systems used to incorporate biologic molecules such as proteins and nucleic acids can be fabricated by several techniques. One of the most common techniques is the use of emulsion processing. Emulsions are prepared by dissolving the polymer in an organic solvent such as dichloromethane or chloroform that is immiscible with aqueous solutions. The molecule to be encapsulated is dissolved in aqueous buffer and mixed with the organic solvent to form a water-in-oil (W/O) emulsion. Such systems are typically mechanically agitated or sonicated to achieve good dispersion of the system. Microparticles can be formed by the removal of the organic solvent through methods such as extraction or evaporation, which is a secondary emulsification. Water-in-oil-in-water (W/O/W) emulsions can be formed by the same approach described, but before evaporation of the organic solvent, the emulsion is added to an aqueous solution of containing another polymer, typically poly(vinyl alcohol) (PVA) or polyethylene oxide (PEO). The solvent can then be removed by evaporation or other techniques. Other polymeric microparticle systems can be formed through these techniques as well.

One challenge for the application of microparticle systems formed with W/O and W/O/W emulsions is the reported loss of activity of proteins and other biologic molecules. Numerous studies have observed a loss of activity of numerous proteins, with most studies looking at loss of activity of enzymes such as lysozyme or alkaline phosphatase as model proteins. However, not all studies indicate loss of protein activity, and the specific mechanisms for loss of activity likely vary depending on the properties of a given biologic molecule (especially enzymatic proteins) and the solvents used.

A number of factors have been considered as sources activity loss associated with emulsification processes. Agitation and sonication present mechanical forces on biologic molecules. However, this mechanism of disruption has been demonstrated to have minimal effect [95,96]. Some systems require the addition of heat, which also may denature biologic molecules. Although the direct dissolution of proteins and polymers in the same solvent system has been reported, some solvents may lead to the direct denaturation of proteins, resulting in loss of activity [97,98].

Another reason for loss of activity is the water–oil phase interface [99,100]. Proteins in particular may denature at interfaces caused by thermodynamic rearrangement as they alter conformation to minimize the free energy of the system as is known to occur with protein adsorption to biomaterial surfaces. For example, whereas hydrophobic motifs may be exposed to the organic phase, hydrophilic motifs associate with the aqueous phase. This mechanism of action seems likely because the aggregation of proteins at the organic–aqueous (or oil–water) interface has been observed [101]. These events occur on a very rapid timescale (seconds to minutes), making it difficult to prevent their occurrence. However, numerous reports also show minimal loss of protein activity in W/O and W/O/W emulsions, indicating that rapid processing may help to overcome these thermodynamic effects. It might be noted that whereas the use of polypeptides are particularly challenging because of their tertiary and quaternary structures, small molecule drugs and nucleic acids that do not have these higher order structures are more favorable in terms of processing.

Most of the synthetic polymers used for regenerative medicine applications are biodegradable polymers. An issue facing these polymers is the effect of degradation products on the stability of encapsulated molecules. Most biodegradable polymers rely on groups within the polymer backbone that can be hydrolyzed such as esters. The resulting degradation products include acid molecules that can lower the local microenvironmental pH and degrade biologic molecules within the microparticulate matrix. Polymers such as poly-ε-caprolactone show less degradation to biologic molecules because they degrade more slowly.

Therefore, the appeal of naturally based polymers (see Table 6-2) is that these polymers are typically more favorable in terms of their degradation products. Many of the protein-based carriers are also capable of supporting cell attachment and can be used for cell encapsulation. In addition, unlike synthetic polymers, most of these systems can be formed under more favorable fabrication conditions not requiring the use of organic solvents. The main drawback to the natural polymers, as can be seen in Table 6-2, is that they typically show release over a shorter timescale than the synthetics.

Electrospun Fibers

Electrospun fibers provide a means by which to recapitulate topographical features of the extracellular matrix and also provide a means for local delivery of bioactive molecules from the nanoscale fibers. The details of forming electrospun scaffolds are described in Chapter 8 and several excellent reviews on the topic [102,103]. In considering the process of electrospinning, it is apparent that there are several components of the process with the potential to degrade biologic molecules. These include the application of high electrical voltage, the use of solvents to dissolve the polymers, gas–liquid interfaces, and mechanical shear through the orifice of the extrusion device. However, the primary challenge to incorporation of biologic molecules into electrospun scaffolds is the ability to achieve dissolution into the solvents typically used for electrospinning. Although several fluorinated alcohol systems (e.g., 1,1,1,3,3,3-hexafluoro-2-propanol) have been identified to allow the electrospinning of natural polymers such as collagen and elastin [104], there is question regarding their ability to preserve the integrity of biologic molecules [105]. Other reports use water-soluble polymers such as poly(vinyl alcohol) (PVA), with desirable fiber diameters (80–250 nm), release profiles (2–3 weeks), and bioactivity. However, this approach limits the number of polymers that can be used for preparing scaffolds [106].

The ability to achieve electrospun scaffolds containing biologic molecules has stemmed from previously demonstrated systems in which chemotherapy, antibiotic

[107], or other small molecule drugs have been incorporated into electrospun scaffolds. Antibiotic delivery is important to many tissue engineering applications in which infection is common, and numerous agents are known to modulate cellular effects, making use of electrospun scaffolds appealing for these approaches. One drawback to electrospinning, particularly with ionic compounds such as many antibiotics and chemotherapy drugs, is that the drugs tend to preferentially locate at the periphery of the fiber [108]. This, in turn, leads to a rapid release of the therapeutic. To overcome this limitation, so-called core-shell or coaxial fibers have been created in which an inner core consisting of a fiber containing the drug is surrounded by an outer layer that prevents the rapid release of the compound [109,110].

This coaxial approach has also proven to be essential for the incorporation of biologic molecules such as growth factors, proteins, and nucleic acids [111] into electrospun scaffolds. In this approach, the biologic molecule is dissolved in aqueous solution, and the polymer is separately dissolved in an appropriate solvent [112,113]. Resulting fibers contain a core aqueous-based layer containing the biologic molecule surrounded by a shell of polymer that controls the rate of release. Numerous modifications to the system can be made to alter the porosity and thickness of the shell layer, thereby modulating the rate of drug release.

Other approaches that have been used to maintain the bioactivity of growth factors and other bioactive molecules include the use of a protein carrier such as albumin [114,115] and the use of emulsifying agents [115,116] during the electrospinning process. The maintenance or loss of biologic activity through these various electrospinning processes (e.g., coaxial, emulsion spinning) is not yet fully characterized and may prove to be a future challenge.

Layer-by-Layer Release

Although not a micro- or nanoparticulate carrier system, LBL approaches make use of similar principles of self-assembly to act as reservoirs for the release of therapeutic agents. This approach forms thin films by depositing alternating layers of oppositely charged polymeric molecules (see Fig. 6-3E). These layers self-assemble through the electrostatic interactions between polymers and are typically built into films 100 to 200 nm in thickness ($\sim$8–10 bilayers 16–20 individual polyionic layers) [117].

These systems are of particular interest for the delivery of biologic molecules, including nucleic acids and growth factors. The most widely studied biologic molecule for LBL technology is DNA as its polyanionic nature can be used in conjunction with numerous polycationic polymers to form the LBL structure. Growth factors with isoelectric points greater than neutral have also been used as the polycation while a synthetic polyanion is used as the alternate layer.

Layer-by-layer approaches have the potential to change methods of achieving biologic structures such as proteins and nucleic acids for several reasons. Most of the polyions used are water soluble, removing the need for the use of organic solvents used to form emulsions and minimizing the loss of activity observed in emulsion microparticles. These systems can also be tailored to release with distinct profiles and under specific conditions. For example, rates of surface erosion can be controlled by polymers such as poly(amino-esters) to allow hydrolytic release of DNA [117,118]. Certainly, timed release based on other intrinsic or extrinsic moduli such as matrix metalloproteinases, temperature, or ultrasound are conceivable as well. Last, the systems are compatible with temporally controlled delivery of multiple components, potentially mimicking native timescales of physiological processes such as angiogenesis in which certain cues or growth factors must be present at the right time and in the correct amounts.

Several parameters must be carefully considered in the design of LBL systems. These systems must provide sufficient stability to allow for the formation of the multilayered construct. However, these systems are also designed to disassemble at a desirable rate to promote the release of DNA or other biologic molecules. One drawback to many polyamine systems is their toxicity to cells. Newer polymer systems are under investigation to minimize the toxicity associated with traditional polyamines.

Another potential problem for LBL systems is that they are typically formed on very smooth surfaces such as glass or silica, potentially limiting their application to tissue engineering scaffolds, which tend to have greater surface topography to promote cell attachment and migration. However, these systems have been described for the release of DNA from stents [119], indicating the potential of these systems for use in the medical device industry and changing the way in which diseases such as atherosclerosis are treated and managed. In addition, the use of multilayer systems has been described as a method to create hollow shell carriers [120,121] as well as micro- and nanoparticles for DNA delivery [122,123]. These particulate systems formed by LBL deposition are suitable for systemic administration, providing mechanisms to achieve timed release of DNA at their site of action as well as improved transfection efficiency. The exact mechanisms by which this approach operates are also yet to be fully elucidated.

Surface-Mediated Delivery

For therapeutic agents such as nucleic acids, barriers to therapeutic activity are as described for systemic delivery: cellular entry, endosomal escape, and transport to the site of action (e.g., the nucleus for DNA). Although microparticles are advantageous for the sustained release of therapeutic agents, nanocarriers are better able to achieve cellular uptake and overcome these barriers. Therefore, approaches to incorporate nanocarriers into or onto biomaterial scaffolds are under investigation. This approach relies on either release of the nanoparticles from the material, leading to a localized cellular uptake, or on the direct uptake of nanoparticles from the material surface. Although components for systemic delivery such as PEG coatings are not required, the other components of nanoparticles highlighted in Figure 6-2C to F may ultimately find use for local delivery (e.g., NLS sequences). These carriers can be adsorbed [124] or tethered [125] to the material surface (see Fig. 6-3D) to promote increased microenvironmental DNA concentration and cellular uptake. Because they are associated with scaffolds and achieve locally high concentrations of DNA, this approach is compatible with most regenerative medicine applications that have a material component.

Stimulus-Responsive Systems

One potential advantage of many of the carrier systems described in this chapter is that because they are self-assembled systems, the introduction of sufficient external energy can disrupt the particles to achieve more rapid release of the contents. This, therefore, provides the opportunity to "dose" these systems for scheduled release of the compounds in a fashion similar to repeated injection of systemically delivered agents. One prerequisite for this approach, however, is that the material must be located such that it can be reached by the energy source. A second requirement is that the applied energy source must be sufficiently focused to avoid damage to cells at the site of the carrier or within the path between the energy source and the particulate carrier system. One form of energy that typically meets these criteria is application of ultrasonic energy to disrupt particulate systems. The use of stimuli-response delivery has been used for systemically delivered agents [26,126]. There are few reports to date on the incorporation of microparticle and nanoparticle systems injected directly to achieve thermo-responsive release. However, this technology has been applied to hydrogel systems [127], and the compatibility of particulate carriers with this technology provides an opportunity to achieve temporal control over therapeutic delivery.

Summary

The techniques and modalities described for controlled-release systems allow a theoretical framework for the provision of chemical and physical cues to regenerating cells and tissues. Although the appropriate use of cell-based therapies offers this same potential, technical and regulatory hurdles make it likely that controlled-release systems will continue to play a role in preclinical development and at the clinical level. Alternatively, these approaches offer the potential to work in concert with cell-based systems to form the environmental conditions necessary to maintain (stem) cells in a multi- or pluripotent state, that is, to act as a proxy to the formation of a stem cell niche.

References

1. Baichwal, A. R. and Neville, D. A. (2001) Adding value to products' life-cycle management: product enhancement through drug delivery systems. *Drug Delivery Technology*, 1(1). Available at: http://www.drug-dev.com/ME2/ (Accessed: 19 October 2012)

2. Dunn, W. A. and Hubbard, A. L. (1984) Receptor-mediated endocytosis of epidermal growth factor by hepatocytes in the perfused rat liver: ligand and receptor dynamics. *J Cell Biol*. 98, 2148–2159

3. Liu, K. X., Kato, Y., Narukawa, M., Kim, D. C., Hanano, M., Higuchi, O., Nakamura, T., and Sugiyama, Y. (1992) Importance of the liver in plasma clearance of hepatocyte growth factors in rats. *Am J Physiol*. 263, G642–649

4. Strebhardt, K. and Ullrich, A. (2008) Paul Ehrlich's magic bullet concept: 100 years of progress. *Nat Rev Cancer*. 8, 473–480

5. Bosch, F. and Rosich, L. (2008) The contributions of Paul Ehrlich to pharmacology: a tribute on the occasion of the centenary of his Nobel Prize. *Pharmacology*. 82, 171–179

6. Caliceti, P. and Veronese, F. M. (2003) Pharmacokinetic and biodistribution properties of poly(ethylene glycol)-protein conjugates. *Adv Drug Deliv Rev*. 55, 1261–1277

7. Pisal, D. S., Kosloski, M. P., and Balu-Iyer, S. V. (2010) Delivery of therapeutic proteins. *J Pharm Sci*. 99, 2557–2575

8. Harris, J. M. and Chess, R. B. (2003) Effect of pegylation on pharmaceuticals. *Nat Rev Drug Discov*. 2, 214–221

9. Harris, J. M., Martin, N. E., and Modi, M. (2001) Pegylation: a novel process for modifying pharmacokinetics. *Clin Pharmacokinet*. 40, 539–551

10. Juliano, R. L., Lopez-Berestein, G., Hopfer, R., Mehta, R., Mehta, K., and Mills, K. (1985) Selective toxicity and enhanced therapeutic index of liposomal polyene antibiotics in systemic fungal infections. *Ann N Y Acad Sci*. 446, 390–402

11. Karathanasis, E., Ayyagari, A. L., Bhavane, R., Bellamkonda, R. V., and Annapragada, A. V. (2005) Preparation of in vivo cleavable agglomerated liposomes suitable for modulated pulmonary drug delivery. *J Control Release*. 103, 159–175

12. Allen, T. M. (1994) Long-circulating (sterically stabilized) liposomes for targeted drug delivery. *Trends Pharmacol Sci*. 15, 215–220

13. Li, S. D. and Huang, L. (2006) Surface-modified LPD nanoparticles for tumor targeting. *Ann N Y Acad Sci*. 1082, 1–8

14. Li, S. D., Chono, S. and Huang, L. (2008) Efficient gene silencing in metastatic tumor by siRNA formulated in surface-modified nanoparticles. *J Control Release*. 126, 77–84

15. Meyer, K. B., Thompson, M. M., Levy, M. Y., Barron, L. G., and Szoka, F. C., Jr. (1995) Intratracheal gene delivery to the mouse airway: characterization of plasmid DNA expression and pharmacokinetics. *Gene Ther*. 2, 450–460

16. Radler, J. O., Koltover, I., Salditt, T., and Safinya, C. R. (1997) Structure of DNA-cationic liposome complexes: DNA intercalation in multilamellar membranes in distinct interhelical packing regimes. *Science*. 275, 810–814

17. Salmaso, S., Pappalardo, J. S., Sawant, R. R., Musacchio, T., Rockwell, K., Caliceti, P., and Torchilin, V. P. (2009) Targeting glioma cells in vitro with ascorbate-conjugated pharmaceutical nanocarriers. *Bioconjug Chem*. 20, 2348–2355

18. Weissig, V., Whiteman, K. R., and Torchilin, V. P. (1998) Accumulation of protein-loaded long-circulating micelles and liposomes in subcutaneous Lewis lung carcinoma in mice. *Pharm Res*. 15, 1552–1556

19. Swanson, S. D., Kukowska-Latallo, J. F., Patri, A. K., Chen, C., Ge, S., Cao, Z., Kotlyar, A., East, A. T., and Baker, J. R. (2008) Targeted gadolinium-loaded dendrimer nanoparticles for tumor-specific magnetic resonance contrast enhancement. *Int J Nanomed*. 3, 201–210

20. Ke, W., Shao, K., Huang, R., Han, L., Liu, Y., Li, J., Kuang, Y., Ye, L., Lou, J., and Jiang, C. (2009) Gene delivery targeted to the brain using an Angiopep-conjugated polyethyleneglycol-modified polyamidoamine dendrimer. *Biomaterials*. 30, 6976–6985

21. Kojima, C., Kono, K., Maruyama, K., and Takagishi, T. (2000) Synthesis of polyamidoamine dendrimers having poly(ethylene glycol) grafts and their ability to encapsulate anticancer drugs. *Bioconjug Chem*. 11, 910–917

22. Wang, D., Kopeckova, J. P., Minko, T., Nanayakkara, V., and Kopecek, J. (2000) Synthesis of starlike N-(2-hydroxypropyl)methacrylamide copolymers: potential drug carriers. *Biomacromolecules*. 1, 313–319

23. Benoit, D. S., Henry, S. M., Shubin, A. D., Hoffman, A. S., and Stayton, P. S. (2010) pH-responsive polymeric sirna carriers sensitize multidrug resistant ovarian cancer cells to doxorubicin via knockdown of polo-like kinase 1. *Mol Pharm*. 7, 442–455

24. Convertine, A. J., Diab, C., Prieve, M., Paschal, A., Hoffman, A. S., Johnson, P. H., and Stayton, P. S. (2010) pH-responsive polymeric micelle carriers for siRNA drugs. *Biomacromolecules*.

25. Gaucher, G., Dufresne, M. H., Sant, V. P., Kang, N., Maysinger, D., and Leroux, J. C. (2005) Block copolymer micelles: preparation, characterization and application in drug delivery. *J Control Release*. 109, 169–188

26. Husseini, G. A., Diaz de la Rosa, M. A., Gabuji, T., Zeng, Y., Christensen, D. A., and Pitt, W. G. (2007) Release of doxorubicin from unstabilized and stabilized micelles under the action of ultrasound. *J Nanosci Nanotechnol*. 7, 1028–1033

27. Boeckle, S., von Gersdorff, K., van der Piepen, S., Culmsee, C., Wagner, E., and Ogris, M. (2004) Purification of polyethylenimine polyplexes highlights the role of free polycations in gene transfer. *J Gene Med*. 6, 1102–1111

28. Zintchenko, A., Philipp, A., Dehshahri, A., and Wagner, E. (2008) Simple modifications of branched PEI lead to highly efficient siRNA carriers with low toxicity. *Bioconjug Chem*. 19, 1448–1455

29. Foster, S., Duvall, C. L., Crownover, E. F., Hoffman, A. S., and Stayton, P. S. (2010) Intracellular delivery of a protein antigen with an endosomal-releasing polymer enhances CD8 T-cell production and prophylactic vaccine efficacy. *Bioconjug Chem*.

30. Discher, B. M., Won, Y. Y., Ege, D. S., Lee, J. C., Bates, F. S., Discher, D. E., and Hammer, D. A. (1999) Polymersomes: tough vesicles made from diblock copolymers. *Science*. 284, 1143–1146

31. Kim, Y., Tewari, M., Pajerowski, J. D., Cai, S., Sen, S., Williams, J. H., Sirsi, S. R., Lutz, G. J., and Discher, D. E. (2009) Polymersome delivery of siRNA and antisense oligonucleotides. *J Control Release*. 134, 132–140

32. Arifin, D. R. and Palmer, A. F. (2005) Polymersome encapsulated hemoglobin: a novel type of oxygen carrier. *Biomacromolecules*. 6, 2172–2181

33. Levine, D. H., Ghoroghchian, P. P., Freudenberg, J., Zhang, G., Therien, M. J., Greene, M. I., Hammer, D. A., and Murali, R. (2008) Polymersomes: a new multi-functional tool for cancer diagnosis and therapy. *Methods*. 46, 25–32

34. Smith, A. M., Gao, X., and Nie, S. (2004) Quantum dot nanocrystals for in vivo molecular and cellular imaging. *Photochem Photobiol*. 80, 377–385

35. Gao, X. and Nie, S. (2003) Molecular profiling of single cells and tissue specimens with quantum dots. *Trends Biotechnol*. 21, 371–373

36. Gao, X. and Nie, S. (2004) Quantum dot-encoded mesoporous beads with high brightness and uniformity: rapid readout using flow cytometry. *Anal Chem*. 76, 2406–2410

37. Gao, X. and Nie, S. (2005) Quantum dot-encoded beads. *Methods Mol Biol*. 303, 61–71

38. Arnold, M. M., Gorman, E. M., Schieber, L. J., Munson, E. J., and Berkland, C. (2007) NanoCipro encapsulation in monodisperse large porous PLGA microparticles. *J Control Release*. 121, 100–109

39. Balmayor, E. R., Feichtinger, G. A., Azevedo, H. S., van Griensven, M., and Reis, R. L. (2009) Starch-poly-epsilon-caprolactone microparticles reduce the needed amount of BMP-2. *Clin Orthop Relat Res*. 467, 3138–3148

40. Jay, S. M. and Saltzman, W. M. (2009) Controlled delivery of VEGF via modulation of alginate microparticle ionic crosslinking. *J Control Release*. 134, 26–34

41. Willmann, J. K., Paulmurugan, R., Chen, K., Gheysens, O., Rodriguez-Porcel, M., Lutz, A. M., Chen, I. Y., Chen, X., and Gambhir, S. S. (2008) US imaging of tumor angiogenesis with microbubbles targeted to vascular endothelial growth factor receptor type 2 in mice. *Radiology*. 246, 508–518

42. Rapoport, N., Gao, Z., and Kennedy, A. (2007) Multifunctional nanoparticles for combining ultrasonic tumor imaging and targeted chemotherapy. *J Natl Cancer Inst*. 99, 1095–1106

43. Treat, L. H., McDannold, N., Vykhodtseva, N., Zhang, Y., Tam, K., and Hynynen, K. (2007) Targeted delivery of doxorubicin to the rat brain at therapeutic levels using MRI-guided focused ultrasound. *Int J Cancer*. 121, 901–907

44. Robbins, G. P., Saunders, R. L., Haun, J. B., Rawson, J., Therien, M. J., and Hammer, D. A. (2010) Tunable leuko-polymersomes that adhere specifically to inflammatory markers. *Langmuir*. 26, 14089–14096

45. Omolola Eniola, A. and Hammer, D. A. (2005) In vitro characterization of leukocyte mimetic for targeting therapeutics to the endothelium using two receptors. *Biomaterials*. 26, 7136–7144

46. Klibanov, A. L., Rychak, J. J., Yang, W. C., Alikhani, S., Li, B., Acton, S., Lindner, J. R., Ley, K., and Kaul, S. (2006) Targeted ultrasound contrast agent for molecular imaging of inflammation in high-shear flow. *Contrast Media Mol Imaging*. 1, 259–266

47. Rychak, J. J., Lindner, J. R., Ley, K., and Klibanov, A. L. (2006) Deformable gas-filled microbubbles targeted to P-selectin. *J Control Release*. 114, 288–299

48. Mennesson, E., Erbacher, P., Kuzak, M., Kieda, C., Midoux, P., and Pichon, C. (2006) DNA/cationic polymer complex attachment on a human vascular endothelial cell monolayer exposed to a steady laminar flow. *J Control Release*. 114, 389–397

49. Jain, R. K. (1987) Transport of molecules across tumor vasculature. *Cancer Metastasis Rev*. 6, 559–593

50. Matsumura, Y. and Maeda, H. (1986) A new concept for macromolecular therapeutics in cancer chemotherapy: mechanism of tumoritropic accumulation of proteins and the antitumor agent smancs. *Cancer Res*. 46, 6387–6392

51. Tuma, P. L. and Hubbard, A. L. (2003) Transcytosis: crossing cellular barriers. *Physiol Rev*. 83, 871–932

52. Lu, W., Zhang, Y., Tan, Y. Z., Hu, K. L., Jiang, X. G., and Fu, S. K. (2005) Cationic albumin-conjugated pegylated nanoparticles as novel drug carrier for brain delivery. *J Control Release*. 107, 428–448

53. Zhang, Y., Schlachetzki, F., and Pardridge, W. M. (2003) Global non-viral gene transfer to the primate brain following intravenous administration. *Mol Ther*. 7, 11–18.

54. Orthmann, A., Zeisig, R., Koklic, T., Sentjurc, M., Wiesner, B., Lemm, M., and Fichtner, I. (2010) Impact of membrane properties on uptake and transcytosis of colloidal nanocarriers across an epithelial cell barrier model. *J Pharm Sci*. 99, 2423–2433

55. Kong, G., Braun, R. D., and Dewhirst, M. W. (2001) Characterization of the effect of hyperthermia on nanoparticle extravasation from tumor vasculature. *Cancer Res*. 61, 3027–3032

56. Koning, G. A., Eggermont, A. M., Lindner, L. H., and ten Hagen, T. L. (2010) Hyperthermia and thermosensitive liposomes for improved delivery of chemotherapeutic drugs to solid tumors. *Pharm Res.* 27, 1750–1754

57. Liu, P., Xu, L. X., and Zhang, A. (2006) Enhanced efficacy of anti-tumor liposomal doxorubicin by hyperthermia. *Conf Proc IEEE Eng Med Biol Soc.* 1, 4354–4357

58. Kong, G., Braun, R. D., and Dewhirst, M. W. (2000) Hyperthermia enables tumor-specific nanoparticle delivery: effect of particle size. *Cancer Res.* 60, 4440–4445

59. Jeppesen, C., Wong, J. Y., Kuhl, T. L., Israelachvili, J. N., Mullah, N., Zalipsky, S., and Marques, C. M. (2001) Impact of polymer tether length on multiple ligand-receptor bond formation. *Science.* 293, 465–468.

60. Wong, J. Y., Kuhl, T. L., Israelachvili, J. N., Mullah, N., and Zalipsky, S. (1997) Direct measurement of a tethered ligand-receptor interaction potential. *Science.* 275, 820–822

61. Champion, J. A., Katare, Y. K., and Mitragotri, S. (2007) Making polymeric micro- and nanoparticles of complex shapes. *Proc Natl Acad Sci U S A.* 104, 11901–11904

62. Gratton, S. E., Ropp, P. A., Pohlhaus, P. D., Luft, J. C., Madden, V. J., Napier, M. E., and DeSimone, J. M. (2008) The effect of particle design on cellular internalization pathways. *Proc Natl Acad Sci U S A.* 105, 11613–11618

63. Fischer, D., Osburg, B., Petersen, H., Kissel, T., and Bickel, U. (2004) Effect of poly(ethylene imine) molecular weight and pegylation on organ distribution and pharmacokinetics of polyplexes with oligodeoxynucleotides in mice. *Drug Metab Dispos.* 32, 983–992

64. Merkel, O. M., Germershaus, O., Wada, C. K., Tarcha, P. J., Merdan, T., and Kissel, T. (2009) Integrin alphaVbeta3 targeted gene delivery using RGD peptidomimetic conjugates with copolymers of PEGylated poly(ethylene imine). *Bioconjug Chem.* 20, 1270–1280

65. Liang, B., He, M. L., Chan, C. Y., Chen, Y. C., Li, X. P., Li, Y., Zheng, D., Lin, M. C., Kung, H. F., Shuai, X. T., and Peng, Y. (2009) The use of folate-PEG-grafted-hybranched-PEI nonviral vector for the inhibition of glioma growth in the rat. *Biomaterials.* 30, 4014–4020

66. Bellocq, N. C., Pun, S. H., Jensen, G. S., and Davis, M. E. (2003) Transferrin-containing, cyclodextrin polymer-based particles for tumor-targeted gene delivery. *Bioconjugate Chem.* 14, 1122–1132

67. Kwon, E. J., Bergen, J. M., and Pun, S. H. (2008) Application of an HIV gp41-derived peptide for enhanced intracellular trafficking of synthetic gene and siRNA delivery vehicles. *Bioconjug Chem.* 19, 920–927

68. Ng, C. P., Goodman, T. T., Park, I. K., and Pun, S. H. (2009) Bio-mimetic surface engineering of plasmid-loaded nanoparticles for active intracellular trafficking by actin comet-tail motility. *Biomaterials.* 30, 951–958

69. Dean, D. A., Strong, D. D., and Zimmer, W. E. (2005) Nuclear entry of nonviral vectors. *Gene Ther.* 12, 881–890

70. Braun, K., von Brasch, L., Pipkorn, R., Ehemann, V., Jenne, J., Spring, H., Debus, J., Didinger, B., Rittgen, W., and Waldeck, W. (2007) BioShuttle-mediated plasmid transfer. *Int J Med Sci.* 4, 267–277

71. de la Fuente, J. M. and Berry, C. C. (2005) Tat peptide as an efficient molecule to translocate gold nanoparticles into the cell nucleus. *Bioconjug Chem.* 16, 1176–1180

72. Ozawa, C. R., Banfi, A., Glazer, N. L., Thurston, G., Springer, M. L., Kraft, P. E., McDonald, D. M., and Blau, H. M. (2004) Microenvironmental VEGF concentration, not total dose, determines a threshold between normal and aberrant angiogenesis. *J Clin Invest.* 113, 516–527

73. Silva, E. A. and Mooney, D. J. (2010) Effects of VEGF temporal and spatial presentation on angiogenesis. *Biomaterials.* 31, 1235–1241

74. Meilander, N. J., Pasumarthy, M. K., Kowalczyk, T. H., Cooper, M. J., and Bellamkonda, R. V. (2003) Sustained release of plasmid DNA using lipid microtubules and agarose hydrogel. *J Control Release.* 88, 321–331

75. Luciani, A., Coccoli, V., Orsi, S., Ambrosio, L., and Netti, P. A. (2008) PCL microspheres based functional scaffolds by bottom-up approach with predefined microstructural properties and release profiles. *Biomaterials.* 29, 4800–4807

76. Wang, X., Wenk, E., Zhang, X., Meinel, L., Vunjak-Novakovic, G., and Kaplan, D. L. (2009) Growth factor gradients via microsphere delivery in biopolymer scaffolds for osteochondral tissue engineering. *J Control Release.* 134, 81–90

77. Guo, X., Park, H., Young, S., Kretlow, J. D., van den Beucken, J. J., Baggett, L. S., Tabata, Y., Kasper, F. K., Mikos, A. G., and Jansen, J. A. (2010) Repair of osteochondral defects with biodegradable hydrogel composites encapsulating marrow mesenchymal stem cells in a rabbit model. *Acta Biomater.* 6, 39–47

78. Richardson, T. P., Peters, M. C., Ennett, A. B., and Mooney, D. J. (2001) Polymeric system for dual growth factor delivery. *Nat Biotechnol.* 19, 1029–1034

79. Basmanav, F. B., Kose, G. T., and Hasirci, V. (2008) Sequential growth factor delivery from complexed microspheres for bone tissue engineering. *Biomaterials.* 29, 4195–4204

80. Yilgor, P., Hasirci, N., and Hasirci, V. (2010) Sequential BMP-2/BMP-7 delivery from polyester nanocapsules. *J Biomed Mater Res A.* 93, 528–536

81. Yilgor, P., Tuzlakoglu, K., Reis, R. L., Hasirci, N., and Hasirci, V. (2009) Incorporation of a sequential BMP-2/BMP-7 delivery system into chitosan-based scaffolds for bone tissue engineering. *Biomaterials.* 30, 3551–3559

82. Trentin, D., Hall, H., Wechsler, S., and Hubbell, J. A. (2006) Peptide-matrix-mediated gene transfer of an oxygen-insensitive hypoxia-inducible factor-1{alpha}variant for local induction of angiogenesis. *Proc Natl Acad Sci U S A*

83. Han, K., Lee, K. D., Gao, Z. G., and Park, J. S. (2001) Preparation and evaluation of poly(L-lactic acid) microspheres containing rhEGF for chronic gastric ulcer healing. *J Control Release.* 75, 259–269

84. Zhao, X., Jain, S., Benjamin Larman, H., Gonzalez, S., and Irvine, D. J. (2005) Directed cell migration via chemoattractants released from degradable microspheres. *Biomaterials.* 26, 5048–5063

85. Lee, J., Oh, Y. J., Lee, S. K., and Lee, K. Y. (2010) Facile control of porous structures of polymer microspheres using an osmotic agent for pulmonary delivery. *J Control Release.* 146, 61–67

86. Cao, X. and Shoichet, M. S. (1999) Delivering neuroactive molecules from biodegradable microspheres for application in central nervous system disorders. *Biomaterials.* 20, 329–339

87. Shenoy, D. B., D'Souza, R. J., Tiwari, S. B., and Udupa, N. (2003) Potential applications of polymeric microsphere suspension as subcutaneous depot for insulin. *Drug Dev Ind Pharm.* 29, 555–563

88. Onishi, H., Machida, Y., and Koyama, K. (2007) Preparation and in vitro characteristics of lactoferrin-loaded chitosan microparticles. *Drug Dev Ind Pharm.* 33, 641–647

89. Solorio, L., Zwolinski, C., Lund, A. W., Farrell, M. J., and Stegemann, J. P. (2010) Gelatin microspheres crosslinked with genipin for local delivery of growth factors. *J Tissue Eng Regen Med.* 4, 514–523

90. Tabata, Y., Hijikata, S., Muniruzzaman, M., and Ikada, Y. (1999) Neovascularization effect of biodegradable gelatin microspheres incorporating basic fibroblast growth factor. *J Biomater Sci Polym Ed.* 10, 79–94

91. Coppi, G., Iannuccelli, V., Bernabei, M., and Cameroni, R. (2002) Alginate microparticles for enzyme peroral administration. *Int J Pharm.* 242, 263–266

92. Hahn, S. K., Kim, S. J., Kim, M. J., and Kim, D. H. (2004) Characterization and in vivo study of sustained-release formulation of human growth hormone using sodium hyaluronate. *Pharm Res.* 21, 1374–1381

93. Kim, S. J., Hahn, S. K., Kim, M. J., Kim, D. H., and Lee, Y. P. (2005) Development of a novel sustained release formulation of recombinant human growth hormone using sodium hyaluronate microparticles. *J Control Release.* 104, 323–335

94. Meilander, N. J., Yu, X., Ziats, N. P., and Bellamkonda, R. V. (2001) Lipid-based microtubular drug delivery vehicles. *J Control Release.* 71, 141–152

95. Kang, F., Jiang, G., Hinderliter, A., DeLuca, P. P., and Singh, J. (2002) Lysozyme stability in primary emulsion for PLGA microsphere preparation: effect of recovery methods and stabilizing excipients. *Pharm Res.* 19, 629–633

96. Sah, H. (1999) Protein behavior at the water/methylene chloride interface. *J Pharm Sci.* 88, 1320–1325

97. Griebenow, K. and Klibanov, A. M. (1997) Can conformational changes be responsible for solvent and excipient effects on the catalytic behavior of subtilisin Carlsberg in organic solvents? *Biotechnology and Bioengineering.* 53, 351–362

98. Knubovets, T., Osterhout, J. J., and Klibanov, A. M. (1999) Structure of lysozyme dissolved in neat organic solvents as assessed by NMR and CD spectroscopies. *Biotechnol Bioeng.* 63, 242–248

99. Fu, K., Klibanov, A. M., and Langer, R. (2000) Protein stability in controlled-release systems. *Nat Biotechnol.* 18, 24–25

100. Sah, H. (1999) Protein instability toward organic solvent/water emulsification: implications for protein microencapsulation into microspheres. *PDA J Pharm Sci Technol.* 53, 3–10

101. van de Weert, M., Hoechstetter, J., Hennink, W. E., and Crommelin, D. J. (2000) The effect of a water/organic solvent interface on the structural stability of lysozyme. *J Control Release.* 68, 351–359

102. Greiner, A. and Wendorff, J. H. (2007) Electrospinning: a fascinating method for the preparation of ultrathin fibers. *Angew Chem Int Ed Engl.* 46, 5670–5703

103. Sill, T. J. and von Recum, H. A. (2008) Electrospinning: Applications in drug delivery and tissue engineering. *Biomaterials.* 29, 1989–2006

104. Matthews, J. A., Wnek, G. E., Simpson, D. G., and Bowlin, G. L. (2002) Electrospinning of collagen nanofibers. *Biomacromolecules.* 3, 232–238

105. Zeugolis, D. I., Khew, S. T., Yew, E. S., Ekaputra, A. K., Tong, Y. W., Yung, L. Y., Hutmacher, D. W., Sheppard, C., and Raghunath, M. (2008) Electro-spinning of pure collagen nano-fibres – just an expensive way to make gelatin? *Biomaterials.* 29, 2293–2305

106. Zeng, J., Aigner, A., Czubayko, F., Kissel, T., Wendorff, J. H., and Greiner, A. (2005) Poly(vinyl alcohol) nanofibers by electrospinning as a protein delivery system and the retardation of enzyme release by additional polymer coatings. *Biomacromolecules.* 6, 1484–1488

107. Kenawy el, R., Bowlin, G. L., Mansfield, K., Layman, J., Simpson, D. G., Sanders, E. H., and Wnek, G. E. (2002) Release of tetracycline hydrochloride from electrospun poly(ethylene-co-vinylacetate), poly(lactic acid), and a blend. *J Control Release.* 81, 57–64

108. Kim, K., Luu, Y. K., Chang, C., Fang, D., Hsiao, B. S., Chu, B., and Hadjiargyrou, M. (2004) Incorporation and controlled release of a hydrophilic antibiotic using poly(lactide-co-glycolide)-based electrospun nanofibrous scaffolds. *J Control Release.* 98, 47–56

109. He, C. L., Huang, Z. M., and Han, X. J. (2009) Fabrication of drug-loaded electrospun aligned fibrous threads for suture applications. *J Biomed Mater Res A.* 89, 80–95

110. Jiang, H., Hu, Y., Li, Y., Zhao, P., Zhu, K., and Chen, W. (2005) A facile technique to prepare biodegradable coaxial electrospun nanofibers for controlled release of bioactive agents. *J Control Release.* 108, 237–243

111. Liang, D., Luu, Y. K., Kim, K., Hsiao, B. S., Hadjiargyrou, M., and Chu, B. (2005) In vitro non-viral gene delivery with nanofibrous scaffolds. *Nucleic Acids Res.* 33, e170

112. Jiang, H., Hu, Y., Zhao, P., Li, Y., and Zhu, K. (2006) Modulation of protein release from biodegradable core-shell structured fibers prepared by coaxial electrospinning. *J Biomed Mater Res B Appl Biomater.* 79, 50–57

113. Sahoo, S., Ang, L. T., Goh, J. C., and Toh, S. L. (2009) Growth factor delivery through electrospun nanofibers in scaffolds for tissue engineering applications. *J Biomed Mater Res A*

114. Chew, S. Y., Wen, J., Yim, E. K., and Leong, K. W. (2005) Sustained release of proteins from electrospun biodegradable fibers. *Biomacromolecules.* 6, 2017–2024

115. Li, X., Su, Y., Liu, S., Tan, L., Mo, X., and Ramakrishna, S. Encapsulation of proteins in poly(L-lactide-co-caprolactone) fibers by emulsion electrospinning. *Colloids Surf B Biointerfaces.* 75, 418–424

116. Yan, S., Xiaoqiang, L., Shuiping, L., Xiumei, M., and Ramakrishna, S. (2009) Controlled release of dual drugs from emulsion electrospun nanofibrous mats. *Colloids Surf B Biointerfaces.* 73, 376–381

117. Zhang, J., Montanez, S. I., Jewell, C. M., and Lynn, D. M. (2007) Multilayered films fabricated from plasmid DNA and a side-chain functionalized poly(beta-amino ester): surface-type erosion and sequential release of multiple plasmid constructs from surfaces. *Langmuir.* 23, 11139–11146

118. Wood, K. C., Boedicker, J. Q., Lynn, D. M., and Hammond, P. T. (2005) Tunable drug release from hydrolytically degradable layer-by-layer thin films. *Langmuir.* 21, 1603–1609

119. Jewell, C. M., Zhang, J., Fredin, N. J., Wolff, M. R., Hacker, T. A., and Lynn, D. M. (2006) Release of plasmid DNA from intravascular stents coated with ultrathin multilayered polyelectrolyte films. *Biomacromolecules.* 7, 2483–2491

120. Caruso, F., Caruso, R. A., and Mohwald, H. (1999) Production of hollow microspheres from nanostructured composite particles. *Chemistry of Materials.* 11, 3309–3314

121. Caruso, F. and Mohwald, H. (1999) Protein multilayer formation on colloids through a stepwise self-assembly technique. *J Am Chem Soc.* 121, 6039–6046

122. Kakade, S., Manickam, D. S., Handa, H., Mao, G., and Oupicky, D. (2009) Transfection activity of layer-by-layer plasmid DNA/poly(ethylenimine) films deposited on PLGA microparticles. *Int J Pharm.* 365, 44–52

123. Saul, J. M., Wang, C.-H. K., Ng, C. P., and Pun, S. H. (2008) Multilayer Nanocomplexes of Polymer and DNA Exhibit Enhanced Gene Delivery. *Advanced Materials.* 20, 19–25

124. Saul, J. M., Linnes, M. P., Ratner, B. D., Giachelli, C. M., and Pun, S. H. (2007) Delivery of non-viral gene carriers from sphere-templated fibrin scaffolds for sustained transgene expression. *Biomaterials.* 28, 4705–4716

125. Segura, T. and Shea, L. D. (2002) Surface-tethered DNA complexes for enhanced gene delivery. *Bioconjug Chem.* 13, 621–629

126. Huang, S. L. and MacDonald, R. C. (2004) Acoustically active liposomes for drug encapsulation and ultrasound-triggered release. *Biochim Biophys Acta.* 1665, 134–141

127. Kikuchi, A. and Okano, T. (2002) Pulsatile drug release control using hydrogels. *Adv Drug Deliv Rev.* 54, 53–77

7

Bioreactor Technologies for Tissue Engineering a Replacement Heart Valve

STEFANIE BIECHLER, MICHAEL J. YOST, RICHARD L. GOODWIN, AND JAY D. POTTS

Introduction

Cardiovascular disease is the leading cause of death in America, and of those deaths, 20,000 are caused by some form of valve disease. Additionally, congenital heart disease, of which valve defects are most common, is the leading cause of death in newborns worldwide [1]. Therefore, a great deal of research has aimed at the development of new treatments and therapies for patients with cardiovascular valve disease. The most common valve diseases include stenosis, or stiffening, and prolapse, or weakening, of valve tissue. Valve diseases such as these result in complete blockage of flow or regurgitation of blood back through the heart, and ultimately, patients experience congestive heart failure and inadequate delivery of nutrients to the body tissue.

These conditions are treated differently depending on the type of valve affected. Typically, atrioventricular (AV) valves are repaired with a conservative surgery performed on the underlying muscle tissue because of the difficulty of a total replacement surgery; however, semilunar (SL) valves, such as the aortic valve, are commonly replaced completely when affected with valve disease [2]. Replacement valves are typically mechanical constructs or are made of biologic tissues such as bovine pericardium, porcine valve tissue, or, less commonly, human valve tissue. Mechanical valves are structurally stable compared with biologic valves; however, patients have an increased risk of thrombosis and must take anticlotting drugs. Conversely, biologic valve replacements are not associated with thrombosis but quickly weaken and degenerate. Therefore, biologic valves commonly have to be replaced and are particularly undesirable in younger patients. Biologic valves directly taken from another human donor (homografts) are rare, so biologic replacements typically originate from a different species (xenografts), and patients still have risk of rejection and infection.

The most ideal treatment option, suitable for both AV and SL valves, would be to engineer a replacement heart valve from autologous tissue; however, before this

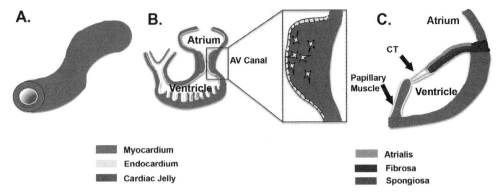

Figure 7-1. Early development of the atrioventricular (AV) valves. (**A**) The early heart tube consists of myocardium (*red*) and endocardium (*yellow*) with a layer of extracellular matrix known as the cardiac jelly (*blue*) between them. (**B**) In the AV canal region of the developing heart, the cardiac jelly expands to form padlike structures that eventually fuse and are filled by migrating stellate-shaped mesenchyme produced as the result of epithelial-to-mesenchymal transformation. (**C**) In the mature heart, this pad is sculpted as a result of fluid dynamics coupled with cellular reprogramming to produce a trilaminar structure. The atrialis (*green*) consists of primarily of elastin fibers, the spongiosa (*blue*) contains glycosaminoglycans, and the fibrosa (*purple*) is mostly collagen type I. This trilaminar structure is maintained in both the AV and semilunar valves. CT = chordae tendinae. (See color plate 13.)

approach can be clinically implemented, all aspects of valve development must be identified. It has been proposed that biochemical factors and physical forces work in concert to control valve morphogenesis [3–5]. Forces associated with hydrodynamic pressure, shear stress, and tissue strain are likely sensed by cells, leading to the initiation of various biochemical signaling cascades in the valve tissue [6]. Up until recent years, the majority of attention paid to valve development focused on understanding the biochemical pathways linked to various stages in development. Specifically, the primitive stages of valve development have become well understood during the time points leading up to a process known as epithelial-to-mesenchymal transformation (EMT) [3,5,6]. Commonly, these stages are associated with the first 3.5 days of chick development and the first 6 weeks of human development. During these stages, there is relatively low blood flow through the embryonic heart. The connected role between biochemical and mechanical factors in the embryonic heart has not been extensively investigated beyond these stages.

The heart initiates as a simple, two-cell layer tube that then becomes slightly constricted at the center to define atrial and ventricular sections. The outer layer, the myocardium, secretes an acellular substance known as cardiac jelly that fills the region between the outer and inner layer (endocardium, Fig. 7-1A). Biochemical signaling molecules produced in the myocardium then induce a phenotypic change in the endocardium during EMT (Fig. 7-1B). The newly transformed mesenchymal cells migrate into the cardiac jelly, and two cardiac cushions begin to form on opposite sides of the tube lumen. Eventually, these inferior and superior cushions grow toward one another and fuse, separating the right and left sides of the heart (future AV valves) and the outflow tract (future SL valves). After the EMT process, smaller subsets of cushions then begin to form as cushion myofibroblasts begin producing collagen on the downstream side of the cushions. These subsets then elongate into leaflets during which point they begin to exhibit three distinct layers (Fig. 7-1C).

The atrialis (in AV valves) or ventricularis (in SL valves) is located on the inflow side of the leaflet. These inflow layers are composed mostly of elastin, which aids to restore leaflet configuration after contraction [6]. The middle layer of valve tissue in both AV and SL valves is the spongiosa, which is composed primarily of proteoglycans that act to absorb shock. The layer situated in the ventricular (outflow) side of both AV and SL valves is the fibrosa, which is composed of collagen [7]. Collagen is the primary extracellular matrix (ECM) component that functions in support. Throughout development, valve leaflets, along with the rest of the heart interior, are covered in a single layer of endothelial cells that aids to prevent thrombosis. These three layers, as well as the endothelial layer, remain intact as development concludes. During the final stages of valve development, the valve leaflets delaminate from the wall. In the case of AV valves, leaflets become anchored to ventricular papillary muscle by connective chordae tendineae. A different yet comparable form of connective tissue acts as a hinge-like anchor at the roots of SL valves [6,7].

Although this overall process of valve morphogenesis has become well defined, much less is known about the role of physical forces such as flow-induced shear stress and pressure or contractile flexure and compression of the tissue. To better understand the role of these factors in valve development, it has been proposed to use bioreactors. The use of such reactors, along with the added benefit of computer-aided simulations, may allow researchers to fully understand valve development and to eventually condition custom replacement valves through tissue engineering. Here, current bioreactor technologies being used to investigate the individual and combined roles of physical forces on valve development are summarized, and their proposed use in tissue engineering of autologous valves is discussed.

Review

Current bioreactors typically fall into two primary categories. Either reactor systems are designed simply to investigate the role of individual physical factors or the system is designed with great complexity to closely mimic every aspect of the physiological environment involved in valve development. Specifically, simple reactor systems typically seek to match the pressure waveform, the flow rate, or the valve flexure of native heart valves undergoing in vivo development. The valve constructs used in these systems may be either completely autologous or composed of autologous cells seeded to a biodegradable polymeric scaffold. Autologous constructs are typically composed of cells seeded to a separately molded acellular matrix component; however, some studies show it is possible to implement bioreactor technologies on wholly dissected autologous valves [8]. All reactor systems discussed here have been used under sterile conditions.

Simple Pressure Duplicator Reactors

The first group of simple reactors includes systems that use air-driven (respirator) pumps to match the pressure waveforms in the developing heart. In a study conducted by Hoerstrup et al., a new reactor was developed that consisted of a Plexiglas flow chamber containing a perfusion section with nutrient media and an air section separated by a moveable membrane [9]. The flow chamber was attached to a respirator pump. An adjustable ventilation rate allowed for various physiological pressures to be maintained which pushed fluid up to the perfusion chamber and into contact with an anchored biodegradable polymeric aortic valve. Specifically, the study aimed at addressing the degradation of the polymeric scaffold because of preconditioning. Before a valve of this type can be inserted in a patient, the polymeric scaffold must completely degrade to prevent host–tissue reactions, and the autologous cells must begin to secrete ECM as the primary support tissue. Although the generated pressures were not complete physiological replicates because they were kept steady over long intervals of time, the valve tissue still showed signs of pressure-induced scaffold degradation. Even though scaffold degradation was witnessed in the study, accompanying ECM generation was not evaluated to classify tissue strength.

In another study that sought to maintain specified pressures in a simple reactor system, Flanagan et al. demonstrated the physiological remodeling of completely autologous valves [10]. The valve in the study was composed of biologic fibrin extracted from the bloodstream. A gelatinous form of the fibrin was used to permeate a scaffold mesh to form a trileaflet (aortic valve) mold, and the mold was then seeded with carotid artery cells. The bioreactor used in the study was comparable to the reactor used by Hoerstrup et al. [9]. The group conditioned valves for several days at a low pressure differential (20 mm Hg) in conjunction with the native environment. During the conditioning period, the reactor pulse rate was increased from 5 to 10 beats/min. After conditioning the valve for several days, immunohistochemistry and protein assays were used to classify valve maturation. Overall, conditioning was found to increase cell proliferation, attachment, and alignment to flow. Additionally, a drastic increase in ECM proteins was found, including collagen (types I and II), glycoproteins (fibronectin and laminin), and glycosaminoacids (GAGs). Although it was hypothesized that this remodeling resulted in increased tissue strength and durability, no material strength tests were performed.

Simple Flexure Duplicator Reactors

The second group of simple reactor systems includes those designed to evaluate flexure and strain on tissue samples. Two studies performed by Engelmayr et al. [11,12] implemented the independent use of three-point, unidirectional cyclic flexure to stiffen biodegradable polymeric scaffolds. In the first study, the bioreactor was used to apply cyclic flexure for several weeks after which time the samples were removed and material properties were evaluated [11]. The sample was marked with a dot, and tensile tests were performed to measure dot displacement and evaluate the effective valve stiffness. Using this method, the group showed that flexed samples demonstrated a decreased stiffness and directional anisotropy. It was proposed that this decreased stiffness might be attributable to inadequate conditioning time. In a second, similar study, Engelmayr et al. showed the effects of the same cyclic flexure on ECM development [12]. Flexed scaffolds were found to contain homogeneous cell distribution and increased collagen deposition. Accordingly, the effective stiffness was found to increase in flexed tissue samples with increased collagen levels. Syedain and Tranquillo performed another study to demonstrate the role of cyclic flexure on fibrin-based, trileaflet scaffolds seeded with human dermal cells [13]. The valve construct was attached to a segment of latex tube, and the tube was then attached to a reactor that allowed close control of tube stretching at the valve base. An additional flow circuit provided slow but adequate delivery of nutrient-enriched media to the tissue. Through use of the ink dot method, leaflets were found to have improved tensile properties after conditioning. Additionally, mature collagen was shown to invade the fibrin mold at the leaflet root while most of the scaffold fibrin degraded.

Simple Flow Duplicator Reactors

The final group of simple bioreactors includes systems that aim to mimic physiological flows. Sodian et al. conducted a study to determine optimal preconditioning parameters of a biodegradable, trileaflet scaffold seeded with carotid artery cells [14]. The valve scaffold geometry was replicated from an adult AV valve. The scaffold was attached to a cylindrical stent and situated in a basic flow reactor with a circulating peristaltic pump. Flow was controlled over 8 days, allowing the valve to synchronously open and close with pump pulses. The longest conditioning interval of 8 days was found to optimize cell proliferation growth into the scaffold. Collagen, elastin, and GAGs were deposited into the scaffold pores, illustrating that flow alone can induce ECM formation. In a study conducted by Weston and Yoganathan, the effects of steady and pulsatile flow (caused by a peristaltic pump) on adult aortic leaflets were compared [15]. The leaflet was attached to a basic flow reactor containing circulating media. Protein levels, proteoglycan levels, and DNA synthesis in both flow groups were comparable to native levels. The study proposed the tensegrity model as a possible mechanism in which bulk stress caused by flow leads to increased tensile forces on the ECM. In biology, the tensegrity model states that mechanical stability in a tensegrity structure is achieved through the interactive distribution and balance of mechanical stresses as opposed to the strength of individual components [16]. Increased tensile forces on the ECM are expected to translate into the cell nucleus where synthesis is directed, thus altering cellular mechanisms.

Karim et al. replicated physiological flows by slightly altering the basic flow reactor design [17]. The group added a rotational component to a cylindrical reactor to determine the optimal parameters in the decellularization and recellularization of SL valves. The group used adult sow SL valves (both AV and SL) in their experiments. The valves were fastened to an inner mounting device inside the cylindrical flow chamber and subjected to rotation followed by nutrient perfusion. Flow rate, rotation rate, and seeding time were optimized to fully decellularize and recellularize the valve construct. A perfusion rate of 18.8 mL/min, a rotation rate of 0.1 turns/min, and a seeding time of 16 hours were found to optimize this process. The group found that with a further increased rotation (higher than 0.1 turns/min) ECM components were degraded.

Another flow mimicking reactor to be discussed is the cone-and-plate viscometer used by Sucosky et al. [18]. Even though this reactor does not exactly replicate flow waveforms, physiological shear stresses were replicated from computational fluid dynamics (CFD) model and Doppler velocimetry flow approximations of the in vivo heart. The cone-and-plate reactor, which was used with aortic valve leaflet tissue, was shown to reduce secondary flow effects and closely mimic in vivo flow-induced shear stress.

Although all of these studies were performed on native adult SL valves or biodegradable scaffold replicates of adult SL valves, new research is being conducted on native embryonic valves [8]. We have developed a basic pulsatile flow bioreactor system composed of a peristaltic pump and a glass bioreactor chamber (Fig. 7-2). The chamber was engineered for use with a custom, three-dimensional collagen tube scaffold. The tubular scaffold is composed of aligned bovine collagen (type I). To allow for proper fibril alignment, collagen is extruded through two counter-rotating cones and into an ammonia-rich polymerization chamber. This process allows for scaffold extrusion of different tube lengths and diameters. The custom tubular scaffold can be easily sutured into the bioreactor glass chamber. Two adjustable nozzle attachments that are mounted to the chamber inflow and outflow sections provide an attachment site for the scaffold. Media from the peristaltic pump is transferred through the inlet nozzle and into the collagen tube. The media then circulates back through the outlet nozzle and returns to the pump, completing a closed flow circuit. The primary advantage of the collagen tube scaffold is the geometric similarity to the early embryonic heart tube. An early valve cushion (chick) can easily be dissected from the embryonic heart and implanted to the lumen of the scaffold. The scaffold can then be connected to

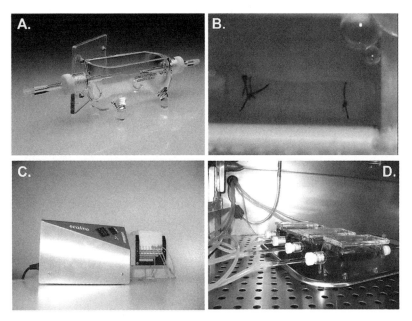

Figure 7-2. Fluid flow bioreactor system. (**A**) The glass bioreactor. (**B**) The collagen tube scaffold attached to the bioreactor. (**C**) The positive displacement pump. (**D**) Fluid flow bioreactor systems inside an incubator. (See color plate 14.)

the flow circuit so that embryonic-like flows can be applied to the cushion and developmental valve morphogenesis can be analyzed over time. Simple two-dimensional CFD models of in vivo flow through the embryonic heart tube can be used to determine the appropriate embryonic-like flows that should be implemented in the bioreactor [19]. Preliminary studies by Goodwin et al. have implemented the predicted in-vivo flow rates from Biechler et al. over embryonic chick AV leaflets implanted to the tubular scaffold. Immunohistochemistry showed that flow culture increased collagen production in the leaflet. Furthermore, force–distance measurements obtained using atomic force microscopy allowed for characterization of tissue stiffness through the Hertz model. Flow culture was found to increase the elastic modulus (stiffness) of the tissue.

Complex Reactors

The second class of bioreactor systems includes complex systems that seek to replicate every aspect of physiological development while maintaining sterility. Additionally, these systems typically use a more sophisticated form of computer-aided control as opposed to manual control and intervention. Hildebrand et al. was one of the first groups to implement this complex technology in the tissue engineering of heart valves [4]. Their system consisted of a vented mechanical atrium that filled a pneumatic ventricle containing a biodegradable aortic valve construct seeded with smooth muscle cells. The compliant ventricle contained an air side and a media side with a mechanical valve at inflow and the bioprosthetic valve at the outflow. The attached pumping system contained a proportional pressure regulator and pressure transducers at inflow and outflow of the ventricle. An ultrasonic flow probe was also situated at the ventricle outflow so both pressure and flow could be highly maintained. Finally, the system contained an afterload setup with adjustable compliance and resistance. The group was able to exactly replicate the flow waveform over time in the ventricular chamber and closely matched the pressure waveform, indicating that with the correct system, multiple aspects of heart development can be replicated simultaneously. There have been several complex bioreactor systems similar to this classic system that mimic preload, afterload, flow rate (and thus shear stress), and pressure [20,21]. Lee et al. [18] recently proposed a system that controlled these variables to decellularize and recellularize autologous porcine aortic valves [22]. The optimal maximum flow rate of 2 L/min was found for endothelialization of the autologous scaffold to yield antithrombotic clinical implications. The flow rate was increased in a stepwise fashion over the course of 7 days until this maximum, optimal flow rate was reached. The mechanical loading caused endothelial cell differentiation and organization into capillary-like structures aligned in the direction of flow. Narita et al. developed a balloon pumping system to highly control pressure, preload, and afterload [23]. The system also consisted of a compliance chamber to generate pulsatility and a clamp resistor to regulate afterload. Canine aortic cells were seeded to a biodegradable aortic scaffold that was placed in the flow chamber. The group monitored pressure and flow rate closely and estimated shear stress computationally. The reactor system was found to operate over a wide range of flow parameters, including flow rates from 0 to 3000 mL/min, systolic pressures of 10 to 200 mm Hg, and diastolic pressures of 0 to 100 mm Hg. Natural flow and pressure waveforms could easily be reached within this range of parameters for many different developmental models (e.g., human, chick). Cell proliferation was greatest for controlled, natural waveforms. Furthermore, proteoglycan and GAG production was found to be greatest for controlled, natural waveforms. The success of this study in achieving such a wide range of controllable flow parameters demonstrates a promising bridge to future clinical applications.

A particular class of complex reactor systems, referred to as diastolic phase duplicators (DPDs), was first introduced by Mol et al. and has since been used among several groups [16,24–26]. The first DPD system consisted of a reactor containing a biodegradable aortic valve scaffold and a media reservoir. A roller pump was used to circulate media. Pressure over the valve was highly controlled (LabView software) to replicate diastolic phase pressures occurring in vivo. To supplement the in-vitro data, finite element analysis was performed for the flow system to evaluate mechanical distributions of strains present on the leaflet. The group went on to add a feedback controller to the DPD system so that local deformations could be monitored and highly controlled during load [21]. Before this development, the main drawback of DPD systems was a lack of load control; however, with this new feedback system, DPD reactors have become capable of maintaining controlled pressure, flow and flexure.

Conclusions

Here, current bioreactor systems used in the tissue engineering of heart valves were summarized and compared. Reactors were classified into two groups including simple systems geared to replicate a single aspect of valve development and complex systems developed to closely mimic several aspects of valve development. The studies presented here showed that individual and combined mechanical factors, such as flow-induced pressure, shear stress, and flexure, can induce valve morphogenesis by improving ECM growth (collagen, elastin, proteogylcans, glycoproteins, and GAGs). Several studies also showed that the increase in ECM components such as collagen led to an increase in overall tissue strength through various tensile tests. Studies were performed on valves composed of seeded cells on a scaffold. Scaffolds were either completely biologic (composed of fibrin or collagen) or biodegradable polymers, both of which are suitable for future clinical use. The collective results of these studies give insight to the mechanical aspects of heart valve development and indicate a promising future in the tissue engineering of autologous heart valves.

References

1. AHA. *Congenital Cardiovascular Defects. Diseases and Conditions.* American Heart Association, Dallas, TX, 2010.
2. Filova, E., Straka, F., Mirejovsky, T., Masin, J., Bacakova, L. Tissue-engineered heart valves. *Physiol Res* 58:S141–S158, 2009.
3. Butcher, J. T., McQuinn, T. C., Sedmera, D., Turner, D., Markwald, R. R. Transitions in early embryonic atrioventricular valvular function correspond with changes in cushion biomechanics that are predictable by tissue composition. *Circ Res* 100(10):1503–1511, 2007.
4. Hildebrand, D. K., Wu, Z. J. J., Mayer, J. E., Sacks, M. S. Design and hydrodynamic evaluation of a novel pulsatile bioreactor for biologically active heart valves. *Ann Biomed Eng* 32(8):1039–1049, 2004.
5. Sacks, M. S., Schoen, F. J., Mayer, J. E. Bioengineering challenges for heart valve tissue engineering. *Ann Rev Biomed Eng* 11:289–313, 2009.
6. Combs, M. D., Yutzey, K. E. Heart valve development regulatory networks in development and disease. *Circ Res* 105(5):408–421, 2009.
7. Hinton, R. B., Lincoln, J., Deutsch, G. H., Osinska, H., Manning, P. B., Benson, D. W., Yutzey, K. E. Extracellular matrix remodeling and organization in developing and diseased aortic valves. *Circ Res* 98(11):1431–1438, 2006.
8. Goodwin, R. L., Nesbitt, T., Price, R. L., Wells, J. C., Yost, M. J., Potts, J. D. Three-dimensional model system of valvulogenesis. *Dev Dynam* 233(1):122–129, 2005.
9. Hoerstrup, S. P., Sodian, R., Sperling, J. S., Vacanti, J. P., Mayer, J. E. New pulsatile bioreactor for in vitro formation of tissue engineered heart valves. *Tissue Eng* 6(1):75–79, 2000.
10. Flanagan, T. C., Cornelissen, C., Koch, S., Tschoeke, B., Sachweh, J. S., Schmitz-Rode, T., Jockenhoevel, S. The in vitro development of autologous fibrin-based

tissue-engineered heart valves through optimised dynamic conditioning. *Biomaterials* 28(23):3388–3397, 2007.

11. Engelmayr, G. C., Hildebrand, D. K., Sutherland, F. W. H., Mayer, J. E., Sacks, M. S. A novel bioreactor for the dynamic flexural stimulation of tissue engineered heart valve biomaterials. *Biomaterials* 24(14):2523–2532, 2003.

12. Engelmayr, G. C., Rabkin, E., Sutherland, F. W. H., Schoen, F. J., Mayer, J. E., Sacks, M. S. The independent role of cyclic flexure in the early in vitro development of an engineered heart valve tissue. *Biomaterials* 26(2):175–187, 2005.

13. Sodian, R., Hoerstrup, S. P., Sperling, J. S., Daebritz, S. H., Martin, D. P., Schoen, F. J., Vacanti, J. P., Mayer, J. E. Tissue engineering of heart valves: In vitro experiences. *Ann Thorac Surg* 70(1):140–144, 2000.

14. Syedain, Z. H., Tranquillo, R. T. Controlled cyclic stretch bioreactor for tissue-engineered heart valves. *Biomaterials* 30(25):4078–4084, 2009.

15. Weston, M. W., Yoganathan, A. P. Biosynthetic activity in heart valve leaflets in response to in vitro flow environments. *Ann Biomed Eng* 29(9):752–763, 2001.

16. Ingber, D. E. The architecture of life. *Sci Am* 278(1):48–57, 1998.

17. Karim, N., Golz, K., Bader, A. The cardiovascular tissue-reactor: A novel device for the engineering of heart valves. *Artif Organs* 30(10):809–814, 2006.

18. Sucosky, P., Padala, M., Elhammali, A., Balachandran, K., Jo, H., Yoganathan, A. P. Design of an ex vivo culture system to investigate the effects of shear stress on cardiovascular tissue. *J Biomech Eng* 130(3) 035001, 2008.

19. Biechler, S. V., Potts, J. D., Yost, M. J., Junor, L., Goodwin, R. L., Weidner, J. W. Mathematical Modeling of Flow-Generated Forces in an In Vitro System of Cardiac Valve Development. *Ann Biomed Eng* 38(1):109–117, 2010.

20. Lee, D. J., Steen, J., Jordan, J. E., Kincaid, E. H., Kon, N. D., Atala, A., Berry, J., Yoo, J. J. Endothelialization of heart valve matrix using a computer-assisted pulsatile bioreactor. *Tissue Eng Part A* 15(4):807–814, 2009.

21. Ruel, J., Lachance, G. A new bioreactor for the development of tissue-engineered heart valves. *Ann Biomed Eng* 37(4):674–681, 2009.

22. Kortsmit, J., Driessen, N. J. B., Rutten, M. C. M., Baaijens, F. P. T. Real time, non-invasive assessment of leaflet deformation in heart valve tissue engineering. *Ann Biomed Eng* 37(3):532–541, 2009.

23. Narita, Y., Hata, K. I., Kagami, H., Usui, A., Ueda, M., Ueda, Y. Novel pulse duplicating bioreactor system for tissue-engineered vascular construct. *Tissue Eng* 10(7–8):1224–1233, 2004.

24. Driessen, N. J. B., Mol, A., Bouten, C. V. C., Baaijens, F. P. T. Modeling the mechanics of tissue-engineered human heart valve leaflets. *J Biomech* 40(2):325–334, 2007.

25. Kortsmit, J., Rutten, M. C. M., Wijlaars, M. W., Baaijens, F. P. T. Deformation-controlled load application in heart valve tissue engineering. *Tissue Eng Part C* 15(4):707–716, 2009.

26. Mol, A., Driessen, N. J. B., Rutten, M. C. M., Hoerstrup, S. P., Bouten, C. V. C., Baaijens, F. P. T. Tissue engineering of human heart valve leaflets: A novel bioreactor for a strain-based conditioning approach. *Ann Biomed Eng* 33(12):1778–1788, 2005.

8

Incorporation of Active Factors (Pharmacological Substances) in Biomaterials for Tissue Engineering

ROCHE DE GUZMAN AND MARK VAN DYKE

In the context of tissue engineering and regenerative medicine, biomaterials are often used as scaffolding implants that act as a surrogate for the extracellular matrix (ECM), supporting local microenvironment-specific populations of cells for the augmentation, repair, or replacement of dysfunctional bodily tissues and organs. Because of the absence of cells and differences in structure, composition, and three-dimensional organization compared with the native tissue target, biomaterial substitutes are biologically and physically tissue mismatched. Thus, they are innately limited in their functional and regenerative capacities. An example is fibers made from the polymer poly(ethylene terephthalate) (PET), commonly known as Dacron, which is still currently being used as a large-diameter blood vessel graft [1]. The only resemblance of Dacron vascular graft to the normal vessel is the tubular solid geometry. On a short-term basis, this conduit works by acting as a means to route the circulation of blood. Protein adsorption at the solid (biomaterial surface)–liquid (blood plasma) interface allows the host cells to recognize the foreign surface and enables the formation of neointimal tissue on the inner wall. However, the newly formed ingrowth is not physiologically similar to the endothelium [2] that naturally covers the inner surface of blood vessels, consequently posing a risk of layer buildup, thrombosis, and occlusion. Repeated mechanical stresses encountered by the implant generates fatigue and material breakdown. Incomplete host cellular integration leads to a nonhealing response and eventual biomaterial implant failure [3].

The intrinsic limitations of biomaterials in their abilities to repair and restore themselves can be circumvented by physically modifying the feature, shape, and architecture of the material. For example, increasing the porosity and introducing nanometer-scale surface roughness is thought to mimic the physical attributes of native ECM. This method is useful for inducing certain direct and indirect beneficial cellular behaviors but does not discriminate between the types of cells that recognize the surface. A more selective and effective approach is to "functionalize" the biomaterial by incorporating bioactive factors or pharmacological substances to form a construct for attracting tissue-specific cells or intermediate cells that reside temporarily and aid in the healing process. Most tissues have the capacity to repair themselves after minor injury, partly because of adult stem cell populations that maintain their multipotency and differentiate to replace the damaged cells. The biomaterial construct may therefore be engineered to provide the necessary conditions for allowing these stem cells to localize and mature into functional specialized cells. Furthermore, the intrinsic restorative capabilities of tissues are in some cases mediated by the local production of growth factors that trigger the pro-regenerative cascade among cells. Thus, functionalization of biomaterials may involve the use of diffusible signaling molecules. Addition of active components may also be used for repulsion of unwanted cells that inhibit and obstruct tissue regeneration (e.g., the use of antibiotics to prevent bacterial infection). This chapter discusses various state-of-the-art methods for biomaterial functionalization, as well as future challenges to developing idealized technologies to initiate and direct the complete regeneration of damaged or deformed anatomic structures.

Desired Properties of an Ideal Biomaterial Construct

To develop the ideal biomaterial construct, the ultimate goal of biomedical engineers and scientists, it is worthwhile to enumerate the qualities that will theoretically give a completely healed tissue end product (Fig. 8-1). The construct should match the gross geometry and mechanical properties of the target tissue structure. Hence, blood vessel replacements are tubular-shaped conduits and can sustain the range of shear stresses generated by the flowing blood. Moreover, they must have adequate tensile strength and elasticity to withstand the constant physiological motion and deformation. Upon implantation, the biomaterial construct must adhere and integrate with adjacent host tissues to avoid dislocation. The initial biointegration is usually facilitated by the use of strong but degradable microsutures or bioadhesive tissue glue that forms tough chemical crosslinks between the host structure and the implanted device. These cohesive materials should not interfere with the biologic effects of the implanted tissue substitute. Host cells from the blood and surrounding structures will immediately be in contact with the material because all implantation procedures involve tissue disruption and wound formation. Accordingly, the biomaterial assembly must not induce these cells to undergo necrosis and apoptosis. The implant will initially be treated as a foreign body by the host immune system and will be subjected to the natural wound healing response of acute inflammation. An ideal construct is biocompatible and immunotolerable; thus, the starting inflammatory reaction should acutely diminish and not progress to the formation of chronic granuloma and activation of cellular and humoral immune rejection.

The ECM determines overall mechanical strength but is largely dependent on resident cells because they maintain the compositional and structural integrity. Cells

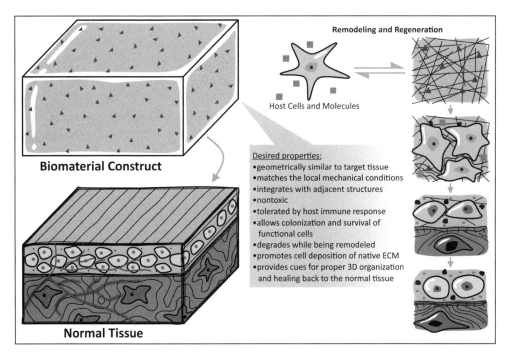

Figure 8-1. An ideal biomaterial construct for tissue engineering incorporates the physical features of the biomaterial with active biological factors. The in vivo regeneration process, dictated by the material and host interplay, replaces the relatively simple temporary structure with the complex normal tissue composed of organized cell populations restricted to their respective extracellular matrices. 3D = three-dimensional. (See color plate 15.)

are in constant feedback communication with their surrounding ECM and dynamically alter the ECM throughout the organism's lifespan. Minor structural damage to the ECM leads to cell-mediated repair and regeneration of the native matrix. To fully remodel an implanted biomaterial scaffold into a native tissue, it should first allow for the active migration, colonization, proliferation, differentiation, and maturation of cells. A population of cells must also be enabled to produce, secrete, and regulate their own natural ECM while embedded in the biomaterial matrix. Then the biomaterial must slowly degrade at the same time as the native ECM is being deposited, such that the tissue mechanical integrity requirements are not compromised. This attribute may be the hardest to satisfy because an optimal balance of resultant forces is needed throughout the remodeling event in which tissue composition is dynamically altered. The Dacron graft fails in this category because of its relative nondegradability, which as a consequence limits the space where native tissue can be formed. Biomaterial degradation is dependent on the chemical structure of the implant and is facilitated by the diffusional movement of interstitial fluid and by infiltrating capillaries.

Table 8-1 summarizes some commonly used degradable polymeric biomaterials for tissue engineering applications [4–12] (subsequent text discussions specifically

Table 8-1. *Degradable polymeric biomaterials for tissue engineering*

Polymer	Short name	Structural formula or repeating units
Aliphatic polyester		
Poly(glycolic acid)	PGA	1
Poly(lactic acid)	PLA PLLA PDLA	2
Poly(lactic-*co*-glycolic acid)	PLGA	3
Poly(ε-caprolactone)	PCL	4
Poly(propylene fumarate)	PPF	5
Poly(dioxanone)	PDO	6
Polyorthoester	POE	7
Polyanhydride	PAH	8

Polymer	Short name	Structural formula or repeating units
Polyurethane	PUR	9
Polyamidoamine	PAA	10
Modified poly(ethylene glycol)	mPEG	11
Polysaccharide Chitosan	CHI	12
Alginate	ALG	13
Agarose	AGA	14
Hyaluronic acid	HYA	15

(*continued*)

Table 8-1 *(continued)*

Polymer	Short name	Structural formula or repeating units
Protein and peptide		
Collagen	COL	[3 alpha subunits with [Pro-Hyp-Gly]$_n$]$_m$
Gelatin	GTN	[3 alpha subunits with [Pro-Hyp-Gly]$_n$]$_m$
Fibrin	FIB	[2 alpha, 2 beta, and 3 gamma subunits]$_n$
Fibroin	FBN	[1 heavy and 1 light subunits with [Gly-Ser-Gly-Ala-Gly-Ala]$_n$]$_m$
Keratin	KRT	[1 acidic and 1 basic subunits]$_n$
Peptide amphiphiles	PAM	[[Xaa]$_n$-alkyl group]$_m$

n, m = repeating units; R = functional group; Xaa = amino acid residue.

focus on some of these materials and their modification through addition of bioactive components). The polymeric nature of these implantable biomaterials suggests that their degradation products are composed of monomeric building blocks. An ideal biomaterial construct must have degradation products that are likewise biocompatible, noncytotoxic, nonpyrogenic, and noncarcinogenic. Additionally, degradation products should be biologically inert; should be easily phagocytosed by macrophages and other scavenger cells; and can be normally cleared through the circulatory, hepatic, and excretory systems of the body. All traces of the exogenous material should be removed when the normal tissue occupies the site of injury.

Cells are fed by oxygen that is carried by circulating erythrocytes. Thus, the biomaterial construct must permit the growth of vasculature for sustained cell viability and for efficient removal of metabolic wastes. The presence of interconnected pores in the scaffold enables both cell infiltration as well as penetration of blood vessels and terminal capillaries. Cartilage, meniscus, and cornea tissue engineering are exceptions because the mature tissues are expected to be avascular. The majority of the body tissues also contain lymphatic vessels and terminal nerve endings for lymph transport and sensation, respectively. The development of these structures, if applicable, should not be hindered by the biomaterial or the incorporated pharmacological substance(s).

Methods for Material Functionalization

Complete tissue healing relies on the biomaterial assembly's ability to direct the proper three-dimensional organization leading to the confinement of specialized cells to their respective ECM microenvironment and avoidance of chronic inflammation or scar tissue formation. Currently, there is limited knowledge on the multipotency of local infiltrating stem cells that mediate the rebuilding of injured tissue structures. However, it is likely that these stem cells, through their interaction with the biomaterial and host signals, can differentiate into multiple specialized cells that consequently deposit and

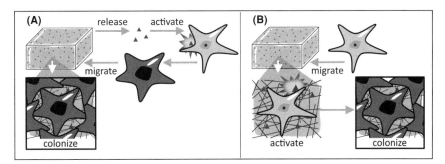

Figure 8-2. (**A**) Active factors incorporated within the biomaterial can be released into the surrounding tissues and subsequently activate target cells to migrate and colonize the scaffold. (**B**) Alternatively, motile target cells that invade the functionalized biomaterial can be induced to attach, differentiate, and populate the construct. (See color plate 16.)

regulate their respective unique ECM resulting in a fully healed anisotropic functional tissue (see Fig. 8-1).

Two general scenarios are likely to take place in allowing regenerative cells from the local microenvironment to penetrate and colonize a functionalized biomaterial construct (Fig. 8-2). The first one is the release of bioactive substances from the construct into the surrounding tissues to generate a gradient effect that activates target cells to move into the construct. Hence, the active components must have chemoattractive and promigratory properties for this event to take place. The target cells here, under normal circumstances, are relatively quiescent and sessile, thus the need for signal activation. This premise also holds for cell structure response toward the released stimuli. In peripheral nerves, for example, the delivered active factors allow for axonal elongation and directed growth into the biomaterial construct while neuronal cell bodies stay in place. In the second case, bioactive components bound to the polymer are retained so that upon encounter with invading cells, these cells are induced to attach, differentiate, and treat the scaffold as their local niche. In this setting, target cells such as leukocytes, fibroblasts, and certain stem cells are motile to begin with and can penetrate the exogenous material during the wound healing response. Therefore, the strategy for incorporation of active factors into biomaterials depends on the type of desired delivery system. Released substances must have a relatively low association with the biomaterial. The mechanism of active factor release may include desorption, diffusion, cleavage, or biomaterial degradation. In contrast, if the bioactive components are required to be immobilized, they must be covalently linked or the binding affinity to the scaffold otherwise assured to be high to prevent escape into the surrounding media before biomaterial breakdown.

A polymeric biomaterial is initially synthesized from repeating units of its monomeric building blocks as displayed in Table 8-1. Naturally occurring polymers such as polysaccharides and proteins are composed of sugar and amino acid residues, respectively, which are already synthesized in long and high-molecular weight chains. Synthetic polymers, however, are assembled via chemical reactions from small monomeric compounds. Hence, they provide more options for polymer modification such as incorporation of degradable components, crosslinkable groups, and other functional monomers. The polymer solution can then be electrospun to generate a thin, dense scaffold with relatively low porosity; thus, it can be considered a surface-acting biomaterial. In contrast to a smooth surface resembling a film, the electrospun construct has a high degree of roughness with a significantly increased surface area. Alternatively, polymers can be formed into a hydrogel via stabilizing the interchain interaction with entrapped water molecules by changing the solute concentration, temperature, pH, ion content, and molecular crosslinks. The gels can be lyophilized to make a spongelike, thick scaffold. Biomaterial scaffolds can also be fabricated through leaching of intermediate components with different solubility than the polymer (e.g., removal of salts crystals that are more soluble in aqueous medium) after casting into a mold. Both the hydrogel and the thick scaffold forms are classified as three-dimensional bulk biomaterials. In each of the steps, bioactive pharmacological substances can be added using different modification strategies (Fig. 8-3).

Bioactive factor incorporation may be performed on the monomer units. Poly(ethylene glycol) (PEG) is normally a nondegradable synthetic polymer. However, by addition of hydrolyzable molecular entities within the network, the modified PEG (mPEG) becomes biodegradable in a controlled fashion and can be used as a temporary matrix for tissue regeneration. In an mPEG-based construct, for example, the bioactive tripeptide Arg-Gly-Asp (RGD) was covalently linked to the amine-reactive monomer N-carbonylimidazole–tethered PEG monoacrylate (PEGMA) before photopolymerization with other monomers to synthesize a tissue-active hydrogel. The chemical reaction involves the substitution of the imidazole group with an RGD peptide [13]. Another type of covalent linkage commonly used for biomaterial functionalization of monomers is the Michael-type reaction involving the addition of a nucleophile (electron donor) to an electrophile (electron acceptor) that is an activated olefin or alkene group (with unsaturated carbon–carbon double bond) to form the Michael adduct product (Fig. 8-4A) [14]. An example using this process was to integrate the RGD-like compound agmatine with bis(acrylamido)acetic acid (BAC) monomer, which is a polyamidoamine (PAA) biomaterial (Fig. 8-4B) [15]. The amino terminus ($-NH_2$) of the agmatine acts as a nucleophile and donates its electrons to an alkene group of the BAC, thus synthesizing the conjugate.

The simplest method of active component incorporation is physical mixing or blending with the polymer solution. In one example, the cell-adhesive trimeric glycoprotein laminin (LM) was mixed with the synthetic biomaterial poly(L-lactic acid) (PLLA) that was dissolved in hexafluoroisopropanol (HFP; a volatile solvent) before

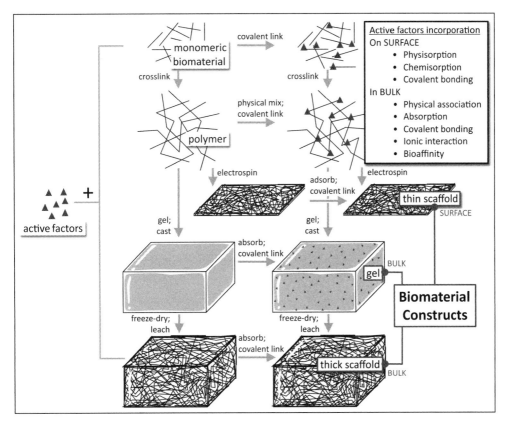

Figure 8-3. Bioactive pharmacological substances can be incorporated at various stages of the biomaterial construct synthesis. They can be added to the monomeric units, unassembled polymers, and final products after electrospinning, gelation, or scaffold formation. (See color plate 17.)

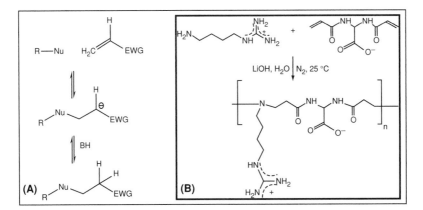

Figure 8-4. (**A**) Michael-type addition reaction adds the nucleophile (Nu) to the alkene electrophile with an electron withdrawal group (EWG) to produce the conjugated product [14]. (**B**) Agmatine with an amino end is added to the bis(acrylamido)acetic acid (BAC) via the alkene group [15].

surface deposition through electrospinning. This process may not always be effective because the organic solvent may denature and alter the biologic activity of the active substance. Alternatively, LM proteins were added to the electrospun mat after deposition. Two distinct surface-incorporation methods were used. The first one involves physisorption of LM on the PLLA construct by incubating overnight at 4°C and allowing the unspecific physical attractive forces to deposit LM on unoccupied surfaces. The second process is via covalent bonding using the crosslinking agents 1-ethyl-3-(3-dimethylaminopropyl) carbodiimide hydrochloride (EDC) and N-hydroxysuccinimide (NHS) to attach the $-NH_2$ termini of LM chains to the carboxyl group (-COOH) of the PLLA to form a stable amide bond [16]. Biomaterial surfaces can also be functionalized by chemisorption, which produces higher binding energy than physisorption because of the strong chemical bond formation between the adsorbate and the substrate. RGD peptide with attached N-terminal cysteine residue (CRGD) for promotion of endothelial cell adhesion was chemisorbed on a gold-coated polyurethane (PUR) biomaterial [17]. The sulfur of the thiol group (-SH) in the cysteine forms a covalent bond with the gold atom for CRGD surface immobilization.

Bulk biomaterial constructs such as hydrogels and scaffolds require physical association, absorption, ionic interaction, covalent linkage, or bioaffinity for bioactive compound functionalization (see Fig. 8-3). Transforming growth factor-β (TGF-β) was blended during the mPEG hydrogel formation. The process did not covalently integrate the growth factor into the biomaterial; instead, TGF-β was physically associated by relatively weaker attractive forces. The release profile of TGF-β from mPEG confirmed the diffusion behavior that is typical of nonbinding interactions [18]. Active components can also be absorbed into the biomaterial network. An example is incubation of a solution of hepatocyte growth factor (HGF) with crosslinked acidic gelatin (GTN) hydrogel to enable growth factor absorption [19]. The absorbed molecules have different binding affinities to the matrix biomaterial. In the case of HGF, it was found to have a high degree of association with GTN [20], thus enabling the growth factor to be retained in the gel with a slow rate of release. The mechanism may be ionic interaction between the positively charged HGF and the negatively charged acidic GTN. Another growth factor with similar behavior towards the GTN biomaterial is fibroblast growth factor 2 (FGF-2). At a pH of 7, FGF-2 with isoelectric point (pI) of 9.6 has a net positive charge, but GTN (pI = 5) is negatively charged. The electrostatic interaction thus produces a polyion complex sufficient for growth factor localization [21].

A more stable method of retention is via covalent bonding. The bioactive peptide solution Tyr-Ile-Gly-Ser-Arg (YIGSR) with an N-terminal-attached cysteine residue was absorbed into the composite scaffold composed of the hydroxyapatite (HA) mineral and polysaccharide shellfish chitin-derived chitosan (CHI) with modified thiol groups. Exposure to an oxygen (O_2) atmosphere led to disulfide bond formation between the cysteine sulfur atoms of the peptide and the modified CHI [22]. Bioaffinity also allows tight interaction between the biomaterial and the active component. Using a peptide amphiphile (PAM) self-assembling biomaterial with the TGF-β–binding peptide sequence His-Ser-Asn-Gly-Leu-Pro-Leu (HSNGLPL), TGF-β was found to associate strongly to the hydrogel matrix and generated a slow growth factor release profile [23].

The succeeding chapter sections enumerate some of the biomaterial constructs that have been functionalized with bioactive pharmacological factors and are currently being developed for tissue repair and regeneration (Table 8-2).

Biomaterials with Extracellular Matrix Proteins and Their Small-Molecule Derivatives

Cells attach to ECM structures primarily via their integrin transmembrane cell-matrix adhesion receptors [38]. The integrin–ECM interaction activates a signal transduction cascade that produces a variety of cell and tissue behavioral responses, including cell migration and tissue remodeling [39]. Hence, one of the most obvious ways to make a functional biomaterial is to incorporate ECM proteins. Collagen, laminin, and fibronectin (FN) are commonly used because they are prevalent throughout the body and thus should support a range of cell types. Poly(caprolactone) (PCL) aliphatic polyester blended with type I collagen (COL1) for skin tissue engineering enabled enhanced cell colonization, basal lamina formation, and stratification of dermal and epidermal layers in vitro after seeding with fibroblasts and keratinocytes; PCL alone did not generate these characteristic skin remodeling responses [24]. In peripheral nerve regeneration experiments, PLLA synthetic polymer with LM promoted longer neurite extensions from neuron-like cells (differentiated PC-12) compared with PLLA without LM [16]. FN, when absorbed in a CHI biomaterial sponge for vascular engineering, allowed adhesion, spreading, and proliferation of cultured endothelial cells. In contrast, an untreated CHI scaffold resulted in poor cell adhesion [25]. The use of a large, multicomponent, and translationally modified native ECM can be a limitation and may lead to varied batch-to-batch outcomes. COL1 has different degrees of hydroxyprolination, hydroxylysination, and glycosylation (responsible for triple-helical formation) [38] depending on the animal tissue source, which ultimately affects its physical properties. LM has 16 different isoforms with three subunits each [40]. The ratios of these LM types can vary with the extraction process and tissue origin. It is therefore important to use ECM additives from the same commercial manufacturer when the experiment is to be replicated.

Extracellular matrix molecules provide the skeletal framework and shape of the tissue. Thus, a majority of ECM protein subunit domains are structural in nature. However, the mechanical role in engineered constructs is already being fulfilled by the polymeric biomaterial scaffold. Accordingly, researchers were able to identify, synthesize, and incorporate only the cell-active regions of ECM for enhanced potency and controllability, resulting in more directed and predictable tissue responses. The

Table 8-2. *Functionalization of polymeric biomaterials with incorporated active factors*

Biomaterial form	Bioactive factor	Regenerative effects compared with untreated biomaterial	Target tissue application	Reference
PCL electro-spun fiber mat	Blended and crosslinked COL1	Increased colonization and proliferation of skin cells Formation of epidermis, dermis, and basal lamina structures	Skin	[24]
PLLA electro-spun fiber mat	Blended LM	Longer neurite outgrowths	Peripheral nerve	[16]
CHI scaffold	Absorbed FN	Enhanced endothelial cell adhesion	Blood vessel	[25]
mPEG hydrogel	Covalently linked RGD	Enhanced fibroblast adhesion Osteoblast deposition of collagen and calcium minerals	Bone	[13]
mPEG hydrogel	Covalently linked RGDS	Increased hMSC viability Improved differentiation of hMSCs into chondrocytes	Articular cartilage	[26]
PLLA electro-spun fiber mat	Blended cRGD	Increased hMSC proliferation Improved differentiation of hMSCs into osteoblasts	Bone	[27]
PAA hydrogel	Covalently linked agmatine	Enhanced attachment and survival of polygonal epithelial cells	Kidney epithelium	[28]
PCL scaffold	Adsorbed GFOGER	Greater bone volume formation in a critical-size long bone defect model	Bone	[29]
CHI–HA composite scaffold	Covalently linked YIGSR	Formation of epineurium in the regenerated nerve	Peripheral nerve	[22]
AGA hydrogel	Covalently linked IKVAV	Longer neurite outgrowths	Peripheral nerve	[12]
mPEG hydrogel	Covalently linked LDV	Enhanced attachment of T cells	Blood vessel	[30]
PUR scaffold	Blended PDGF	More granulation tissue formation Accelerated scaffold degradation	Skin	[31]

Biomaterial form	Bioactive factor	Regenerative effects compared with untreated biomaterial	Target tissue application	Reference
mPEG hydrogel	Blended TGF-β	Increased amount of chondrocytes and GAGs	Articular cartilage	[18]
mPEG hydrogel	Blended IGF-1 in GTN microparticles	Better overall regeneration of the chondral region of the new articular cartilage tissue	Articular cartilage	[18]
PAM hydrogel	Bioaffinity-bound TGF-β	Better cartilage repair scores in a full-thickness defect model	Articular cartilage	[23]
ALG hydrogel	Blended VEGF-A	Increased endothelial cell proliferation and sprouting More blood vessel formation and higher blood flow in ischemic model	Vascularized tissues	[32]
FBN–PEG composite electro-spun fiber mat	Blended EGF	Accelerated wound reepithelialization and closure in an in vitro wound healing model	Skin	[33]
GTN hydrogel	Absorbed HGF	More organized collagen, elastin, and HYA Vocal fold thickness and vibration function restored in scarred lamina propria	Vocal folds	[19]
HYA–CMC composite scaffold	Absorbed FGF-2	Increased chondrocyte proliferation More organized tissue structure, better epithelial closure, and less inflammation	Tracheal cartilage	[34]
FIB–heparin composite hydrogel	Bioaffinity-bound GDNF	More successful grips Stronger muscle forces and lower muscle atrophy Increased retrograde transport	Peripheral nerve	[35]
FIB–heparin composite hydrogel	Bioaffinity-bound NGF	Stronger muscle forces Increased retrograde transport	Peripheral nerve	[35]

(*continued*)

Table 8-2 *(continued)*

Biomaterial form	Bioactive factor	Regenerative effects compared with untreated biomaterial	Target tissue application	Reference
AGA–COL hydrogel	Blended BDNF	Longer axons in a spinal cord hemitransection injury	Spinal cord	[36]
KRT hydrogel	Blended BMP-2	New bone formation in a critical-size rat segmental defect model	Bone	[37]

AGA = agarose; ALG = alginate; BDNF = brain-derived neurotrophic factor; BMP-2 = bone morphogenetic protein 2; CHI = chitosan; CMC = carboxymethyl cellulose; COL = collagen; COL1 = type I collagen; cRGD = cyclic Arg-Gly-Asp; EGF = epidermal growth factor; FBN = fibroin; FGF-2 = fibroblast growth factor 2; FIB = fibrin; FN = fibronectin; GAG = glycosaminoglycan; GDNF = glial cell line-derived neurotrophic factor; GFOGER = Gly-Phe-Hyp-Gly-Glu-Arg; GTN = gelatin; HA = hydroxyapatite; HGF = hepatocyte growth factor; hMSC = human bone marrow mesenchymal stem cell; HYA = hyaluronic acid; IGF-1 = insulin-like growth factor 1; IKVAV = Ile-Lys-Val-Ala-Val; KRT = keratin; LDV = Leu-Asp-Val; LM = laminin; mPEG = modified poly(ethylene glycol); NGF = nerve growth factor; PAA = polyamidoamine; PAM = peptide amphiphile; PCL = poly(caprolactone); PDGF = platelet-derived growth factor; PEG = poly(ethylene glycol); PLLA = poly(L-lactic acid); PUR = polyurethane; RGD = Arg-Gly-Asp; RGDS = Arg-Gly-Asp-Ser; TGF-β = transforming growth factor-β; VEGF-A = vascular endothelial growth factor A; YIGSR = Tyr-Ile-Gly-Ser-Arg.

tripeptide RGD, found in numerous ECM proteins as the main cell-adhesion sequence, is probably the most used ECM derivative for biomaterial functionalization [41 ,42]. Using a photopolymerized mPEG hydrogel composed of PEG diacrylate (PEGDA), fumarated PEG diglycidyl ether (PEGDGE), and PEGMA linked to RGD, it was determined that the presence of RGD enabled the cultured fibroblasts to attach and spread on the material surface. Moreover, osteoblasts from differentiated human bone marrow mesenchymal stem cells (hMSCs) recognized the PEG-based biomaterial with conjugated RGD as a suitable substrate for collagen deposition and mineralization (indirectly evidenced by elevated elemental nitrogen and calcium, respectively), suggesting that the construct can be applied to bone regeneration applications [13].

Cell attachment on the biomaterial surface can be enhanced by increasing the affinity between the receptor (integrin expressed on cells) and ligand (RGD on biomaterials). Addition of extra amino acid residues to RGD allows ligand conformational change and chain lengthening for optimal cell–biomaterial interaction, as well as selectivity for specific integrin types present on distinct population of cells. Some of the experimental RGD-based peptides that have been used to promote cell adhesion include RGDS, GRGD, GRGDG, GRGDS, GRGDY, YRGDS, YRGDG, GRGDSP,

GRGDSY, and GRGDSPK [41]. RGDS incorporated in another PEG-based hydrogel supported increased cell viability and improved chondrogenic differentiation of cultured hMSCs for cartilage tissue engineering. More specifically, production of glycosaminoglycans (GAGs), aggrecan, and type II collagen (COL2) was elevated compared with the PEG biomaterial without RGDS [26].

Another modification for better functionality is by converting the linear RGD peptide to a cyclic RGD (cRGD) structure because cRGD may mimic the native integrin-binding domain better and has a more fixed conformation than linear RGD [43]. Electrospun PLLA nanofibers with cRGD in the form of cyclo(-RGDfK) (RGD plus amino acids: D-Phe and Lys) enabled the growth of hMSCs in osteogenic media containing dexamethasone, ascorbic acid-2-phosphate, and β-glycerophosphate. The differentiation of hMSCs into osteoblastic lineage was more pronounced in PLLA nonwoven matrix with cRGD, as determined by COL1 and osteocalcin expression [27].

The binding of cell integrins to the biomaterial can also be achieved by mimicking the RGD motif. Agmatine that is covalently linked to BAC PAA biomaterial exhibits structural and biofunctional resemblance to RGD [15]. A kidney epithelial cell line with polygonal morphology attached and survived better on the RGD-like material surface compared with the construct without the guanidinium side chain of RGD. Cell culture in the presence of soluble GRGD peptide inhibited cell adhesion, indicating that the primary mode of cell–biomaterial interaction is through the integrin receptor binding to the agmatine–BAC RGD-like domains [28]. Other RGD peptidomimetic molecules that were synthesized based on the tyrosine template and immobilized on PET polymer demonstrated enhanced colon epithelial cell line adhesion [44].

Extracellular matrix derivatives such as RGD are not always superior to the native ECM. Whereas COL1 and LM on PEG hydrogel for cardiac muscle tissue engineering enabled cardiomyocyte maturation, the RGD-modified hydrogel did not [45]. In this case, it is possible that other cell-active domains of COL1 and LM are essential for the proper activity of cells. The motif Gly-Phe-Hyp-Gly-Glu-Arg (GFOGER) in COL1 binds to specific integrin α2β1 expressed on a subset of cells. GFOGER adsorbed on rigid PCL scaffold enabled significant bone formation in a critical-size defect model compared with uncoated PCL control [29], indicating that the GFOGER-initiated signaling activates osteogenesis for bone healing. Other COL1-derived peptide sequences that interact with integrin α2β1 for bone tissue engineering include Asp-Gly-Glu-Ala (DGEA) and Gly-Thr-Pro-Gly-Pro-Gln-Gly-Ile-Ala-Gly-Gln-Arg-Gly-Val-Val (P15) [46].

Short motifs in LM such as YIGSR and Ile-Lys-Val-Ala-Val (IKVAV) have also been used for biomaterial functionalization. YIGSR (with Cys-Asp-Pro-Gly peptide attached to its amino terminus), when combined with the composite CHI and HA, produced regenerated nerve tissue with epineurium-like structure in a transected rat sciatic nerve model [22]. IKVAV covalently attached to agarose (AGA) hydrogel induced more extensive neurite outgrowth from cultured PC-12 cells than the untreated AGA for peripheral nerve tissue engineering applications [12]. Leu-Asp-Val (LDV) found in the ECM molecule FN is another cell-active peptide used with biomaterials. LDV linked to PEG polymer enabled a higher level of Jurkat T lymphocyte cell line adhesion compared with PEG with nonadhesive peptide Leu-Glu-Val [30]. Additionally, LDV binds selectively to integrin α4β1 and thus is capable of targeting specific cells of interest. The Pro-His-Ser-Arg-Asn (PHSRN) motif found in FN is specifically recognized by integrin α5β1 [47], which may also be used for populating scaffolds with distinct cell types.

Biomaterials with Growth Factors

The natural ECM of tissues and organs are reservoirs of growth factors and bioactive molecules [48,49]. These cell-secreted signaling substances are needed by resident tissue-specific cells for maintenance of activity and function. In the peripheral nervous system, for example, neurotrophic factors produced by supporting glial cells are delivered to the neuronal cell body through retrograde transport to promote homeostasis and survival [50]. Heparan sulfate proteoglycans, which are ECM components of the peripheral nerves, bind and sequester neurotrophic factors to facilitate local retention as well as to mediate their signaling and activity [51]. Extracellularly released growth factors generally have short half-lives because they are tightly regulated to prevent unwanted phenotypic downstream effects. They are also targets of proteases for degradation. Accordingly, growth factors have specific binding domains to the ECM. ECM interaction thus prevents their immediate breakdown and extends their bioavailability and potency toward target cells. Biologic signals are transduced to recipient cells via cell-surface receptors that are activated upon growth factor binding and interaction. During tissue injury and subsequent initiation of healing and repair, the expression of these growth factors are upregulated because they also function as regenerative molecules for activating cells to synthesize new ECM and for inducing stem cells to migrate into the site of injury and differentiate to replace the damaged cells. Additionally, growth factors that are locally bound to the ECM are released during tissue damage and breakdown and consequently jumpstart the regeneration process. Decellularized grafts are effective regenerative materials because they can still contain residual growth factors that are entrapped within the ECM network.

Key players in wound healing responses are responsible for locally delivering some of the growth factors that promote tissue regeneration after structural damage. For example, activated platelets that are entrapped in the temporary fibrin mesh of a hemostatic blood clot release numerous growth factors with tissue-healing effects, including platelet-derived growth factor (PDGF), TGF-β, insulin-like growth factor 1 (IGF-1), vascular endothelial growth factor A (VEGF-A), and epidermal growth factor (EGF) [52–54]. ECM growth factor systems can be mimicked synthetically by

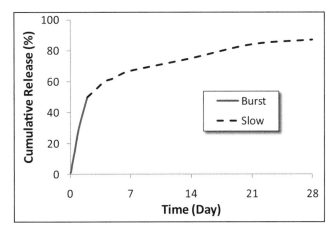

Figure 8-5. A typical two-stage drug release profile composed of an initial burst and then a slow, sustained release. This release mechanism is common for growth factors incorporated in a biomaterial carrier for tissue engineering applications.

incorporating purified commercially available growth factors to polymeric biomaterial gels and scaffolds.

Platelet-derived growth factor (PDGF-BB homodimer form) blended with a PUR biomaterial scaffold for skin tissue engineering enabled a faster wound healing response because more granulation tissue formation was observed in the full-thickness excisional wound site compared with the PUR without any growth factor [31]. The in vitro PDGF release from the scaffold displayed a typical profile (Fig. 8-5) consisting of an acute burst effect followed by a sustained slow release over time. The kinetics of initial high-dose delivery was hypothesized to attract mesenchymal stem cells, and the subsequent low-level growth factor release enabled the promotion of tissue remodeling. Furthermore, the scaffold degradation rate was remarkably increased in the PDGF-treated group, which may have been caused by more scaffold-penetrating cells such as neutrophils, macrophages, and fibroblasts that allowed for better tissue regeneration.

In articular cartilage tissue engineering, TGF-β (specifically, the TGF-β1 isoform) mixed with a chemically initiated PEG-based hydrogel also generated a characteristic initial burst effect as bioactive molecules eluted out of the hydrogel matrix. Implantation into a defect site led to increased chondrocytes and GAG content at the chondral region of the neo-tissue compared with the hydrogel control without growth factor [18]. The outcome of articular cartilage regeneration was drastically improved when the hydrogel was loaded with IGF-1. Instead of direct mixing with the polymer matrix, the growth factor was first absorbed in degradable GTN microparticle gels before incorporation to make the final construct. The microparticle–growth factor delivery system enabled a more sustained release over the course of time and produced a regenerated tissue with hallmarks of normal articular cartilage [18]. Additionally, this delayed release strategy enabled the growth factor to be more effectively protected from degradation and deactivation. A PAM biomaterial with HSNGLPL (a peptide that binds to TGF-β1) in combination with the growth factor TGF-β1 enhanced the healing of an articular cartilage defect site better than the hydrogel with no TGF-β1. Tissue regeneration was characterized by more organized tissue layers and higher levels of GAGs and COL2 [23]. The bioaffinity of TGF-β1 to the HSNGLPL sequence in PAM allowed for higher growth factor retention within the site of injury over the time span, which may have improved the overall result of cartilage healing.

Another growth factor that is important in tissue regeneration and remodeling is VEGF-A, which specifically induces the growth of new blood vessels that integrate the tissue with the organism's circulatory system. In vitro analysis showed that higher levels of VEGF-A translate to an increased primary endothelial cell proliferation. Moreover, the temporal delivery of the growth factor played a significant functional role as an initial high dose followed by decreasing levels generated the highest endothelial cell sprouting compared with a constant high-quantity delivery or to a gradual increasing VEGF-A treatment [32]. Using an injectable in situ polymerizable seaweed-derived polysaccharide alginate (ALG) matrix, the incorporated VEGF-A (165–amino acid splice variant VEGF-A$_{165}$) was shown to release in a typical diffusional burst, then sustained mode. This release profile led to more capillary formation and faster recovery of regional blood flow over time in an ischemic muscle model compared with growth factor–free ALG gel [32].

Skin regeneration and wound healing use growth factors for improved structural outcome. In one study, EGF released from an electrospun nanofiber mat composite of silkworm fibroin (FBN) and PEG enabled the migration of epithelial cells at the wound margin in an in vitro wound healing model compared with the composite mat with no EGF. Similar to the previously described growth factor–biomaterial combinations, the delivery of EGF followed the initial burst and a linear slow release model [33].

Activated neutrophils that migrate to the site of injury during the acute inflammatory response are also natural sources of growth factors that promote tissue regeneration. Among the neutrophil-secreted growth factors are VEGF-A and HGF [55]. HGF, a heparin-binding glycoprotein that regulates cell growth and motility, was shown to enable better collagen, elastin, and hyaluronic acid (HYA) organization when absorbed in glutaraldehyde-crosslinked injectable GTN hydrogel in a dog vocal fold scarring model compared with the growth factor–free biomaterial. The presence of growth factor also led to the formation of native-thickness vocal folds. Moreover, HGF delivery over a 2-week time period allowed restoration of normal mucosal vibrations characterized by low pressure to initiate phonation and high amplitude waves [19].

Macrophages differentiate from circulating blood monocytes and infiltrate injured tissue after the influx of neutrophils. They then release several growth factors such as TGF-β, PDGF, VEGF-A, and FGF-2 to induce cell proliferation and ECM deposition from skin cells [53]. FGF-2 absorbed to a scaffold composite composed of the nonsulfated GAG HYA and the cellulose derivative thickener carboxymethyl cellulose (CMC) enabled more proliferation of chondrocytes in a tracheal cartilage defect compared with the construct with no FGF-2. Semiquantitative scoring also showed that FGF-2 incorporation increased connective tissue organization, provided better epithelial layer closure, and reduced tracheal tissue inflammation [34].

Injury to specialized tissues of the body such as the nerve, spinal cord, and bone triggers the release of growth factors. Glial cell line-derived neurotrophic factor (GDNF) secreted by Schwann cells is known to aid in peripheral nerve regeneration. Fibrin (FIB) gel with heparin (linked via a bi-domain heparin-binding peptide) allowed the affinity binding of GDNF to prolong its bioavailability. Animals treated with the GDNF-biomaterial construct recovered better than the no growth factor control group using a hindlimb grid-grip test 12 weeks after sciatic nerve transection. Also, the nerve guides with GDNF led to stronger extensor digitorum longus muscle tetanic and twitch forces and reduced muscle atrophy. When nerve growth factor was incorporated in the FIB–heparin hydrogel, greater muscle forces were recorded compared with the control group. Retrograde transport activity was enhanced in nerve guides with growth factors [35]. In spinal cord tissue engineering, brain-derived neurotrophic factor (BDNF) blended with COL1 and gelled with AGA scaffold promoted better repair of the rat spinal cord lesions. The number of axons traversing the implanted construct was significantly increased compared with the control group lacking BDNF [36].

One of the most potent growth factors for bone tissue repair after injury is bone morphogenetic protein 2 (BMP-2). BMP-2 secretion is increased significantly from invading and proliferating mesenchymal progenitor cells and periosteal cells that are responsible for bone regeneration [56,57]. Keratin (KRT) biomaterial hydrogel loaded with BMP-2 enabled the formation of new bone tissue that completely bridged the critical-size rat femur defect. The presence of BMP-2 also generated bone with mechanical properties (ultimate torsional torque, rotational stiffness, and shear modulus) comparable to the uninjured bone, but KRT gel alone did not induce significant bone formation at the 16-week endpoint [37].

Summary

Biomaterials used for tissue engineering and restoration of normal structures are biocompatible polymeric molecules that are naturally derived or artificial. They serve as temporary, degradable ECM to initially substitute the damaged tissue structure, as well as to promote healing. To enable progenitor cells to colonize, proliferate, and differentiate into normal tissue-specific resident cells, biomaterials are functionalized by addition of bioactive factors or pharmacological substances. Bioactive ECM proteins and cell-adhesion peptides are generally incorporated into the biomaterial matrix via stable chemical bonds that prevent their release before substrate degradation.

Selective short peptides are preferred to target only the cell populations that are involved in tissue regeneration. In contrast, added growth factors need to be dissociated from the biomaterial and delivered to local surrounding tissues to activate the quiescent scaffold-infiltrating stem cells. The system can be improved by mimicking the temporal delivery of multiple growth factors in the natural healing process. To develop an ideal cell-free biomaterial construct that can remodel into a fully functional normal tissue, a multicomponent device composed of different biomaterial matrices and bioactive factors may be needed.

References

1. Zilla P, Bezuidenhout D, Human P. Prosthetic vascular grafts: wrong models, wrong questions and no healing. Biomaterials 2007;28(34):5009–5027.
2. Walles T, Gorler H, Puschmann C, Mertsching H. Functional neointima characterization of vascular prostheses in human. Ann Thorac Surg 2004;77(3):864–868.
3. Van Damme H, Deprez M, Creemers E, Limet R. Intrinsic structural failure of polyester (Dacron) vascular grafts. A general review. Acta Chir Belg 2005;105(3):249–255.
4. Vert M. Degradable and bioresorbable polymers in surgery and in pharmacology: beliefs and facts. J Mater Sci Mater Med 2009;20(2):437–446.
5. Falco EE, Patel M, Fisher JP. Recent developments in cyclic acetal biomaterials for tissue engineering applications. Pharm Res 2008;25(10):2348–2356.
6. Holland TA, Mikos AG. Biodegradable polymeric scaffolds. Improvements in bone tissue engineering through controlled drug delivery. Adv Biochem Eng Biotechnol 2006;102:161–185.
7. Ifkovits JL, Burdick JA. Review: photopolymerizable and degradable biomaterials for tissue engineering applications. Tissue Eng 2007;13(10):2369–2385.
8. Zhu J. Bioactive modification of poly(ethylene glycol) hydrogels for tissue engineering. Biomaterials 2010;31(17):4639–4656
9. Middleton JC, Tipton AJ. Synthetic biodegradable polymers as orthopedic devices. Biomaterials 2000;21(23):2335–2346.
10. Kasper FK, Tanahashi K, Fisher JP, Mikos AG. Synthesis of poly(propylene fumarate). Nat Protoc 2009;4(4):518–525.
11. Svenson S. Dendrimers as versatile platform in drug delivery applications. Eur J Pharm Biopharm 2009;71(3):445–462.
12. Bellamkonda R, Ranieri JP, Aebischer P. Laminin oligopeptide derivatized agarose gels allow three-dimensional neurite extension in vitro. J Neurosci Res 1995;41(4):501–509.
13. Akdemir ZS, Akcakaya H, Kahraman MV, Ceyhan T, Kayaman-Apohan N, Gungor A. Photopolymerized injectable RGD-modified fumarated poly(ethylene glycol) diglycidyl ether hydrogels for cell growth. Macromol Biosci 2008;8(9):852–862.
14. Mather BD, Viswanathan K, Miller KM, Long TE. Michael addition reactions in macromolecular design for emerging technologies. Prog Polym Sci 2006;31(5):487–531.
15. Franchini J, Ranucci E, Ferruti P, Rossi M, Cavalli R. Synthesis, physicochemical properties, and preliminary biological characterizations of a novel amphoteric agmatine-based poly(amidoamine) with RGD-like repeating units. Biomacromolecules 2006;7(4):1215–1222.
16. Koh HS, Yong T, Chan CK, Ramakrishna S. Enhancement of neurite outgrowth using nano-structured scaffolds coupled with laminin. Biomaterials 2008;29(26):3574–3582.

17. McMillan R, Meeks B, Bensebaa F, Deslandes Y, Sheardown H. Cell adhesion peptide modification of gold-coated polyurethanes for vascular endothelial cell adhesion. J Biomed Mater Res 2001;54(2):272–283.

18. Holland TA, Bodde EW, Cuijpers VM, Baggett LS, Tabata Y, Mikos AG, et al. Degradable hydrogel scaffolds for in vivo delivery of single and dual growth factors in cartilage repair. Osteoarthritis Cartilage 2007;15(2):187–197.

19. Kishimoto Y, Hirano S, Kitani Y, Suehiro A, Umeda H, Tateya I, et al. Chronic vocal fold scar restoration with hepatocyte growth factor hydrogel. Laryngoscope 2010;120(1):108–113.

20. Ozeki M, Tabata Y. Interaction of hepatocyte growth factor with gelatin as the carrier material. J Biomater Sci 2006;17(1–2):163–175.

21. Muniruzzaman, Tabata Y, Ikada Y. Complexation of basic fibroblast growth factor with gelatin. J Biomater Sci 1998;9(5):459–473.

22. Itoh S, Matsuda A, Kobayashi H, Ichinose S, Shinomiya K, Tanaka J. Effects of a laminin peptide (YIGSR) immobilized on crab-tendon chitosan tubes on nerve regeneration. J Biomed Mater Res B Appl Biomater 2005;73(2):375–382.

23. Shah RN, Shah NA, Del Rosario Lim MM, Hsieh C, Nuber G, Stupp SI. Supramolecular design of self-assembling nanofibers for cartilage regeneration. Proc Nat Acad Sci U S A 2010;107(8):3293–3298.

24. Powell HM, Boyce ST. Engineered human skin fabricated using electrospun collagen-PCL blends: morphogenesis and mechanical properties. Tissue Eng Part A 2009;15(8):2177–2187.

25. Amaral IF, Unger RE, Fuchs S, Mendonca AM, Sousa SR, Barbosa MA, et al. Fibronectin-mediated endothelialisation of chitosan porous matrices. Biomaterials 2009;30(29):5465–5475.

26. Salinas CN, Cole BB, Kasko AM, Anseth KS. Chondrogenic differentiation potential of human mesenchymal stem cells photoencapsulated within poly(ethylene glycol)-arginine-glycine-aspartic acid-serine thiol-methacrylate mixed-mode networks. Tissue Eng 2007;13(5):1025–1034.

27. Schofer MD, Boudriot U, Bockelmann S, Walz A, Wendorff JH, Greiner A, et al. Effect of direct RGD incorporation in PLLA nanofibers on growth and osteogenic differentiation of human mesenchymal stem cells. J Mater Sci Mater Med 2009;20(7):1535–1540.

28. Jacchetti E, Emilitri E, Rodighiero S, Indrieri M, Gianfelice A, Lenardi C, et al. Biomimetic poly(amidoamine) hydrogels as synthetic materials for cell culture. J Nanobiotechnol 2008;6:14.

29. Wojtowicz AM, Shekaran A, Oest ME, Dupont KM, Templeman KL, Hutmacher DW, et al. Coating of biomaterial scaffolds with the collagen-mimetic peptide GFOGER for bone defect repair. Biomaterials 2010;31(9):2574–2582.

30. Taite LJ, Rowland ML, Ruffino KA, Smith BR, Lawrence MB, West JL. Bioactive hydrogel substrates: probing leukocyte receptor-ligand interactions in parallel plate flow chamber studies. Ann Biomed Eng 2006;34(11):1705–1711.

31. Li B, Davidson JM, Guelcher SA. The effect of the local delivery of platelet-derived growth factor from reactive two-component polyurethane scaffolds on the healing in rat skin excisional wounds. Biomaterials 2009;30(20):3486–3494.

32. Silva EA, Mooney DJ. Effects of VEGF temporal and spatial presentation on angiogenesis. Biomaterials 2010;31(6):1235–1241.

33. Schneider A, Wang XY, Kaplan DL, Garlick JA, Egles C. Biofunctionalized electrospun silk mats as a topical bioactive dressing for accelerated wound healing. Acta Biomater 2009;5(7):2570–2578.

34. Parker NP, Bailey SS, Walner DL. Effects of basic fibroblast growth factor-2 and hyaluronic acid on tracheal wound healing. Laryngoscope 2009;119(4):734–739.

35. Wood MD, MacEwan MR, French AR, Moore AM, Hunter DA, Mackinnon SE, et al. Fibrin matrices with affinity-based delivery systems and neurotrophic factors promote functional nerve regeneration. Biotechnol Bioeng 2010;106(6):970–979.

36. Stokols S, Tuszynski MH. Freeze-dried agarose scaffolds with uniaxial channels stimulate and guide linear axonal growth following spinal cord injury. Biomaterials 2006;27(3):443–451.

37. de Guzman RC, Saul JM, Ellenburg MD, Merrill MR, Coan HB, Smith TL, et al. Bone regeneration with BMP-2 delivered from keratose scaffolds. *Biomaterials* 2012 (accepted).

38. Alberts B, Johnson A, Lewis J, Raff M, Roberts K, Walter P. Molecular biology of the cell. 4th ed. New York: Garland Pub., 2002.

39. Berrier AL, Yamada KM. Cell-matrix adhesion. J Cell Physiol 2007;213(3):565–573.

40. Aumailley M, Bruckner-Tuderman L, Carter WG, Deutzmann R, Edgar D, Ekblom P, et al. A simplified laminin nomenclature. Matrix Biol 2005;24(5):326–332.

41. Hersel U, Dahmen C, Kessler H. RGD modified polymers: biomaterials for stimulated cell adhesion and beyond. Biomaterials 2003;24(24):4385–4415.

42. Heckmann D, Kessler H. Design and chemical synthesis of integrin ligands. Methods Enzymol 2007;426:463–503.

43. Kumagai H, Tajima M, Ueno Y, Giga-Hama Y, Ohba M. Effect of cyclic RGD peptide on cell adhesion and tumor metastasis. Biochem Biophys Res Commun 1991;177(1):74–82.

44. Biltresse S, Attolini M, Dive G, Cordi A, Tucker GC, Marchand-Brynaert J. Novel RGD-like molecules based on the tyrosine template: design, synthesis, and biological evaluation on isolated integrins alphaVbeta3/alphaIIbbeta3 and in cellular adhesion tests. Bioorg Med Chem 2004;12(20):5379–5393.

45. LaNasa SM, Bryant SJ. Influence of ECM proteins and their analogs on cells cultured on 2-D hydrogels for cardiac muscle tissue engineering. Acta Biomater 2009;5(8):2929–2938.

46. Hennessy KM, Pollot BE, Clem WC, Phipps MC, Sawyer AA, Culpepper BK, et al. The effect of collagen I mimetic peptides on mesenchymal stem cell adhesion and differentiation, and on bone formation at hydroxyapatite surfaces. Biomaterials 2009;30(10):1898–1909.

47. Satriano C, Messina GM, Marino C, Aiello I, Conte E, La Mendola D, et al. Surface immobilization of fibronectin-derived PHSRN peptide on functionalized polymer films–effects on fibroblast spreading. J Colloid Interface Sci 2010;341(2):232–239.

48. von der Mark K, Park J, Bauer S, Schmuki P. Nanoscale engineering of biomimetic surfaces: cues from the extracellular matrix. Cell Tissue Res 2010;339(1):131–153.

49. Discher DE, Mooney DJ, Zandstra PW. Growth factors, matrices, and forces combine and control stem cells. Science 2009;324(5935):1673–1677.

50. Terenghi G. Peripheral nerve regeneration and neurotrophic factors. anatomy Anat 1999;194 (Pt 1):1–14.

51. Silvian L, Jin P, Carmillo P, Boriack-Sjodin PA, Pelletier C, Rushe M, et al. Artemin crystal structure reveals insights into heparan sulfate binding. Biochemistry 2006;45(22):6801–6812.

52. Barrientos S, Stojadinovic O, Golinko MS, Brem H, Tomic-Canic M. Growth factors and cytokines in wound healing. Wound Repair Regen 2008;16(5):585–601.

53. Eming SA, Hammerschmidt M, Krieg T, Roers A. Interrelation of immunity and tissue repair or regeneration. Semin Cell Dev Biol 2009;20(5):517–527.

54. Velnar T, Bailey T, Smrkolj V. The wound healing process: an overview of the cellular and molecular mechanisms. J Int Med Res 2009;37(5):1528–1542.
55. McCourt M, Wang JH, Sookhai S, Redmond HP. Activated human neutrophils release hepatocyte growth factor/scatter factor. Eur J Surg Oncol 2001;27(4):396–403.
56. Marsell R, Einhorn TA. The role of endogenous bone morphogenetic proteins in normal skeletal repair. Injury 2009;40 Suppl 3:S4–7.
57. Cho TJ, Gerstenfeld LC, Einhorn TA. Differential temporal expression of members of the transforming growth factor beta superfamily during murine fracture healing. J Bone Miner Res 2002;17(3):513–520.

9

Enabling Drug Discovery Technologies for Regenerative Pharmacology

G. SITTA SITTAMPALAM

Although the process of drug discovery today is a product of organic chemistry, cell biology, clinical observations of disease pathology, and pharmacology, its early history is quite primitive and rests in the use of food and herbal remedies from plant products by ancient Asian, Egyptian, and Greek civilizations [1]. This was known as the *age of botanicals* when plant extracts were extensively used to treat common illnesses. The next phase of drug development started in the late nineteenth century with the isolation of plant extracts by physiologists and chemists in Europe, but these were used to treat common diseases by physicians since the 1500s. Isolation of salicylic acid (aspirin), quinine, digitalis, atropine and other alkaloids, ephedrine, and so on occurred between 1850s and the early 1900s [2]. These developments spurred the birth of pharmacology as a distinct discipline by physiologists who pioneered the study of drugs on animals.

The isolation of morphine from plant products by F.W. Serturner in the early nineteenth century followed by the availability of coal-tar products from industrialization in Europe led to modern roots of medicinal chemistry and pharmacology by the work of legendary physiologists Francois Magendie and Claude Bernard. In the 1870s, Oswald Schmiedeberg established the first Department of Pharmacology at the University of Strasbourg, which laid the foundation for modern pharmacology. Paul Ehrlich, considered the undisputed father of modern drug discovery, pioneered the use of synthetic organic dye molecules to study cellular activity in the 1870s at the University of Strasbourg. A superb summary of early drug discovery and the modern developments can be found in a seminal paper by Jürgen Drews that traces this history [2] and in more detail in his book on this topic [3].

Ehrlich's early experiments involved staining cells with organic dyes for microscopic examination, which led to his curiosity as to the nature of the interaction of these dyes with cellular components. He discovered that the dye methylene blue bound to nerve cells and used it to stain nerve cells in rodents. Interestingly, he also discovered that dyes also bind to parasitic organisms such as trypanosomes (trypan blue) and the malarial parasite *Plasmodium* (methylene blue) and inhibited their growth and survival in culture. In fact, Ehrlich was the first to treat patients with mild malaria with methylene blue, a distinct chemical entity, or a "drug," demonstrating successful results in two patients. This was probably the earliest example of scientific method of drug discovery and clinical trials, all in one laboratory!

As the pharmacies of the early twentieth century evolved into small and large pharmaceutical industries, the influence of isolated natural medicinal products and the advent of modern organic synthesis began in the textile dye industry to generate small molecule collections that could be tested to treat not only infectious diseases but also other ailments such as hypertension, ulcers, and pain. World Wars I and II further demonstrated the need for medications for infectious diseases and injuries among troops engaged globally. The 1950s saw the advent of vaccines, surgical techniques improved with the use of pills, and the discovery of DNA. In the next decade, scientists began to accept technologic advances in analytical and synthetic chemistry coupled with advances in pharmacological sciences and drove the belief that diseases could be treated and controlled. Development of this concept of synthetic drugs to treat many diseases is a critical leap, leading to translational and applied sciences becoming important in medicine along with hygienic practices developed through public health initiatives. The war on cancer emerged in the 1970s as a national priority along with breakthroughs in molecular biology, biologic chemistry, and the birth of biotechnology. The natural evolution from these events is the drive toward chemical biology and modern drug discovery driven by high-throughput screening (HTS) in the 1980 and 1990s.

The early approach of painstakingly testing new chemical entities (NCEs), *one molecule* at a time, with diseased tissues and animal models was successfully practiced in academic and pharmaceutical laboratories until the mid-1970s. Such an approach was slow because complex druglike molecules are hard to synthesize, and depending on their structural complexity, it takes months to make in high purity in milligram to gram quantities for sophisticated biologic and pharmacological testing. Combined with the need to understand the pathophysiological nature of human diseases, the need to demonstrate safety and efficacy, and the development of animal models to test NCEs, modern drug discovery has evolved into a complex and demanding discipline. Therefore, a typical drug would take 15 to 20 years to be discovered and tested for safety and efficacy in clinical trials with patients. Because the unexpected side effects in humans cannot be easily predicted by genetically homogeneous mouse and rat animal models used in drug development, the marketed drug uptake by clinicians was slow and deliberate. In addition, clinical trials were conducted in relatively small populations of healthy volunteers (phase I) and patient populations (phases II and III) to adequately establish safety and efficacy. Because the number of molecules tested was small, the launch of new drugs was also few up until the 1970s.

In the late 1970s and 1980s, several new technologies were emerging. Although Watson and Crick described the DNA structure in the early 1950s, molecular biology techniques did not progress rapidly until the early 1970s. This development strongly contributed to the ability to sequence and clone target genes associated with diseases. Advances in cell biology with improved cell culture and expression of cloned genes in bacterial and mammalian cells for protein expression came into practice to study disease biochemistry, pathology, and physiology. Powerful optical and electron microscopic and imaging techniques to investigate cellular organelles further contributed to understanding cellular dynamics and tissue function. Rapid developments in computer and information technology, powerful analytical instrumentation, automation, biochemical and cellular assay reagents, and combinatorial synthesis of peptides and organic molecules to generate libraries of hundreds of molecules further accelerated drug discovery research in the 1980s and 1990s. Highly efficient protein purification techniques (analytical and preparative chromatography) were developed to meet this demand. The stage was set for an explosion in high-throughput drug discovery technologies using these technologic and scientific developments [4]. Contrary to common belief [5], the high-throughput technologies have contributed immensely to the human genome sequencing the discovery and development of significant number of novel drugs and therapies in the past 15 years [6].

Recent advances in stem cell biology, tissue engineering, and material sciences are beginning to open up new approaches to drug discovery and regenerative medicine, marking the advent of regenerative pharmacology [7–9]. Advancement in regenerative medicine and pharmacology in the next decade promises to improve quality of life by using stem cells and molecular modulators of cell and tissue growth to treat degenerative diseases and organ repair in unprecedented manner [10,11]. Figure 9-1 illustrates the systematic evolution of the advent of modern drug discovery and regenerative medicine through the past two centuries.

The following sections address modern drug discovery technologies developed in the 1990s and the early twenty-first century that promise to revolutionize the future of drug discovery and development and patient outcomes. Many of these technologies have contributed to the development of a large high-throughput drug discovery and development industry. These include sophisticated and robotics automation, bio- and cheminformatics, assay reagents, high-throughput bioanalytical instrumentation, and data management software development companies estimated to have annual sales of $20 billion by 2017 (http://www.StrategyR.com/). The advent of high-throughput cell culture technologies, stem cells, including induced pluripotent stem (iPSs) cells and chemical biology, further expands the combinatorial use of drugs and cells for new treatment modalities. This approach of using novel cells, tissues, and drugs forms the basis of regenerative pharmacology and may revolutionize health care in the twenty-first century. These developments point to contributions from regenerative medicine and tissue engineering that, combined with pharmacology, may lead to a new era of treatments for approximately 90 percent of devastating ailments that fall currently

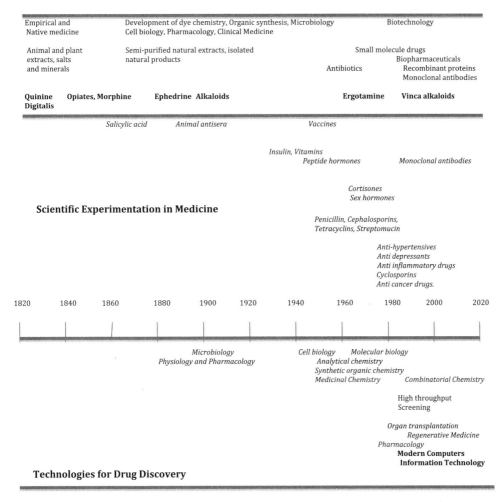

Figure 9-1. Evolution of modern drug discovery. (Adapted from Drews [2].) (See color plate 18.)

in the category of rare and neglected diseases (Therapeutics for Rare and Neglected Diseases Web site: http://www.ncats.nih.gov/research/rare-diseases/trnd/trnd.html).

Chemical Biology and Drug Discovery Technologies

Chemical biology is an interdisciplinary field that uses chemical and biological methods to understand life processes [12–14]. It cuts across multiple fields of molecular and structural chemistry, biochemistry, chemical synthesis, and cell and molecular biology. The use of chemical entities to modulate cellular functions and study the effects in normal and diseased cells and tissues is key to understanding pharmacology and toxicology of new drugs. Hence, pharmacology has moved from its classical study of drug actions in animals to more detailed investigations of the mechanisms

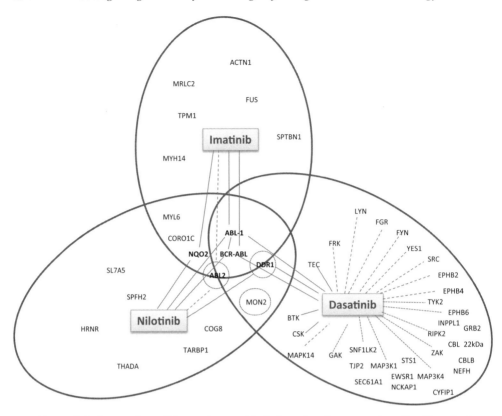

Figure 9-2. Interaction of kinase drugs with their molecular targets in cells. Chemical modulation of cellular function. *Solid lines* denote target–drug interactions that are well established, and the *dotted lines* represent potential or probable interactions. No connections indicate suspected interactions yet to be confirmed. (Reproduced with permission from Royal Society of Chemistry [13].) (See color plate 19.)

of biological activity of druglike molecules in disease processes. Chemical biology in action is nicely depicted in Figure 9-2, where the inhibitor network for tyrosine kinases involved in cancer is described. The interaction diagram shows the tyrosine kinase target network of the cancer drugs imatinib, nilotinib, and dasatinib. Using complex proteomic technologies, including affinity chromatography and mass spectrometry, these interactions of the individual drugs were elucidated. Note that all three drugs (for chronic myelogenic leukemia) share only a few common tyrosine kinase targets – Bcr-Abl, Abl1, Abl2, and DDR1 – but show dramatically different target interactions. These differences may account for side effects and their differential efficacy in subsets of patient populations. Such differences are possibly attributable to the high genetic diversity in human populations and are the subject of the emerging field of pharmacogenomics [2,14].

Understanding the different interactions in the cellular milieu is at the early stages of drug development and is critical to conceive novel approaches to drug discovery.

High-throughput technologies applied to biology and chemistry work at the cutting edge, generating massive datasets, with considerable need for information technology required to analyze and predict the cellular pathways modulated by new molecular entities (NMEs). However, a major gap in this continuum today is the ability to predict drug activities with high confidence from in vitro cellular function to animal models of disease and subsequent translation into human clinical efficacy. Genetic and proteomic profiling of disease pathologies in animals and humans is extremely complex but is a necessary approach to bridging the gap between chemical biology and clinical efficacy in humans. Other issues such as the effects of temporal, mechanical, and spatial (three-dimensional) tissue on drug efficacy and safety are still in early stages of development [15].

In regenerative medicine and pharmacology, much of the applications would be directed to repairing and regenerating damaged tissue using pharmacological agents. This can be accomplished using primary cells, progenitors, and adult stem cell–based assay systems to screen for molecules that would modulate stem cell phenotype to maintain pluripotency for tissue engineering applications or chemically induce favorable differentiation to beneficial cellular lineages when administered therapeutically. For example, in treatments involving degenerative diseases, one can envision using stem and progenitor cells to regenerate damaged nerves, muscles, skin, bone, and other tissues to repair damage and restore function. Molecular "adjuvants," such as small molecule drugs, peptides, proteins, or combinations can be administered simultaneously to enhance stem cell survival and controlled differentiation to appropriate tissue components and can be envisioned as important steps toward successful regenerative treatments in the future. Hence, chemical biology and regenerative pharmacology of multiple cell types, including stem cells, would be a significant field in the future of personalized and regenerative medicine.

Combinatorial Chemistry and High-Throughput Screening

The 1980s and early 1990s saw a major shift in the science of drug discovery caused by advances in molecular biology that enabled the cloning of and expression of disease targets and the understanding cellular signaling pathways [14]. Simultaneously, the advent of human genome sequencing in the mid- to late 1990s added pressure to test larger number of molecules in newly discovered targets and pathways in human disease that led to the development of combinatorial chemistry [16].

Combinatorial chemistry is the automated parallel synthesis of large number of diverse organic molecules using standardized synthetic methods. The rationale was to explore the large chemical space around a pharmacophore that could selectively activate or inhibit the biologic activities of target protein molecules. A typical combinatorial synthesis design is shown in Figure 9-3. In the mix-and-split technique using solid phase synthesis, molecular units represented by X, Y, and Z are functional groups

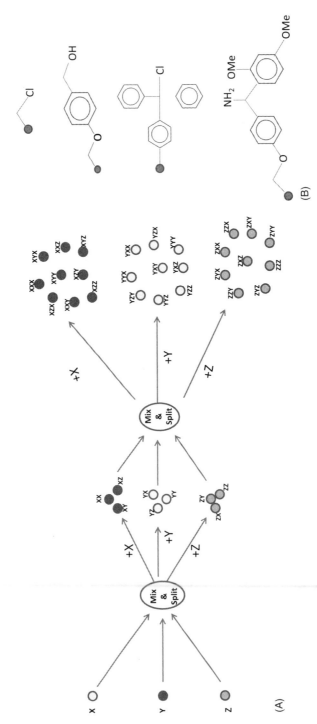

Figure 9-3. Basic combinatorial chemistry design. (**A**) Mix and split solid phase synthesis to synthesize trimeric molecules with three building blocks: X, Y, and Z. Solid phase methods allow to wash away excess reagents and unwanted by-products at every step. (**B**) Types of commercial resins used for solid phase synthesis. (Reproduced with permission from Drews [14]). (See color plate 20.)

Current HTS Technologies-1

Binding & Cell-Based Assays in HTS/MTS/LTS

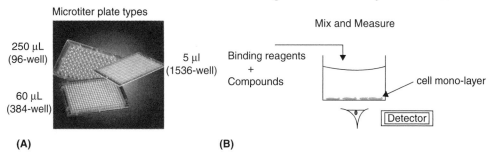

Microtiter plate types

250 μL
(96-well)

60 μL
(384-well)

5 μl
(1536-well)

Binding reagents
+
Compounds

Mix and Measure

cell mono-layer

Detector

(A)   **(B)**

Figure 9-4. (**A**) Microtiter plate types used in high-throughput screening (HTS) and lead optimization studies. Maximum reaction volume capacities are shown for each well type. (**B**) Assay in a microtiter plate well. LTS = low-throughput screen; MTS = medium-throughput screen. (See color plate 21.)

that would react to produce multiple combinations of NMEs with distinct chemical and pharmacological properties. With three functional groups and two mix-and-split reactions, 27 different molecules can be produced and cleaved from the beads and purified. Multiple types of these beads with different chemical starting points are now available commercially for use in highly automated chemical reactors to produce of hundreds of compounds in a single reaction. An elegant example of novel steroid molecules synthesized using combinatorial chemistry is described by Maltais et al. [17].

This was a major development since the early part of the twentieth century when new molecules were synthesized and purified by a series of chemical reactions *one molecule at a time*. Such an approach was too slow and inefficient for drug discovery and screening applications in the 1990s. By the end of the 1990s and early 2000s, most pharmaceutical companies synthesized large libraries of compounds to cover druglike chemical space using combinatorial chemistry, accumulated 2 to 3 million discrete chemical compounds, and needed to test thousands of molecules per day. Advances in combinatorial technologies combined with molecular biology, human genome sequencing, structural biology, and computational modeling studies drove the explosion of research in the understanding of the pathophysiology of diseases and the need to develop high-through put testing systems.

To meet this demand generated by the availability of large molecular libraries and advances in cell culture techniques, genomic targets and pathways, and HTS emerged, which involved the use of robotics to automate therapeutically relevant bioassays for drug discovery. The microtiter plates (96,384, and 1,536 wells; Fig. 9-4A) are the mainstay today for carrying out biochemical and cell-based assays to test compounds of thousands of molecules per day. The history of the development of microtiter plates to carry out cellular and biochemical assays is out of scope for this chapter but makes an interesting reading [18]. The microtiter plates accommodated testing different compounds in each well on the plate in the *same* biochemical or cellular assay systems. The same cell-based and biochemical assay is carried out in each well precisely, with an analytical measurement that read out perturbations to the assay system by the unique molecules added to the wells (Fig. 9-4B). The assay systems were designed to interrogate a target protein or signaling pathway that was critical to the disease pathology. This meant that the assay systems performed reproducibly, precisely, and reliably *in each well* so as to measure the differences in biologic or biochemical activity of each compound. This is a stringent requirement with a need to have large quantities of well-characterized reagents that included enzymes, substrates, cell membranes with receptors, different types of cell lines genetically engineered for specific readouts of signaling pathways, and so on [63].

A large industry sprung up in the 1990s that developed assay reagents (proteins and cells), multiple plate types, and sophisticated quantitative plate readers to measure enzymatic activities and binding interactions using spectroscopic (absorbance and fluorescence, luminescence) and radiometric measurements in the microtiter plates [19]. Large number of assay systems and thousands of compounds to be tested, and to process the large datasets, *automation* of both the assay systems and data analysis rapidly developed. Combining with automated plate and liquid handling robots to handle hundreds of plates dispense cells, reagents, and compound collections, HTS rapidly gained ground as a major drug discovery tool in the mid-1990s, and is a powerful tool in all drug discovery operations in the industry, government, and academia [20]. Much of the automation and information technologies that were developed have become quite useful in high-throughput genomics, proteomics, agricultural screening, and screening for biomaterials and catalysts [21–23] and have spurred the growth of multibillion dollar industry worldwide. An integrated approach to drug discovery and development was thus emerging, and the contribution of HTS technologies to discovery of known marketed drugs today is discussed in a recent publication by Macarron et al. [6].

High-Throughput Assays to Measure Biological Response

One of the most exciting developments in the past two decades is the advent of sensitive and selective bioanalytical techniques to measure protein and cell functions on high-throughput platforms listed in Table 9-1. These techniques, although well known in previous decades, were not easily amenable to high-throughput applications in microtiter plates. One has to measure diverse biologic responses of cells and protein systems when treated with druglike molecules related to disease pathology and normal function. Inglese et al. published an excellent review on high-throughput assay systems in 2007 for the identification of chemical probes and hits [19].

The advent of powerful high content screening (HCS) microscopes compatible with microtiter plates has greatly contributed to live cellular imaging (live and fixed cells) [36] along with automated cell culture systems and liquid handlers. Automated

Table 9-1. *Common high-throughput screening–compatible assay platforms*

Assay technology	Principle and use
Atomic absorbance spectroscopy	Ions such as Na, K, Rb, and others are vaporized from cell or tissue samples and analyzed by light absorbed by the vaporized ions that is proportional to concentration. HT instruments ICR 8000, ICR 12000. Na and K channel targets in drug discovery.
Optical absorbance	Absorbance of chromaphores that are products of enzymatic and other biologic reactions. Follows Beer-Lambert law.
Amplified proximity luminescent homogeneous assay (ALPHA)	Uses singlet oxygen generated by donor bead detected by the acceptor bead when the beads are in proximity because of protein–protein or protein–Ab binding ($\lambda_{ex} = 680$ nm; $\lambda_{em} = 530$–630 nm).
Bioluminescence	Luciferase reporter gene assays. Uses D-luciferin as substrates to quantify gene expression in cell-based and biochemical assays.
Bioluminescent resonance energy transfer (BRET) assay	Uses the Renilla luciferase luminescence that couples and excites green and yellow fluorescence protein emission. Generally used for protein–protein interaction in cell-based assays. Dipole interaction dependence ($1/r^6$).
Dissociation-enhanced fluorescent immunoassay (DELFIA)	An immunoassay in which the Ab is labeled with lanthanite chelates. Common lanthanides are Eu, Sm, and Tb with excitation ~340 nm and time-resolved emission ~610 nm. Very sensitive because of time-resolved emission at longer wavelengths.
Electrochemiluminescence (ECL) assay	Uses Ru-bipyridyl complexes that oxidize at electrodes and emit at visible wavelengths. Used as labels for antibodies in ECL-n based immunoassays.
Enzyme fragment complementation	Enzyme fragments attached to potentially interacting proteins, leading to complementation activation of enzyme activity (e.g., β-galactosidase).
Protein complementation assay	Complementation of fluorescent proteins, luciferases, and β-galactosidase fragments used in protein–protein interaction assays. Low-affinity complementation assays.
Fluorescence lifetime assays	Measures changes in fluorescent lifetime (nanoseconds lifetimes) of labeled fluorophores caused by biomolecular interactions. Useful in eliminating background fluorescence and molecular modifications.

(continued)

Table 9-1 (*continued*)

Assay technology	Principle and use
Fluorescence polarization	Changes in intensity of polarized light caused by binding of a fluorophore-labeled probe to a receptor. Ratiometric measurement of vertically and horizontally polarized light intensity and requires ~10-fold change in molecular weight to detect changes. Widely used in immunoassays and enzyme activity–based screens.
Fluorescence resonance energy transfer	Nonradiative dipole–dipole coupling and energy transfer occurs between fluorophores at proximity (Forster Resonance Energy transfer). Used extensively to study protein–protein, protein–peptide, and protein–nucleic acid interactions (e.g., EDANS-DABCYL).
Time-resolved fluorescence energy transfer (FRET)	Time-resolved FRET also known commercially as HTRF. Non–separation-based assays using lanthanide cryptates with long fluorescence lifetimes (~400–500 μS).
Fluorescence intensity (endpoint)	Measurement of prompt fluorescence intensity in enzymatic activity and other biochemical reactions. Fluorescence intensity enhancements and quenching are also used to measure biomolecular interactions. Large collections of fluorophores are available for labeling macromolecules.
Fluorescence intensity (kinetics)	Changes in fluorescence intensity tracking ion flux (Ca, K, and Cl ions) in cells. Dyes that bind these ions and become fluorescent are commercially available. Also requires specialized instruments such as FLIPR and FDSS6000 for rapid kinetic measurements in 96- and 384-well plates.
Fluorescence protein imaging	Cell-based imaging assays to monitor protein expression, interactions, translocation, and localization. Sophisticated confocal fluorescent microscopy–based instruments are needed. Multicolor fluorescent proteins are the mainstay for these measurements in reporter formats.
High-throughput (HT) electrophysiology	Measurement of ion-channel currents using planer microarray electrodes in a patch clamp mode. Many HT instruments are available on the market for microplate-based electrophysiology screens.
Scintillation proximity assay	Scintillation signals from radiolabels (^{3}H, ^{33}P, ^{35}S) detected in a nonseparation mode in which scintillants are incorporated in beads (or plates – FlashPlates) coated with capture reagents (Ab, receptors). Radiolabeled ligand binding to the bead stimulates scintillation.

EDANS = 5-((2-Aminoethyl)amino)naphthalene-1-sulfonic acid. DABCYL = 4-([4-(Dimethylamino)phenyl]-azo)-benzoic acid. FLIPR = fluorescent imaging plate reader.

Adapted with permission from Inglese [19].

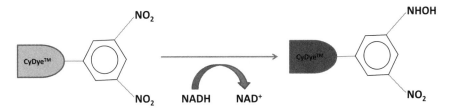

A non-fluorescent cell-permeable substrate is converted to fluorescent product in the cell by nitroreductase enzyme co-expressed with a gene of interest. This is a reporter system in which cells are intact for the readout while having enzymatic amplification for high sensitivity.

Figure 9-5. Reporter systems: chemiluminescence. (From [24].) (See color plate 22.)

cell culture systems that were developed in the late 1990s and early 2000s were key to the advancement in this field since reproducible culture techniques to mass produce cells for screening were not readily available. For example, when cells are plated at a density of 3,000 cells/well, almost 300,000 cells/plate are required. At the rate of screening approximately 80 compounds/plate, screening 100,000 compounds will require 1,250 plates and 3.75×10^8 cells for the screen. Many laboratories screen 500,000 compounds or more in a week regularly and in a cell-based assay it may require about 2 billion cells in reproducible and stable condition to complete the screen in addition to the cell culture reagents and compounds in appropriate quantities and concentrations.

Special reagents had to be developed for protein and enzyme targets for in vitro biochemical and cell-based assays. New and efficient enzyme substrates, labeled drugs and peptides, cell lines with fluorescent (green fluorescent protein [GFP], red fluorescent protein [RFP], M-Cherry) or luminescent reporter elements (luciferase, β–galactosidase), and genetic transfection agents are examples of new reagents developed in the past two decades (Table 9-1 and Fig. 9-5). The next step was to configure the assays in a scalable format to test hundreds and thousands of molecules in an automated system followed by the development of data analysis tools and storage informatics methods to handle massively parallel data output. For example, screening 100,000 compounds in a single high-content imaging assay with multiple readout could generate millions of data points in a week. Many HTS laboratories today implement 20 to 50 screening campaigns per year, generating billions of data points that should be analyzed, interpreted, and stored.

Of the assay systems developed in the 1990s (see Table 9-1), selected methods involving stable cell-based signal production systems based on luciferase, aequorin, and fluorescent proteins (FPs) are discussed later. (Note: It is impossible to address all assay systems described in Table 9-1, and readers are encouraged to access relevant references cited for additional details.) It is important to note that NMEs active in biochemical systems need to demonstrate activities in relevant cells where the targets exist. Hence, cellular systems that detect the therapeutically relevant biological reactions also indirectly demonstrate the cell permeability of the molecules tested, particularly if the disease targets are part of the intracellular functions. NMEs that are poorly water soluble or do not penetrate cells cannot be detected as actively modulating the disease target and are of no interest for further development or for chemical modification to engineer useful activity (structure–activity relationships). This property is important even if the targets that are on the cell surface (e.g., G protein–coupled receptors) because molecules that do not pass the cell membrane barrier would be difficult to deliver orally or even by intravenous or intramuscular injections. Therefore, it was critical that the cellular systems were constructed so that biologic pathways that were modulated by the NMEs will also result in the modulation of the signaling proteins in cells and can be readily detected with high sensitivity, selectivity, and linearity in assay systems.

The Luciferase System

The enzyme luciferase in bacteria (*Photobacterium fisherii*), fireflies (*Photinus pyralis*), and sea pansy (*Renilla reniformis*) emerged as excellent chemiluminescent reporter system to be genetically coupled to signaling pathways in engineered cells. The firefly and *Renilla* are the most common luciferases used in current practice [24,25].

Genetic events coupled to the expression of specific proteins in response to drug treatments can be monitored in cells using these reporter enzymes. These events include mRNA and protein expression; protein–protein interaction; protein folding; protein translocations; signal transduction; metabolic reaction cascades and DNA and RNA processing; and a multitude of cellular functions, including cell proliferation and cell death. To monitor transcriptional and translational events, the Firefly gene is coupled to the promoters that induce the desired biologic process and transfected into appropriate host cells for assay development. Commercially available Firefly enzyme kits contain reagents to lyse cells and add luciferin substrate, ATP and Mg^{2+} in the appropriate buffer systems to measure luciferase activity in treated cells. The reaction produces intense light signal (Fig. 9-6) with a flash of light (emission 550–575 nm) measured in sensitive luminometers. The firefly luciferase is a popular reporter because (1) the light signal is produced in seconds, (2) with high quantum efficiency for light production and (3) active enzyme is translated without the need for posttranslational modifications, and (4) the linearity of the signal spans over eight orders of magnitude. Very small amounts of the enzyme (10^{-18}–10^{20} moles) can be detected in cell lysates. Current commercial kits also include coenzyme A to increase turn over and other reagents that stabilize longer time for light emission for easy automation in HTS applications.

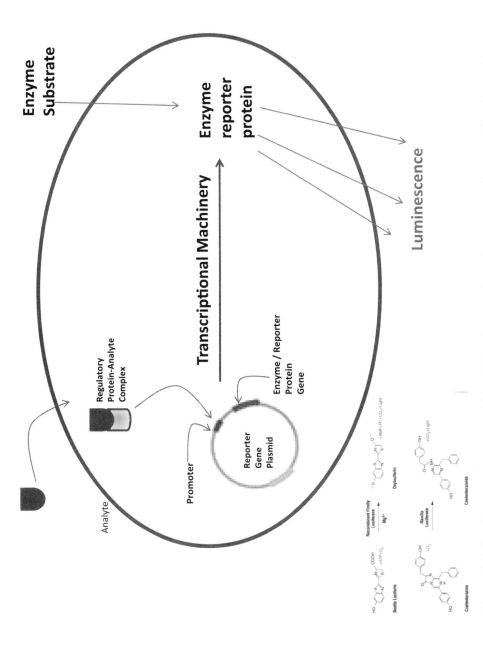

Figure 9-6. Luciferase reporter system for cell-based assays. A nonfluorescent cell-permeable substrate is converted to fluorescent product in the cell by nitroreductase enzyme coexpressed with a gene of interest. This is a reporter system in which cells are intact for the readout while having enzymatic amplification for high sensitivity. (Adapted from Amersham Biosciences.) (See color plate 23.)

The *Renilla* luciferase uses a different substrate, coelentrazine, which is oxidized to coelentramide, emitting light in the blue (480 nm). Although this luciferase is useful, it is limited in use because of lower sensitivity of nonenzymatic autoluminescence in a hydrophobic environment of the cellular milieu. Generally, *Renilla* luciferase is not used as a preferred reporter except when a dual reporter system is required in a cell-based assay. In this case, sequential measurements of two separate genetic events can be measured because these enzymes can be cloned to independent promoter and enhancer systems in the same cells. The activity of firefly enzyme is measured first, and the reaction is quenched followed by the measurement of *Renilla* enzyme activity. An excellent example of measuring the constitutive activity of telomerase, and inducible nuclear factor kappa-B (NFκB) expression in zebra fish embryos was illustrated in a recent paper [26]. A commercially available dual reporter system is available [27] and has significantly contributed to HTS applications in many drug discovery applications.

Recently, several multicolor luciferase systems were reported [28,29] for cell-based assays that could be used to monitor the expression of three separate genes simultaneously using Firefly luciferin as the common substrate. The authors constructed a NIH-3T3 murine fibroblast cell line with a green luciferase (*Rhagophthalmus ohbai*), an orange luciferase (a point mutant T226N of the green luciferase), and a red luciferase (*Phrixothrix hirtus*) using three separate plasmids. The dynamic range of this novel system ranges about three orders of magnitude and is suitable for the simultaneous monitoring of any gene expression pattern. The authors used this elegant system to demonstrate the regulation of clock gene Bmal1 through its RORE (retinoic acid receptor-related response elements) promoter region by transcription factor RORα4. In another elegant paper, Hida et al [29] reported the use of split luciferases from firefly (*Photinus pyralis*), click beetle in green luciferase (*Cratomorphus distinctus*), and click beetle in red luciferase (*Pyrophorus plagiophthalamus*) in a protein complementation assay. The system was used to study protein–protein interactions between transcription factors called Smads: the studies involved interactions between Smad 1–Smad 4 and Smad 2–Smad 4 in *Xenopus laevis* embryos and living mice. These examples clearly demonstrate the power of luciferase systems not only in cell-based assays for applications in HTS but also in animal studies in which these systems are used to image tissues and organs [26].

Other Enzyme Reporters

It is important to mention that several other enzyme systems have been used as reporters in cell-based assays, including chloramphenicol assay transferase, β-galactosidase, β-lactamase, and nitroreductase (NTR) enzymes are examples. In recent years, the luciferase [25–27], β-lactamase [30], and NTR system [31] developed by General Electric have replaced other enzymes. The general principles are the same, in which different enzyme reporters are coupled to a promoter system controlling the expression of a protein of interest and are detected using various colorimetric, luminescent, and fluorescent substrates.

The Nitroreductase NTR enzyme is an FMN-dependent enzyme that converts nitro groups on specially modified fluorescent dyes to hydroxyl amines in the presence of NADH (reduced form of nicotinamide adenine dinucleotide) or NADPH (reduced form of nicotinamide adenine dinucleotide phosphate). For example, the introduction of dinitrophenyl moiety into highly fluorescent Cy5 chromophore results in a highly quenched dye precursor (Cy5Q). This dye precursor is also modified to incorporate lipophilic character to promote cell permeability and remains nonfluorescent in the cell until NTR induced by transcriptional activity converts the dye to a fluorescent product (see Fig. 9-5). The NTR and the substrate are nontoxic to mammalian cell systems. The fluorescence of the Cy5 systems is in the Far-infrared region (600–700 nm range) with minimal interference from fluorescent compounds encountered in many HTS collections and cellular autofluorescence.

Note that the choice of a reporter system depends on a variety of considerations that include the biologic pathway interrogated in the screen, cell systems used, assay performance requirements, available imaging instrumentation, cost of reagents, properties of the compound collection, and affordability.

Fluorescent Protein Technology

Fluorescent proteins (FP) have become standard tools to track cellular functions, particularly when fused with functional cellular proteins that are expressed in response to various stimuli. FPs are now widely used in HTS applications to track and quantify protein translocations from cellular compartments (membrane to cytoplasm, cytoplasm to nucleus, and other organelles), cell cycle events, cell shape, and motility [32]. These proteins are also used in in vivo animal imaging in addition to the luciferase reporter systems.

Work on FPs started with the original discovery of blue FP aequorin and GFP in jellyfish, *Aequoria victoria* in the 1960s. It was cloned in the early 1990s [33,34] and used for gene expression studies in *Escherichia coli* under the control of T7 promoter and in *Caenorhabditis elegans*. In the latter, GFP (absorbance = 395 nm; emission = 470 nm) was under the control of the promoter of tubulin gene (mec-7) to study the expression of β-tubulin [34]. One advantage of GFP is that it does not require cofactors or other substrates because the fluorescence emission is photostable and not toxic to the cells. The intrinsic fluorescence of GFP (and other known FPs) is caused by a compact and very rigid β-barrel structure (Fig. 9-7A) formed by 11 β-sheets that surround a central α-helix in which only four amino acids are absolutely conserved in the chromophore (G67, Y66, E222, and R96). Kremers et al. [35] recently published an excellent review of the FPs useful in in vitro and

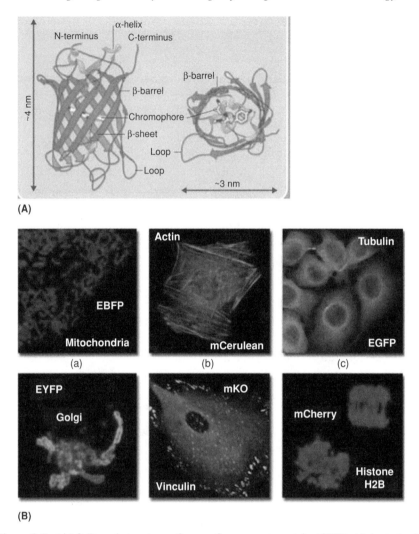

Figure 9-7. (**A**) β-Barrel structure of green fluorescent protein (GFP). (Adapted with permission from D. Piston, 2011.) (**B**) Subcellular localization of fluorescent proteins. EBFP = engineered blue fluorescent protein; EGFP = engineered green fluorescent protein; EYFP = engineered yellow fluorescent protein. (See color plate 24.)

in vivo imaging that discusses in detail the properties and biochemistry of available FPs.

Since the early1990s, several mutants of the GFP protein have been produced with chromophores that fluoresce in blue, cyan, and yellow. The color palette has also recently been expanded to orange, red, and far-infrared regions. These point mutations have not only increased the proteins available for various spectral regions for fluorescence measurements but have also provided means to significantly improve other properties such as stability, folding rates, thermal sensitivity, and maturation rates. A sampling of the available multicolor proteins and their fluorescence properties are shown in Table 9-2. Subcellular localization of various proteins covalently fused with FPs is shown in Figure 9-7B. Note that the clarity and intensity of the colors are quite impressive, and with modern automated microscopes and detection systems designed for scanning microtiter plates, one could conduct high-content imaging assays of compounds that perturb or modulate intracellular functions and the phenotype. A comprehensive review of the high-content screening systems comparing instrumentation available on the market was published recently [36].

Another interesting development is the advent of infrared fluorescent proteins (IFPs) developed from a bacterial phytochrome described by Shu et al. [37]. These proteins have high extinction coefficients ($\sim$90,000 M^{-1} cm^{-1}) and have an excitation maximum at 684 nm and emission at 708 nm. The DrCBD proteins of bacterial origin ([Protein Data Bank (PDB) ID: 1ztu]) contain biliverdin surrounded by 14–amino acid residues that form the fluorescent chromophore. However, the quantum efficiency of these proteins appears to be low ($\sim$0.07). Thus, mutations of the surrounding amino acids are important handles to generate engineered IFPs with improved fluorescent properties. Because of fluorescence in the infrared region, these proteins would be valuable tools in whole-body imaging.

Photoactivatable FPs have also been developed recently [38,39]. These proteins can change emission intensity with preexposure to light stimulation. These are known as optical or molecular highlighters producing high-contrast images to follow dynamic changes in macromolecules within cells. For example, photoactive version of the GFP (PA-GFP after activation at 400 nm) shows an almost 100-fold increase in excitation peak at 488 nm compared with the wild type GFP, but the excitation wavelength (395–400 nm) of the unconverted PA-GFP remains unchanged [39].

Overall, research in FPs is moving rapidly toward developing orange, red, and infrared proteins through specific mutations for multicolor imaging in tissues and whole animals. Work continues to fine tune the monomeric GFP and blue FPs to bright and fast maturing mutants and photoactivatable variants described earlier. A large number of FP color palettes are already available to customize both in vitro and in vivo imaging studies in drug discovery and diagnosis.

Measurement of Second Messengers

Second messengers or small intercellular mediators are small molecules that transmit and amplify extracellular signals received by receptors on the cell surface. An activated or stimulated receptor produces large amounts of these molecules that diffuse away from the cell membrane to various intracellular compartments and transmit the signal by binding and altering the conformation and function of intracellular signaling proteins, thus modifying cellular, tissue response to external stimuli [40]. Examples of the second messengers include water-soluble Ca^{2+} ions; inositol-(1,4,5)-triphosphate

Table 9-2. *Fluorescent proteins, their properties, and their associated mutations*

Protein	Excitation maximum (nm)	Emission maximum (nm)	Molar extinction coefficient (cm−1)	Quantum yield	Relative brightness (% of EGFP)	Functional structure/ mutation
Green Proteins						
Green fluorescent protein (wtGFP)	395/475	509	21,000	0.77	48	Monomer
Enhanced GFP* (E-GFP)	484	507	56,000	0.60	100	Monomer
Emerald	487	509	57,500	0.68	116	Monomer
Turbo-GFP	482	502	70,000	0.53	110	monomer
Cyan Proteins						
Enhanced cyan fluorescent protein (E-CFP)	439	476	32,500	0.40	39	Monomer
mTFP1 (Teal)	482	492	64,000	0.85	162	Monomer
Cerulean	433	475	43,000	0.62	79	Monomer
Midori-Ishi cyan	472	495	27,300	0.90	73	Dimer
Blue Proteins						
Enhanced blue fluorescent protein (E-BFP)	383	445	29,000	0.31	27	Monomer
Sapphire	399	511	29,000	0.64	55	Monomer
T-sapphire	399	511	44,000	0.60	79	Monomer

Yellow Proteins

Enhanced yellow fluorescent protein (E-YFP)	514	527	83,400	0.61	151	Monomer
Topaz	514	527	94,500	0.60	169	Monomer
YPet	517	530	104,000	0.77	238	Monomer

Orange and Red Proteins

mOrange	548	562	71,000	0.69	146	Monomer
dTomato	554	581	69,000	0.69	142	Dimer
tdTomato	554	581	138,000	0.69	283	Monomer
DsRed	558	583	75,000	0.79	176	Tetramer
DsRed2	563	582	43,800	0.55	72	Tetramer
mCherry†	587	610	72,000	0.22	47	Monomer
mPlum	590	649	41,000	0.10	12	Monomer
mApple	568	592	75,000	0.49	109	Monomer
mRuby	558	605	112,000	0.35	117	Monomer
mStrawberry	574	596	90,000	0.29	78	Monomer

* mEGFP is a monomeric variant that was derived by introducing the A206K mutation into EGFP.
† mCherry is the second-generation monomeric red fluorescent proteins that have improved brightness and photostability.
EGFP = enhanced green fluorescent protein.
Adapted from http://www.olympusfluoview.com/applications/fpcolorpalette.html.

(IP_3); cyclic nucleotides such as cyclic adenosine monophosphate (cAMP), cyclic guanosine monophosphate (cGMP), and cyclic guanosine triphosphate (cGTP); and hydrophobic molecules such as diacylglycerol (DAG), ceramides, and phosphatidylinositols. Gases such as nitric oxide (NO), hydrogen sulfide (H_2S), and carbon monoxide (CO) also play this role in the cell.

Small molecule drugs that modulate the level and activity of the second messengers through G protein–coupled receptors; ion channels; and intracellular enzymes such as adenylate cyclases, phospholipases, and protein kinases also play a significant role in normal and disease pathology. Sophisticated bioanalytical methods for screening for molecular modulators on the second messengers have also been developed in recent years [41].

One of the earliest assays developed for the measurement of Ca^{2+} ion mobilization in cells for high throughput applications was the Fluorescent Imaging Plate Reader (FLIPR) technology. Originally developed in the early 1990s for membrane potential measurements [42], it was later adopted to measure Ca^{2+} ions [43] released from intracellular stores or entering cells from the environment. A dye that is nonfluorescent within cells is preloaded into the cell as an ester, which is cleaved by cellular esterases. When free Ca^{2+} ion release is stimulated by drugs and bind to the dye, fluorescence emission in visible region was measured by the FLIPR. Typical Ca^{2+} sensitive dyes used in such application include Fluo-3 AM, Fluo4-AM, and Fura-AM version. Today more than 30 such Ca^{2+}-sensitive dyes are available for use [44] for customized HTS applications.

The uniqueness of the FLIPR technology in the 1990s was due to its unique ability to measure fluorescence signals with a spatial resolution of about 200 μm at the bottom of all wells in 96-well microtiter plates in less than 1 sec using a specially designed optical system and a charge-coupled device (CCD) camera. This meant that the instrument could accomplish kinetic measurements of intracellular Ca^{2+} mobilization caused by external or internal stimuli. This technology has been used extensively in HTS and lead generation applications in the past 15 years [45]. Modern instrumentation in this technology now includes Functional Drug Screening Systems (FDSS) from Hamamatsu that can read both fluorescence and luminescence signals from cells in kinetic mode using the standard fluorescent with high speed and precision [46] and includes built-in liquid dispensing systems for rapid automation of cell-based assays.

cAMP measurement technologies have also been developed recently using enzyme fragment complementation assay that uses fragments of β-galactosidase [47]. In this format (Fig. 9-8), two inactive fragments of the enzyme are used: enzyme acceptor (EA) and enzyme donor (ED) fragments. The ED is coupled to cAMP (cAMP-ED), which competes with free cAMP produced in the cell to bind an anti-cAMP antibody in solution. In the absence of free cAMP in solution, the cAMP-ED is sequestered by the anti-cAMP, thus preventing active enzyme formation in solution. When free

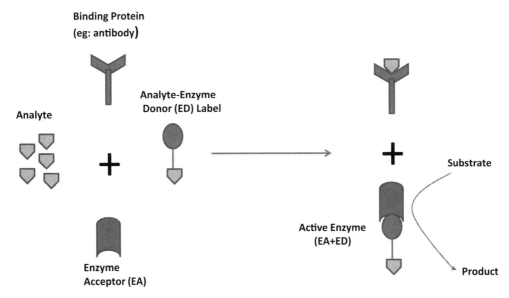

Figure 9-8. Enzyme complementation assay for a second messenger. EA = enzyme acceptor; ED = enzyme donor. (Adapted from DiscoveRx Inc: http://www.discoverx. com/technology/technology-hithunter.php.) (See color plate 25.)

cAMP from cells is present, the cAMP-ED is displaced from the antibody to bind EA fragment and form active tetrameric β-galactosidase enzyme. The active enzyme can be detected by colorimertic, fluorometric, or luminescent products generated by the enzyme. This technology can be modified to detect other intracellular messengers, including IP_3, cGMP, and so on, with use of appropriate antibodies and the labeled ED fragment.

Informatics for Drug Discovery

Bio- and cheminformatics are two related fields that provide tools to systematically process massive amounts of biological and chemical data generated using modern high-throughput technologies. The advent of miniaturized bioassay methods for HTS of small molecules, combinatorial chemical synthesis proteins and peptides, DNA and RNA sequencing, protein purification and crystallization, and robotic technologies to implement these formats in the 1990s created the need for high-throughput informatics that address biologic and chemical information.

Bioinformatics is a discipline in which information technology, biology, statistics, and computer science merge to device tools to interrogate the massive databases and to obtain relevant information to specific questions. In cheminformatics, chemical information such as protein structure, chemical and biochemical information are dealt with in the biological context using computer science and information technology. Both of these address important biologic and biochemical questions from two slightly different vantage points using the same technologies. This is possible because of the advances in computing power developed in the past 20 years [48,49]. The significance is the ability to mine large databases to develop testable hypotheses and generate scientific insights into complex biological problems.

For example, the molecular basis of disease can be deduced from genetic information in normal and patient gene sequences and by examining the homologous gene sequences in animal models. These comparisons provide insights into the evolutionary history of the disease process and the contributions of mutations [2,14]. Proteins are the main "effecter molecules" in cells and organelles encoded by specific DNA and mRNA sequences. The structure of these molecules elucidated by protein crystallization, NMR and molecular modeling can be of immense significance in understanding cellular function and dysfunction in disease [3].

A large number of informatics databases are available in biological sciences today. If one does an Internet search on the term "bio- and cheminformatics databases," one can easily get more than 100,000 hits with varying significance! This demonstrates the need for and proliferation of such tools to mine a variety of databases with diverse information. These data tools not only identify genes, mutations, genetic identity and similarity, and evolutionary relationships but also superimpose, visualize, and design molecules; identify pharmacophores; and model protein–small molecule interactions to name a few. These tools are playing important role in modern drug discovery and medicine.

Molecular Modulators of Cell Proliferation and Differentiation

Many small and large molecules of biologic origin modulate biological function. These include small molecules such as second messengers (e.g., cAMP, cGMP, IP_3); nucleotides (e.g., adenosine monophosphate [AMP], adenosine triphosphate [ATP], adenosine diphosphate [ADP]); neurotransmitters (e.g., serotonin, dopamine, NO); sugars; fatty and amino acids; and a myriad of proteins, hormones, growth factors, cytokines, lipids, and carbohydrates, to name a few. However, there are extrinsic molecules, including drugs, toxins, trace metals, and nutrients, that also influence function such as cell growth, proliferation, death, and differentiation that are hallmarks of life and biological function. These latter processes are essential to maintain homeostasis, aging, and regeneration of organs and tissues in biologic systems. Hence, these extrinsic molecules form an important repertoire in regenerative medicine and pharmacology.

Small Molecule Drugs That Determine Cell Signaling and Function

From the days of Paul Ehrlich's experiment with methylene blue to the discovery of aspirin and antibiotics and the modern age of drug discovery, a wealth of data has accumulated on the biologic modulation of tissue and organ function by small molecule drugs. These lifesaving drugs have contributed immensely to public health in the twenty-first century. All known drugs and well-designed small molecule collections can affect cell growth and proliferation and, more importantly, cell differentiation and transdifferentiation. Profiling these phenotypic activities is an important step in identifying new targets and eventual treatments for complex diseases [50,62]. In addition, the understanding of global biologic functions in cells, in the context of tissues and organs (regenerative potential), is beginning to be recognized as a significant advance in regenerative medicine: here the possibility that modulating primary and stem and progenitor cells (and even primary cells via transdifferentiation) from patients can be induced to differentiate in to useful transplantable tissues such as skin is a real possibility. Furthermore, they can also be valuable in inducing stem and progenitor cells in endogenous tissues to repair tissue and organ damage caused by disease and injury.

Table 9-3 shows a sampling of known drugs and small molecules that are reported to influence stem and progenitor cells [51]. It is not known if the modulation of activities of stem and progenitor cells is important for the therapeutic actions of these molecules, but these are significant observations on the regenerative potential of these molecules. Note that the examples in Table 9-3 show that the molecules are of diverse chemical structures and biologic functions that are important in cellular growth and differentiation. Hence, these molecules can be used as starting points to design drugs to regenerate and repair tissues, particularly in degenerative diseases.

For example, dexamethasone, vitamin C, and 5-azacytidine have been reported to induce differentiation of embryonic and mesenchymal stem cells. The latter, 5-azacytidine, was used to investigate myogenic differentiation and the discovery of the transcription factor Myo-D in 1986 [9,51]. Another interesting example is reversine, which de-differentiates myoblasts into progenitor cells that can be driven to adipogenesis and osteogenesis pathways. Hence, considerable opportunities are available to use HTS with phenotypic cell-based assays to identify small molecule modulators of cell fate, either alone or in cocktails of molecular adjuvants such as cytokines, growth factors, and hormones in regenerative pharmacology.

Perspectives and Challenges

Today's medicine has evolved from old natural product concoctions, extracts, crude surgical treatments, bloodletting, and transfusions to well-defined drug molecules that comprise small organics, vaccines, and powerful biopharmaceuticals. Many of these treatments are still combined with sophisticated modern surgical technologies that clearly provide higher quality of life. Still, many of the degenerative ailments such as Alzheimer's disease, Lou Gehrig's disease, spinal muscular atrophy, old age–related muscle wasting, arthritis, cancer-related cachexia, metabolic diseases such as

Table 9-3. *Examples of molecules reported to control the fate of stem and progenitor cell fate and function*

Drug	Type of molecule	Known function
Ascorbic acid	Vitamin C	Essential vitamin
5-Azacytidine	Nucleoside analog	Inhibitor of DNA methylation
Bortezomib	Tripeptide boronic acid derivative	Proteasome inhibitor
Cardiogenol C	Diamine pyrimidine analog	ES cells to cardiomyocytes
Cyclopamine	Steroidal alkaloid	Inhibits Hedgehog signaling
Dexamethasone	Steroidal drug	Anti-inflammatory
Dimethyl sulfoxide	Organic sulfur compound	Analgesic, cryoprotectant, universal organic solvent
Forskolin	Bicyclic diterpene	Activates adenylyl cyclase
Fluoxetine	Diphenyl hydramine derivative	SSRI
Gleevec (STI571)	2-phenylamino pyrimidine derivative	Bcr-Abl tyrosine kinase inhibitor
Geldenamycin	Benzoquinone ansamycin antibiotic	HSP90 inhibitor
LY294002	Morpholino-benzopyran derivative	Selective PI3 kinase inhibitor
Myoseverin	2,6,9-Trisubstitutued purine	Microtubule binding and reversible myotube fission
Purmorphamine	2,6,9-Trisubstitutued purine	Differentiation of mesenchymal progenitor cells
Retinoic acid (all-trans)	Vitamin A metabolite	Embryonic development: regulates gene expression
Reversine	2,6-Dissubstitutued purine derivative	Dedifferentiation of myoblasts
Rosiglitazone	Thiazolidinedione derivative	Insulin sensitizer, PPAR receptor modulator
SAHA	Suberoylanilide hydroxamic acid	HDAC inhibitor
TWS119	4,6-Disubstituted pyrrolopyrimidine	Potent GSK-3β kinase inhibitor

ES = embryonic stem; GSK = glycogen synthase kinase 3β; HDAC = histone deacetylase; PPAR = peroxisome proliferator-activated receptor; SSRI = selective serotonin reuptake inhibitor.
Adapted from Ding and Schultz [51].

diabetes and obesity, osteoporosis, and congenital organ defects do not have effective treatments [60]. Even in the case of myocardial infarction and spinal cord injuries, damaged tissue cannot be easily regenerated, resulting permanent scar tissues and lifelong disability. Surgical techniques such as heart bypass surgery and organ transplantation (heart, liver, skin, kidney, and so on) were pioneered in the last half of the twentieth century were major breakthroughs but have their own risks and complications such as immune rejection. One of the major impediments was the availability of suitable and healthy organs and tissues for transplant along with the need for immune suppressive drugs. Cyclosporine A was the one of the first immunosuppressive drugs (discovered in 1969) [61] that started the field of immunopharmacology. Today the challenge is getting the right patient-matched organs and tissues at the right time and place for chronic and emergency surgery. Hence, advances in pharmacology and tissue engineering are poised to make the next leap in modern therapies for difficult complex degenerative diseases.

In the 1980s, bone marrow transplants using hematopoietic stem cells made significant advance in treating many childhood and adult leukemias [52]. This was the beginning of true stem cell therapies. Very little progress was made in the last half of the century in using embryonic and adult stem cells because of technical and sociopolitical reasons. Embryonic and adult stem cells were hard to isolate, grow, and expand. In the past 10 years, stem cell culture techniques have made significant advances, enabling the isolation, growth, characterization, and expansion of embryonic and adult mesenchymal stem cells. Many of these cells are in clinical trials for the treatment of spinal cord injuries and tissue injuries. In 2007, Takahashi et al. [53] described a revolutionary procedure to induce mouse and human adult primary cells, such as fibroblasts, to de-differentiate into stem cells. These cells, known as iPS cells, can be made by virally transfecting four transcription factors (*C-myc*, *Sox-2*, *KLf4*, and *Oct 4*) that reprogram adult cells to embryonic stage. Recently, it has been shown that iPS cells from patients [54] with disease mutations can be used in drug discovery. Today technologies are also being explored to directly modify mature fibroblasts and keratinocytes to other cellular lineages such as cardiomyocytes and neurons without going through the pluripotent stem cell stage [55,56]. Even with all of these developments, the current challenge is to successfully integrate modern drug discovery technologies such as HTS, cell and molecular and computational biology, biochemistry, chemical and structural biology, tissue engineering, pharmacology, and so on to impact regenerative medicine and pharmacology for effective treatments [57–59].

References

1. Lesney M. "Patents and potions: entering pharmaceutical industry." *The Pharmaceutical Century: Ten Decades of drug Discovery Supplement to the American Chemical Society;* 2000, p. 18–31. American Chemical Society Publications, Washington DC.
2. Drews J. "Drug discovery: a historical perspective." *Science.* 2000; 287, 1960–1964.
3. Drews J. "In quest of tomorrow's medicines." New York: Springer 1998.
4. Mayr LM, Fuerst P. "The future of high throughput screening." *J Biomol Screen.* 2008; 13, 443–448.
5. Garnier J. "Rebuilding the R&D engine in big pharma." *Harvard Bus Rev.* 2008; 86, 68–76.
6. Macarron R, Banks MN, Bojanic, D, Burns, DJ, Cirovic DA, Garyantes T, Green DVS, Hertzberg RP, Janzen WP, Paslay JW, Schopfer U, Sittampalam GS. "Impact of high throughput screening in biomedical research." *Nat Rev Drug Disc.* 2011; 10, 188–195.
7. Andersson K-E, Christ GJ. Regenerative pharmacology: the future is now." *Mol Interv.* 2007; 7, 79–86.

8. Nirmalanandhan VS, Sittampalam GS. "Stem cells in drug discovery, tissue engineering, and regenerative medicine: emerging opportunities and challenges." *J Biomol Screen.* 2009; 14, 755–768.

9. Furth, ME, Christ GJ. "Regenerative pharmacology for diabetes mellitus." *Mol Interv.* 2009; 9, 171–174.

10. "2020: A New Vision – A Future for Regenerative Medicine." Washington, DC: US Department of Health and Human Services. http://www.hhs.gov/reference/newfuture .shtml.

11. Nelson TJ, Behfar A, Terzic A. "Stem cells: biologics for regeneration." *Clin Pharm Ther.* 2008; 84, 620–623.

12. Eggert US, Superti-Furga G. "Drugs in action." *Nat Chem Biol.* 2008; 4(1), 7–11.

13. Royal Society of Chemistry. Advances in Chemical Sciences. "Chemical Biology – A Vital Partnership for Progress." 2006. http://www.rsc.org/ScienceAndTechnology/ Policy/Bulletins/Issue3/Chemicalbiology.asp.

14. Drews J. "Genomic sciences and the medicine of tomorrow." *Nat Biotechnol.* 1996; 14, 1516–1518.

15. DuFort CC, Paszek MJ, Weaver VM. "Balancing forces: architectural control of mechanotransduction." *Nat Rev Mol Cell Biol.* 2011; 12, 308–319.

16. Crooks SL, Charels LJ. "Overview of combinatorial chemistry." *Curr Protoc Pharmacol.* 2000; 9(3), 1–16.

17. Maltais R, Tremblay MR, Ciobanu LC, Poirier D. "Steroids and combinatorial chemistry." *J Comb Chem.* 2004; 6(4), 443–456.

18. Drecker S. "Necessity is the mother of invention." *BioTEK Technical Bulletin.* 2004. GIT Labor-Fachzeitschrift 12/2004, S. 1120-1121, GIT VERLAG GmbH & Co. KG, Darmstadt, www.gitverlag.com/go/git.

19. Inglese I, Johnson RL, Simeonov A, Xia M, Zheng W, Austin CP, Auld DA. "High-throughput screening assays for the identification of chemical probes." *Nat Chem Biol.* 2007; 3(8), 466–479.

20. Traulau-Stewart CJ, Wyatt CA, Kleyn DE, Alex A. "Drug discovery: new models for industry-academic partnerships." *Drug Discov Today.* 2009; 14 (1/2), 95–101.

21. Tyers M, Mann M. "From genomics to proteomics." *Nature.* 2003; 422, 193–197.

22. Simon CG, Lin-Gibson S. "Combinatorial high throughput screening of biomaterials." *Adv Mater.* 2011; 23(3), 369–387.

23. Ylliperttula M, Chung, BG, Navaladi A, Manbachi A, Urtti A. "High-throughput screening of cell responses to biomaterials." *Eur J Pharm Sci.* 2008; 35, 151–160.

24. Daunert S, Barrett G, Feliciano JS, Shetty R, Shresth S, Smith-Spence W. "Genetically engineered whole cell sensing systems: coupling biological recognition with reporter genes." *Chem Rev.* 2000; 100, 2705–2738.

25. Wood KV: "The chemistry of bioluminescent reporter assays." *Promega News.* 1998, No.65; p. 14.

26. Perez FA, Mulero V, and Cayuela ML: "Application of dual-luciferase reporter assay to the analysis of promoter activity in zebra fish embryos." *BMC Biotec.* 2008; 8:81; pp-1–8.

27. *Promega Dual Luciferase Reporter System Technical Manual.* Revised August 2006: Part No. TM046, Promega Corp. Madison, WI, USA.

28. Nakjama Y, Kimura T, Sugata K, Enomoto T, Askawa A, Ikeda M, Ohmiya Y. "Multicolor luciferase assay system: one step monitoring of multiple gene expressions with a single substrate." *BioTechniques.* 2005; 38, 891–894.

29. Hida N, Awais M, Takeuchi M, Ueno N, Tashiro M, Takagi C, Singh T, Hayashi M, Ohmiya Y, Ozawa T. "High-sensitivity real-time imaging of dual protein-protein

interactions in living subjects using multicolor luciferases."*PLoS One*. 2009; 4(6), e5868.

30. Hallis TM, Kopp AL, Gibson J, Lebakken CS, Hancock M, Van Den Heuvel-Kramer K, Turek-Etienne T. "An improved b-lactamase reporter assay: multiplexing with cytotoxicity readout for enhanced accuracy for hit detection." *J Biomol Screen*. 2007; 12(5), 635–644.

31. Stein DC, Carrizosa E, Dunham S. "Use of *nfsB*, encoding nitroreductase, as a reporter gene to determine the mutational spectrum of spontaneous mutations in *Neisseria gonorrhoeae*." *BMC Microbiol*. 2009; 9, 239.

32. Auld DS, Zhang YQ, Veith H, Jadhav, A, Yasgar A, Simeonov A, Zheng W, Martinez ED, Westwick JK, Austin CP, Inglese J. "Fluorescent protein bases cellular assays analyzed by laser scanning microplate cytometry in 1536-well format." *Methods in Enzymo*. 2006; 414, 566–589.

33. Prasher DC, Eckenrode VK, Ward WW, Prendergast FG, Cormier MJ. "Primary structure of the *Aequorea victoria* green-fluorescent protein." *Gene*. 1992; 111, 229–233.

34. Chalfie M G, Euskirchen G, Ward WW, Prasher DC. "Green fluorescent protein as a marker for gene expression." *Science*. 1994; 263, 802–805

35. Kremers G-J, Gilbert SG, Cranfill PJ, Davidson MW, Piston DW. "Fluorescent proteins at a glance." *J Cell Sci*. 2011; 124(2), 157–160.

36. Zanella F, Lorens JB, Ink W. "High content screening: seeing is believing." *Trends Biotechnol*. 2010; 28(5), 237–245.

37. Shu X, Roynat A, Lin MZ, Aguilera TA, Lev-Ram V, Steibach PA, Tsien RY. "Mammalian expression of infrared fluorescent proteins engineered from a bacterial phytochrome." *Science*. 2009; 234, 804–807.

38. Piston DW, Patterson GH, Lippincott-Swartz J, Claxton NS, Davidson MW. "Introduction to fluorescent proteins." 2010. http://www.microscopyu.com/articles/livecellimaging/fpintro.html.

39. Lukyanov KA, Chudakov DM, Lukyanov S, and Verkhusha VV. "Innovation: photoactivatable fluorescent proteins." *Nat Rev Mol Cell Biol*. 2005; 6, 885–891.

40. Alberts B, Johnson A, Lewis J, Raff M, Roberts K, Walter P. *Molecular Biology of the Cell*, 5th edition. New York: Garland Science, Taylor & Francis; 2008.

41. Gregory KJ, Sexton PM, Christopoulos A. Hick CA. 2010 second messenger assays for G protein-coupled receptors: cAMP, Ca^{2+}, inositol phosphates, ERK1/2. In *G Protein-Coupled Receptors: Essential Methods*, edited by D.R. Poyner, M. Wheatley. Oxford, UK: Wiley-Blackwell.

42. Schroeder KS, Neagle BD. "FLIPR: a new instrument for accurate, high throughout optical screening." *J Biomol Screen*. 1996; 1(2), 75–80.

43. Whitaker KL, Sullivan JP, Gopalakrishnan M. " Cell-based assays using Fluorometric Imaging Plate Reader (FLIPR)." *Curr Protoc Pharmacol* 2000; 9.2.1–9.2.23.

44. Summary of molecular probes fluorescent Ca2+ indicators. In *The Molecular Probes*® *Handbook*, 11th edition. 2011. Life Technologies, Grand Island, NY.

45. "FLIPR Assays to measure GPCR and ION Channel Targets" 2011. http://www.ncgc.nih.gov/guidance/section9.html.

46. Titus SA, Beacham D, Shahane SA, Southall N, Xia M, Huang R, Hooten E, Zhao Y, Shou L, Austin CP, Zheng W. "A new homogeneous high-throughput screening assay for profiling compound activity on the human ether-a-go-go-related gene channel." *Anal Biochem*. 2009; 394(1), 30–38.

47. Golla R, Seethala R. "A homogeneous enzyme fragment complementation cyclic AMP screen for GPCR agonists." *J Biomol Screen*. 2002; 7(6), 515–525.

48. Claverie JM, Notredame C. *Bioinformatics for Dummies*. Wiley; Hoboken, NJ, 2003.

49. Baxevanis AD, Ouellette BFF. (eds.) *Bioinformatics: A Practical Guide to the Analysis of Genes and Proteins*, third edition. Wiley, 2005. ISBN 0–471-47878–4.

50. Congreve M, Murray CW, Blundell TM. "Structural biology and drug discovery." *Drug Discov Today*. 2005; 10(13), 895–907.

51. Ding S, Schultz PG. "A role for chemistry in stem cell biology." *Nat Biotech*. 2004; 22(7), 833–840.

52. Korbling M, Przepiorka D, Huh YO, Engel H, van Besien K, Giralt S, Andersson B, Kleine HD, Seong D, Deisseroth AB. "Allogeneic blood stem cell transplantation for refractory leukemia and lymphoma: potential advantage of blood over marrow allografts." *Blood*. 1995; 85(6), 1659–1665.

53. Takahashi K, Tanabe K, Ohnuki M, Narita M, Ichisaka T, Tomoda K, Yamanaka S. "Induction of pluripotent stem cells from adult human fibroblasts by defined factors." *Cell*. 2007; 131(5), 861–872.

54. Soldner F, Hockemeyer D, Beard C, Gao Q, Bell GW, Cook EG, Hargus G, Blak A, Cooper O, Mitalipova M, Isacson O, HJaenisch R. "Parkinson's disease patient-derived induced pluripotent stem cells free of viral reprogramming factors." *Cell* 2009; 136(5), 964–977.

55. Kim, S-K. "Converting human skin cells to neurons: a new tool to study and treat brain disorders?" *Cell Stem Cell*. 2011; 9, 179–180.

56. Ieda M, Fu J-D, Delgado-Olguin P, Vedantham V, Hyashi Y, Bruneau B, Srivastava D. "Direct reprogramming if fibroblasts into functional cardiomyocytes by defined factors." *Cell*. 2010; 142, 375–386.

57. Christ GJ, Chen AF. "The grand challenge for integrative and regenerative pharmacology." *Front Pharmacol*. 2011; 2 (5), 1–2.

58. Christ GJ, Furth ME. "Regenerative pharmacology for diabetes mellitus." *Mol Interven*. 2009; 9(4), 171–174.

59. Mozetta C, Minetti G, Puri PL. "Regenerative pharmacology in the treatment of genetic disorders: the paradigm for muscular dystrophy." *Int J Biochem Cell Biol*. 2009; 41, 701–710.

60. Begley S, Carmichael M. "Desperately seeking cures: how the road from promising scientific breakthrough to real-world remedy has become all but a dead end." *Newsweek*. 2010; May 31, pp. 38–42.

61. Borel JF. "History of the discovery of cyclosporine and of its early pharmacological development." *Wien Klin Wochenschr*. 2002; 114(12), 433–437.

62. Lee JA, Uhlick MT, Moxham CM, Tomandl D, Sall DJ. "Modern phenotypic drug discovery is a viable, neoclassic pharma strategy." *J Med Chem*. 2012; 55, 4527–4538.

63. Inglese J, Shamu CE, Guy RK. "Reporting data from high-throughput screening of small-molecule libraries." *Nat Chem Biol*. 2007; 8(3), 438–441.

10

Animal Models of Regenerative Medicine

J. KOUDY WILLIAMS, JAMES YOO, AND ANTHONY ATALA

In the process of scientific discovery and eventual translation of this information to the clinic, a fundamental step is exploration of the safety and efficacy of these discoveries in preclinical studies. These questions are addressed in animal models that provide a sufficient level of reproducibility. Fundamental discovery also demands animal systems in which reagents (e.g., antibodies and probes) are readily available and turnover of individuals and the occurrence of biologic events are rapid. Therefore, the study of animals with short development and life cycles (days to months) provides the best opportunities for initial detection and observation of the process under study. Common choices for initial feasibility research include *Drosophila melanogaster* (fruit fly), *Caenorhabditis elegans* (nematode worm), *Danio rerio* (zebra fish), and many varieties of *Mus musculus* (mouse) and *Rattus norvegicus* (rat). Development of knockout and transgenic animals has greatly increased the rate of fundamental biologic discovery in the past decade.

Feasibility testing is almost always performed in small mammals, specifically mice and rats, in which outcomes can be determined after relatively short periods of observation; reagents are readily available; and the variations in radiographic, imaging, histologic, or biochemical outcomes among individuals are small. Many standard models for the assessment of implant materials in small mammals have been described in standard protocol documents published by major standards and regulatory organizations, including the American Society for Testing and Materials (ASTM), International Standards Organization (ISO), U.S. Food and Drug Administration (FDA), and European Commission.

After initial feasibility studies have been completed or in cases in which the size of rodents precludes sufficient evaluation of the technology, studies must be advanced into larger animals, such as rabbits, dogs, sheep, nonhuman primates, or pigs. In these studies, every attempt is made to create an environment that is as close as possible to the clinical setting. As such, studies using these models are designed to deliver potential therapeutics in the manner in which they will be delivered in a clinical setting, and surgical techniques that match clinical methods are used. In addition, it is important to use an animal model that provides a metabolic background and physiological responsiveness comparable to those of humans and to use a formulation of active agent that has the same composition, dose, release, retention, and degradation properties as the formulation that will be used clinically.

Assessing the safety and efficacy of a novel therapeutic in any animal model and the eventual translation to human beings is confounded by species differences in biology. Some immunologic barriers make successful transplantation of human cells into animals as xenografts difficult. Additionally, there is an assumption that the starting composition and intrinsic biologic potential of tissue-derived cell populations from animal species are comparable to those of cell populations that may be harvested from human subjects. Special challenges are presented when the clinical cell processing or validation methods can only be applied to human cells because of the need to use species-specific reagents. In this case, preclinical studies may require use of a surrogate reagent or process that provides comparable processing effect to the missing reagent. Another critical challenge occurs in in vitro cell culture and expansion in which the optimal culture conditions for animal cells may not be comparable to those achieved by highly refined systems developed for human clinical application. Preclinical systems must also be established to assess the long-term fate of culture-expanded cells and to detect and limit the potential for selection or development of clones with undesirable or potentially harmful biologic properties during periods of rapid expansion outside of the normal systems of systemic immune surveillance.

The following review outlines progress made in the types of stem and progenitor cells isolated from commonly used animal species and their uses in regenerative medicine approaches to tissue engineering.

Rodent Models

As stated, rodent models of regenerative medicine are widely used because of the size, cost, and relatively easy husbandry requirements of these animals. In addition, the genome of rodents can be altered to study specific gene contributions to disease. Much of the initial work isolating various stem and progenitor cell populations has been done in rodents.

Rodent Mesenchymal Stem Cells

Numerous studies using mesenchymal stem cells (MSCs) have been performed at preclinical level to assess their in vivo behavior and suitability for the treatment of a number of injuries and diseases. Ortiz and colleagues evaluated the ability of intra-venously infused MSCs to engraft in the lung tissue in bleomycin-exposed mice, which represents a lung injury model [1]. Additionally, intravenous administration of

MSCs has been used for recovery of small intestine structure in NOD/SCID (nonobese nondiabetic/severe combined immune deficient) mice after abdominal irradiation [2]. Green fluorescent protein–labeled MSCs have been used to examine kidney engraftment and tubular epithelial differentiation after renal failure in mice [3], for chronic wound closure and angiogenesis [4], for diabetes applications [5], and for corneal reconstruction [6]. Recently, MSCs have also been shown to improve hematopoietic transplantation [7,8]. Enhanced hematopoietic engraftment has been reported upon infusion of a limiting number of umbilical cord blood stem cells with unrelated MSCs in mice. Co-transplanting MSCs with hematopoietic stem cells (CD34$^+$ cells) has been shown to improve engraftment in the bone marrow in mice, although the underlying mechanism needs to be elucidated. Migration of MSCs to the sites of injury and disease has also been well documented in animal models for myocardial infarction (MI) and cerebral ischemia [9,10]. Further studies using disease models need to be carried out to elucidate the molecular mechanism involved in MSC homing for the improvement of current therapies.

Genetically modified MSCs have also been used for a wide variety of cell- and tissue-based engineering techniques. After transplantation, the fate of MSCs may be dependent on the niches they fill; therefore, not all transplanted cells might contribute to the repair of the damage. As recently demonstrated in mice, transplanted MSCs differentiate into osteoblasts in the heart [11]. Thus, site-specific transplantation of functional, differentiated cells would be advantageous under certain conditions. Although differentiated cells can be generated by chemical stimulants or differentiation factors in vitro, the differentiation state may not be stable upon transplantation. Therefore, genetically modifying stem cells may help to achieve directed and complete differentiation into the desired lineage. Studies on the therapeutic applicability of genetically modified MSCs have been done in rodent species for several applications. MSCs transfected with PDX-1 (pancreatic and duodenal homeobox 1) have been used for treatment of diabetes in immunodeficient mice [12,13]. MSCs transduced with bone morphogenetic proteins 2 and 4 (BMP-2 and BMP-4) have been shown to successfully repair a variety of musculoskeletal defects [14]. Angiopeptin-1–modified MSCs have been shown to improve heart function and enhance angiogenesis when delivered into the myocardium after experimentally produced MI [15]. MSCs transduced with BMP-9 have been used to enhance spinal fusion in athymic mice [16], and intravenous interleukin-10–transduced MSCs have been used to reduce the inflammatory response in graft-versus-host disease (GVHD) [17]. Apart from modifying the differentiation potential of MSCs, genetic modification can also be used to target cells to specific tissues. For instance, MSCs transduced with CXCR4 (CXC-chemokine receptor 4) exhibited enhanced homing to infarcted myocardium in rats after intravenous delivery [18,19].

Rodents are also widely used for tissue engineering approaches using MSCs. Various approaches such as protein-impregnated scaffolds [20], gene vector–incorporated matrices [21], and combinations of cells and scaffolds have been designed. Autologous MSCs seeded on hydrogels have been used to enhance ingrowth of axons in nerve lesions and improve function in a rat model of spinal cord injury [22]. Modified MSCs, seeded in type I collagen sponges, have been used to enhance bone formation in a mouse model of bone defects [23]. Similarly, gene-modified MSCs seeded onto collagen scaffolds have been used to repair tendons in rats [24].

Rodent Embryonic Stem Cells

Rodents were also one of the first animals from which researchers were able to extensively use embryonic stem (ES) cells for regenerative medicine purposes. Mouse embryonic stem (mES) cells were first isolated in the early 1980s [25,26]. These cells generated great expectations as a potential resource for gene and cell therapy because of their ability to differentiate into various types of cells. The use of genetic manipulation in ES cells has provided an invaluable tool for research into gene functions and disease pathogenesis [27,28]. Each of these approaches is used routinely in murine ES cells to generate transient genetic alterations, as well as random and targeted alterations at many genetic loci. As more genes implicated in lineage-specific commitment are identified, there will be a concomitant increase in the potential to both actively direct lineage-specific differentiation of ES cells and the ability to track this process through the expression of reporter genes under the control of lineage-specific promoters [27].

Induced Pluripotent Stem Cells

In mouse models, induced pluripotent stem (iPS) cells have now been used successfully for tissue regeneration and cell therapy. Researchers have demonstrated that sickle cell anemia can be cured [29] and that iPS cell–derived neural cells can ameliorate experimental Parkinson's disease (PD) [30]. There are, however, several cautionary notes to contemplate before clinical use of iPS cells can be considered. In the first generation of iPS cell experiments, the four genetic factors used to induce pluripotency in the cells (Sox2, Nanog, Klf4, and c-Myc [or lin-28]) were expressed by retroviral vectors and permanently integrated into the genome. In addition, a selection marker was simultaneously integrated. Viral integrations are considered to be potentially dangerous because they occur randomly and may affect the transcription of genes close to the integration sites. This problem has been successfully tackled in a recent publication in which transient expression of these same genes (without viral integration) has been shown to be similarly effective [31]. There are also concerns over using the proven oncogene c-Myc in the generation of iPS cells. James Thomson's group showed that c-Myc was not critically required but could be replaced by lin-28 [32], and later Rudolf Jaenisch and Shinya Yamanaka showed that c-Myc could be dispensed with altogether [33,34]. Removal of c-Myc has indeed reduced problems with tumor formation in mice generated from iPS cells [33]. There are also considerable efforts to develop small molecules that will activate endogenous genes and to use starting cells with endogenously high expression of some of the critical genes. Recently, addition of only one gene, Oct4, was shown to convert neuronal stem (NS) cells to iPS cells [35], but other studies have shown that two factors, Oct4 and Klf4, are required for conversion of NS cells to iPS cells [36,37]. Integration of the selection marker has also been avoided by using morphologic criteria rather than genetic selection for drug resistance [38,39].

Rabbit Models

Because of their intermediate size, relatively easy husbandry, and low cost, rabbits are commonly used to study regenerative medicine and tissue engineering approaches to disease. One of the most common uses for rabbits is in the study of regeneration of the musculoskeletal system. Additionally, rabbits have been used extensively for regeneration of cartilage and intervertebral disks. Anderson et al. review the uses of stem cells for disk repair [40]. Nayak et al. report the expression of gap-junctional communication of rabbit bone marrow stem cells with two adherent cell lines of musculoskeletal system in vitro and confirmed that incorporation of stem cells augments fibrocartilage regeneration [41]. Injectable gellan gum hydrogels containing autologous cells have been used to regenerate fibrocartilage in rabbits [42]. Masuda and Lotz discuss the use of animal models, including rabbits, for future regenerative medicine applications for intervertebral disk treatment [43].

Cardiovascular applications of regenerative medicine have also used rabbits. In particular, rabbits have been used to study tissue-engineered heart valves [44] and blood vessels [45,46].

Finally, rabbits have been used to develop regenerative medicine approaches to the genitourinary system. De Filippo et al. used the rabbit model for tissue engineering approaches to vaginal reconstruction [47]. Eberli et al. reported a method to improve cellular content for penile corporal tissue engineering [48]. Additionally, Minuth et al. report the uses of certain cells to regenerate renal tubules [49].

Parthenogenesis, the process by which an egg can develop into an embryo in the absence of sperm, may be a potential source of ES cells that may avoid some of the political and ethical concerns surrounding ES cells. Koh et al. reported the use of rabbits for ES cell isolation followed by expansion from the parthenogenetic activation of oocytes [50]. These cells were characterized for their stem cell properties. In addition, these cells were induced to differentiate to the myogenic, osteogenic, adipogenic, and endothelial lineages and were able to form muscle-like and bony-like tissue in vivo. Furthermore, parthenogenetic stem cells were able to integrate into injured muscle tissue.

Sheep Models

Sheep and other ungulates are used for regenerative medicine and tissue engineering applications because their size permits implantation of bioengineered constructs into near "human-size" recipients. This is especially true for cardiovascular applications in which sheep have been used often as recipients of bioengineered heart valves and vessels. Studies by Koch et al. reported the use of sheep in receipt of fibrin-polylactide–based tissue-engineered vascular grafts in the arterial circulation [51]. Sheep are useful for testing a wide variety of scaffold materials. Yazdani et al. reported the use of autologous cells to bioengineer arterial grafts [52]. Salvucci et al. describe the various requirements needed to bioengineer arteries and veins for implantation [53]. One of the most common uses for the sheep model is for receipt of bioengineered heart valves. Their size permits access to the pulmonary and aortic valve site, and their blood volume permits heart bypass. Autologous cells can be collected from various sites without depleting the blood volume of bone marrow. Gottlieb et al. [54] and Ramaswamy et al. [55] describe the use of autologous cells for engineering pulmonary valves. Additionally, endothelial progenitor cells can be readily isolated from peripheral blood and seeded on heart valve scaffolds for transplantation into the pulmonary valve position [56].

Sheep are also useful for bone and cartilage applications of regenerative medicine. Van der Pol et al. report the use of biocomposite scaffolds for healing bone defects in sheep [57]. An interesting application of bone engineering is the use of large-volume calcium phosphate bone substitute to aid in vascularization of bone in a sheep model [58]. Similarly, small intestinal submucosa has been used for anular defect closure in a sheep model [59]. Sheep are also used for a variety of tissue engineering approaches to joint repair [60,61].

Again, because of their large size and blood volume, sheep are commonly used as animal models of skin bioengineering [62], to produce animal-derived pharmaceuticals [63], and for esophageal repair [64].

Dog Models

Dogs have been used for many years and models of human diseases [65]. For example, the physiology, disease presentation, and clinical responses of dogs are very similar to those of human beings. For instance, of the 400 known hereditary canine diseases, more than half have an equivalent human disease, including cardiomyopathies, muscular dystrophy, and prostate cancer. Many common inherited human diseases, including asthma, diabetes, epilepsy, and cancer, are caused by complex interactions among multiple genes and environmental factors that are shared by dogs and human beings [65]. The sequencing of the dog genome [66,67] and related genomic resources position dogs as important models for understanding the genetic basis of disease.

In stem cell transplantation, dogs have been used for more than thirty years. Dogs are biologically more comparable to human beings with respect to stem cell kinetics, hematopoietic demand, and responsiveness to cytokines [68]. Much information has been gained from canine studies with regard to the conditioning for transplantation, selection of donors by histocompatibility typing, prevention of GVHD by depletion of T cells, and adoptive immunotherapy in mixed chimeras [69]. In addition, a variety of disease models are available in dogs, including hemolytic anemias, granulocytic disorders, storage diseases, and immunodeficiencies [68]. Taken together, dogs represent promising models for the study of regenerative medicine approaches to human disease.

Embryonic stem cells have been isolated from dog models by several different groups. Hatoya et al. reported the isolation of two cell lines from canine blastocysts showing characteristic ES-like morphology and expression of pluripotency markers such as OCT4 (octamer-binding transcription factor 4) and stage-specific embryonic antigen-1 (SSEA-1) [70]. These cells formed embryoid bodies in suspension culture, which differentiated into neuron-like, epithelium-like, fibroblast-like, and myocardium-like cells. Unfortunately, it was not possible to maintain the undifferentiated phenotype of the cell lines beyond passage 8. Additional studies by Schneider et al. confirmed that canine embryo-derived cell lines can be established and that these cells can be differentiated into hematopoietic stem cells [71]. Very recently, the generation of several canine blastocyst-derived cell lines satisfying most of the criteria for ES cells has been described by Hayes et al. [72]. One of these lines was maintained through passage 34 and characterized in further detail.

Nonhuman Primate Models

Clinical Relevance

The main premise of using nonhuman primates (NHPs) in regenerative medicine research is that isolation of a novel class of stem cells from nonhuman primate species would hasten the development of replacement tissues and organs for human beings. Old-world primate species, such as cynomolgus monkeys (*Macaca fascicularis*), share an extremely close phylogenetic relationship with human beings and develop heritable, age- and gender-related diseases that could benefit from regenerative medicine approaches for their treatment and cure [73–78]. Specifically, cynomolgus monkeys are an established animal model of age- and gender-related risk for coronary, cerebral, and peripheral vascular disease; types I and II diabetes; cancer; dementia; and genitourinary, bone, and joint diseases [79–83]. As such, this species of monkey is a well-established model for many of the chronic diseases that account for a vast majority of the morbidity, mortality, and medical cost in the United States. Several types of stem and progenitor cells have been isolated from NHPs and used for regenerative medicine approaches to tissue and organ replacement. These studies are reviewed here.

Embryonic Stem Cells

Monkey ES cell lines have been established from monkey blastocysts [84], and these lines have been reviewed by Nakatsuji et al. [85]. So far, ES cell lines have been established from rhesus monkey (*Macaca mulatta*), common marmoset (*Callithrix jacchus*), and cynomolgus monkey (*Macaca fascicularis*) using blastocysts produced naturally or by in vitro fertilization (IVF) and intracytoplasmic sperm injection (ICSI). These cell lines seem to have very similar characteristics. They express alkaline phosphatase activity and SSEA-4 and, in most cases, SSEA-3. Their pluripotency was confirmed by the formation of embryoid bodies and differentiation into various cell types in culture and by the formation of teratomas that contained many types of differentiated tissues, including derivatives of all three germ layers after transplantation into severe combined immunodeficiency (SCID) mice. However, unlike in ES cells from rodents, leukemia inhibitory factor signaling does not maintain primate ES cells in a pluripotent state, making cultures of primate and human ES cell lines prone to spontaneous differentiation. Thus, it is difficult to maintain these stem cell colonies. Also, these ES cells are more susceptible to various stresses, leading to difficulties with subculturing using enzymatic treatment and cloning from single cells. However, with various improvements in culture methods, it is now possible to maintain stable colonies of monkey ES cells using a serum-free medium that can be subcultured with trypsin treatment. Under such conditions, cynomolgus monkey ES cell lines can be maintained in an undifferentiated state with a normal karyotype and pluripotency even after prolonged periods of culture (longer than 1 year). Such progress should facilitate many aspects of stem cell research using both nonhuman primate and human ES cell lines. Other fetal cells have been isolated from the brain of a cynomolgus monkey [86].

Spermatogonial Stem Cells

Herman et al. have described the isolation of spermatogonial stem cells (SSCs) from primates [87]. This report recounts the development of a xenotransplant assay for functional identification of primate SSCs that has led to progress in understanding the molecular and clonal characteristics of the primate spermatogenic lineage. Because these primates have similar reproductive cycles to human beings, these studies can be used to develop and test new hypotheses about the biology and regenerative capacity of primate SSCs.

Bone Marrow–, Peripheral Blood–, and Amnion-Derived Stem Cells

Masuda et al. describe the isolation and use of bone marrow–derived MSCs to improve the efficacy of transplantation of gene-modified hematopoietic stem cells in primates, with enhanced engraftment in bone marrow as well as increased chimerism in peripheral blood through migration and homing [88]. Additionally, Williams et al. report isolation of peripheral blood- and bone marrow-derived endothelial progenitor cells [89]. Finally, amniotic fluid, which is readily available and known to contain multiple cell types derived from developing fetuses, could provide a large source of stem cells for research [90].

Tissue Engineering Applications in Nonhuman Primates

Nonhuman primates have been used for a variety of tissue engineering applications. Rosson et al. report the use of NHP models to restore motor nerve function across a conduit [91]. Leschik et al. report the utility of NHP ES cells in regenerating cardiac tissue [92]. Additionally, NHPs have been used for tissue engineering approaches to diabetes [93], bone reconstruction[94], reconstructive craniofacial surgery [95], arterial injury repair [96], and xenotransplantation [97].

Porcine Models

Xenotransplantation

Tissues from pigs are often used for xenotransplantation into human beings [71]. Because of this and their size, they are a useful animal model for testing regenerative medicine approaches to a wide variety of diseases. In the ongoing search for a reliable source of tissue to replace lost cells, tissues, and organs, research in the area of xenotransplantation (cross-species transplantation) has grown tremendously in the past twenty years [98]. Overcoming the immunologic hurdle of cross-species transplantation as well as the problem of cross-species pathogen infectivity are the scientific challenges facing the field. The ability to genetically modify species such as the pig through transgenesis and nuclear transfer still holds promise for engineered tissues and organs for human transplantation. An example of this is the production of galα1,3gal transferase null transgenic pigs, which represents a development toward reducing both hyperacute and acute vascular rejection. Additionally, there have been several pig-to-human xenotransplantation clinical experiments for the treatment of diabetes and FDA-approved clinical trials for the treatment of neurologic disorders using outbred pig tissue [99–101]. Although there was some evidence of cell engraftment in both indications [100,102], no efficacy was established. To date, a phase I clinical trial was completed using transgenically engineered pig livers to detoxify the blood of fulminant hepatic failure patients via extracorporeal perfusion [103]; however, there is yet to be an FDA-approved transgenic animal tissue for use in human transplantation. Although the theoretical risk of xenozoonosis represents a significant psychosocial issue, several studies investigating the possibility of cross-species infectivity, including a retrospective analysis of 160 human transplant recipients exposed to porcine tissues, have yet to reveal transmission of porcine viruses to humans or primates in vivo [104–107].

Uses of Porcine Stem Cells

Similar to nonhuman primates, ES cells have been isolated from pigs [108]. These cells and others have been used in pigs for transplantation of corneal epithelial cells [109], treatment of intrabony periodontal defects [110], engineered livers [111], regenerative bladder augmentation [112], matrix engineering [113], and cardiovascular tissue [114].

Conclusions

Regardless of the animal model, the fundamental question remains: how similar are animal models to the human condition they are designed to represent? Each animal model must be selected to answer specific questions. Specific molecular pathway information may best be obtained in mice but should be interpreted only as far as the mouse model is applicable. Studies in nonhuman primates may lead to an almost directly translatable finding to human beings but lack the precision of rodent models. As regenerative medicine research continues to advance at ever-increasing speeds, the role of animal models in this research will need to be continuously assessed and reexamined.

Acknowledgments

The authors would like to thank Dr. Jennifer Olson for editorial assistance with this manuscript.

References

1. Ortiz L A, Gambelli F, McBride C, et al. (2003) Mesenchymal stem cell engraftment in lung is enhanced in response to bleomycin exposure and ameliorates its fibrotic effects. Proc Natl Acad Sci U S A 100: 8407–11
2. Semont A, Francois S, Mouiseddine M, et al. (2006) Mesenchymal stem cells increase self-renewal of small intestinal epithelium and accelerate structural recovery after radiation injury. Adv Exp Med Biol 585: 19–30
3. Herrera M B, Bussolati B, Bruno S, et al. (2004) Mesenchymal stem cells contribute to the renal repair of acute tubular epithelial injury. Int J Mol Med 14: 1035–41
4. Wu Y, Chen L, Scott P G, et al. (2007) Mesenchymal stem cells enhance wound healing through differentiation and angiogenesis. Stem Cells 25: 2648–59
5. Boumaza I, Srinivasan S, Witt W T, et al. (2009) Autologous bone marrow-derived rat mesenchymal stem cells promote PDX-1 and insulin expression in the islets, alter T cell cytokine pattern and preserve regulatory T cells in the periphery and induce sustained normoglycemia. J Autoimmun 32: 33–42
6. Ma Y, Xu Y, Xiao Z, et al. (2006) Reconstruction of chemically burned rat corneal surface by bone marrow-derived human mesenchymal stem cells. Stem Cells 24: 315–21
7. Maitra B, Szekely E, Gjini K, et al. (2004) Human mesenchymal stem cells support unrelated donor hematopoietic stem cells and suppress T-cell activation. Bone Marrow Transplant 33: 597–604
8. Le Blanc K, Frassoni F, Ball L, et al. (2008) Mesenchymal stem cells for treatment of steroid-resistant, severe, acute graft-versus-host disease: a phase II study. Lancet 371: 1579–86

9. Barbash I M, Chouraqui P, Baron J, et al. (2003) Systemic delivery of bone marrow-derived mesenchymal stem cells to the infarcted myocardium: feasibility, cell migration, and body distribution. Circulation 108: 863–8

10. Mahmood A, Lu D, Lu M, et al. (2003) Treatment of traumatic brain injury in adult rats with intravenous administration of human bone marrow stromal cells. Neurosurgery 53: 697–702; discussion 702–3

11. Breitbach M, Bostani T, Roell W, et al. (2007) Potential risks of bone marrow cell transplantation into infarcted hearts. Blood 110: 1362–9

12. Li Y, Zhang R, Qiao H, et al. (2007) Generation of insulin-producing cells from PDX-1 gene-modified human mesenchymal stem cells. J Cell Physiol 211: 36–44

13. Xu J, Lu Y, Ding F, et al. (2007) Reversal of diabetes in mice by intrahepatic injection of bone-derived GFP-murine mesenchymal stem cells infected with the recombinant retrovirus-carrying human insulin gene. World J Surg 31: 1872–82

14. Chang S C, Chuang H L, Chen Y R, et al. (2003) Ex vivo gene therapy in autologous bone marrow stromal stem cells for tissue-engineered maxillofacial bone regeneration. Gene Ther 10: 2013–9

15. Sun L, Cui M, Wang Z, et al. (2007) Mesenchymal stem cells modified with angiopoietin-1 improve remodeling in a rat model of acute myocardial infarction. Biochem Biophys Res Commun 357: 779–84

16. Dumont R J, Dayoub H, Li J Z, et al. (2002) Ex vivo bone morphogenetic protein-9 gene therapy using human mesenchymal stem cells induces spinal fusion in rodents. Neurosurgery 51: 1239–44; discussion 1244–5

17. Min C K, Kim B G, Park G, et al. (2007) IL-10-transduced bone marrow mesenchymal stem cells can attenuate the severity of acute graft-versus-host disease after experimental allogeneic stem cell transplantation. Bone Marrow Transplant 39: 637–45

18. Cheng Z, Ou L, Zhou X, et al. (2008) Targeted migration of mesenchymal stem cells modified with CXCR4 gene to infarcted myocardium improves cardiac performance. Mol Ther 16: 571–9

19. Zhang D, Fan G C, Zhou X, et al. (2008) Over-expression of CXCR4 on mesenchymal stem cells augments myoangiogenesis in the infarcted myocardium. J Mol Cell Cardiol 44: 281–92

20. Burkus J K, Transfeldt E E, Kitchel S H, et al. (2002) Clinical and radiographic outcomes of anterior lumbar interbody fusion using recombinant human bone morphogenetic protein-2. Spine (Phila Pa 1976) 27: 2396–408

21. Fang J, Zhu Y Y, Smiley E, et al. (1996) Stimulation of new bone formation by direct transfer of osteogenic plasmid genes. Proc Natl Acad Sci U S A 93: 5753–8

22. Sykova E, Jendelova P, Urdzikova L, et al. (2006) Bone marrow stem cells and polymer hydrogels–two strategies for spinal cord injury repair. Cell Mol Neurobiol 26: 1113–29

23. Tu Q, Valverde P, Li S, et al. (2007) Osterix overexpression in mesenchymal stem cells stimulates healing of critical-sized defects in murine calvarial bone. Tissue Eng 13: 2431–40

24. Hoffmann A, Pelled G, Turgeman G, et al. (2006) Neotendon formation induced by manipulation of the Smad8 signalling pathway in mesenchymal stem cells. J Clin Invest 116: 940–52

25. Evans M J, Kaufman M H (1981) Establishment in culture of pluripotential cells from mouse embryos. Nature 292: 154–6

26. Martin G R (1981) Isolation of a pluripotent cell line from early mouse embryos cultured in medium conditioned by teratocarcinoma stem cells. Proc Natl Acad Sci U S A 78: 7634–8

27. Conley B J, Young J C, Trounson A O, et al. (2004) Derivation, propagation and differentiation of human embryonic stem cells. Int J Biochem Cell Biol 36: 555–67

28. Desbaillets I, Ziegler U, Groscurth P, et al. (2000) Embryoid bodies: an in vitro model of mouse embryogenesis. Exp Physiol 85: 645–51
29. Hanna J, Wernig M, Markoulaki S, et al. (2007) Treatment of sickle cell anemia mouse model with iPS cells generated from autologous skin. Science 318: 1920–3
30. Wernig M, Zhao J P, Pruszak J, et al. (2008) Neurons derived from reprogrammed fibroblasts functionally integrate into the fetal brain and improve symptoms of rats with Parkinson's disease. Proc Natl Acad Sci U S A 105: 5856–61
31. Yu J, Hu K, Smuga-Otto K, et al. (2009) Human induced pluripotent stem cells free of vector and transgene sequences. Science 324: 797–801
32. Yu J, Vodyanik M A, Smuga-Otto K, et al. (2007) Induced pluripotent stem cell lines derived from human somatic cells. Science 318: 1917–20
33. Nakagawa M, Koyanagi M, Tanabe K, et al. (2008) Generation of induced pluripotent stem cells without Myc from mouse and human fibroblasts. Nat Biotechnol 26: 101–6
34. Wernig M, Meissner A, Cassady J P, et al. (2008) c-Myc is dispensable for direct reprogramming of mouse fibroblasts. Cell Stem Cell 2: 10–2
35. Kim J B, Sebastiano V, Wu G, et al. (2009) Oct4-induced pluripotency in adult neural stem cells. Cell 136: 411–9
36. Kim J B, Zaehres H, Wu G, et al. (2008) Pluripotent stem cells induced from adult neural stem cells by reprogramming with two factors. Nature 454: 646–50
37. Silva J, Barrandon O, Nichols J, et al. (2008) Promotion of reprogramming to ground state pluripotency by signal inhibition. PLoS Biol 6: e253
38. Blelloch R, Venere M, Yen J, et al. (2007) Generation of induced pluripotent stem cells in the absence of drug selection. Cell Stem Cell 1: 245–7
39. Meissner A, Wernig M, and Jaenisch R (2007) Direct reprogramming of genetically unmodified fibroblasts into pluripotent stem cells. Nat Biotechnol 25: 1177–81
40. Anderson D G, Risbud M V, Shapiro I M, et al. (2005) Cell-based therapy for disc repair. Spine J 5: 297S–303S
41. Nayak B P, Goh J C, Toh S L, et al. (2010) In vitro study of stem cell communication via gap junctions for fibrocartilage regeneration at entheses. Regen Med 5: 221–9
42. Oliveira J T, Gardel L S, Rada T, et al. (2010) Injectable gellan gum hydrogels with autologous cells for the treatment of rabbit articular cartilage defects. J Orthop Res 28(9): 1193–9
43. Masuda K, Lotz J C (2010) New challenges for intervertebral disc treatment using regenerative medicine. Tissue Eng Part B Rev 16: 147–58
44. Nakayama Y, Yamanami M, Yahata Y, et al. (2009) Preparation of a completely autologous trileaflet valve-shaped construct by in-body tissue architecture technology. J Biomed Mater Res B Appl Biomater 91: 813–8
45. Watanabe T, Kanda K, Ishibashi-Ueda H, et al. (2010) Autologous small-caliber "biotube" vascular grafts with argatroban loading: a histomorphological examination after implantation to rabbits. J Biomed Mater Res B Appl Biomater 92: 236–42
46. Tillman B W, Yazdani S K, Lee S J, et al. (2009) The in vivo stability of electrospun polycaprolactone-collagen scaffolds in vascular reconstruction. Biomaterials 30: 583–8
47. De Filippo R E, Bishop C E, Filho L F, et al. (2008) Tissue engineering a complete vaginal replacement from a small biopsy of autologous tissue.[erratum appears in Transplantation. 2008 Sep 15;86(5): 751. Note: De Philippo, Roger E [corrected to De Filippo, Roger E]]. Transplantation 86: 208–14
48. Eberli D, Susaeta R, Yoo J, et al. (2008) A method to improve cellular content for corporal tissue engineering. Tissue Engineering: Part A 14: 1581–1589
49. Minuth W W, Denk L, Meese C, et al. (2009) Ultrastructural insights in the interface between generated renal tubules and a polyester interstitium. Langmuir 25: 4621–7
50. Koh C J, Delo D M, Lee J W, et al. (2009) Parthenogenesis-derived multipotent stem cells adapted for tissue engineering applications. Methods 47: 90–7

51. Koch S, Flanagan T C, Sachweh J S, et al. (2010) Fibrin-polylactide-based tissue-engineered vascular graft in the arterial circulation. Biomaterials 31: 4731–9

52. Yazdani S K, Tillman B W, Berry J L, et al. (2010) The fate of an endothelium layer after preconditioning. J Vasc Surg 51: 174–83

53. Salvucci F P, Bia D, Armentano R L, et al. (2009) Association between mechanics and structure in arteries and veins: theoretical approach to vascular graft confection. Conf Proc IEEE Eng Med Biol Soc 2009: 4258–61

54. Gottlieb D, Kunal T, Emani S, et al. (2010) In vivo monitoring of function of autologous engineered pulmonary valve. J Thorac Cardiovasc Surg 139: 723–31

55. Ramaswamy S, Gottlieb D, Engelmayr G C, Jr., et al. (2010) The role of organ level conditioning on the promotion of engineered heart valve tissue development in-vitro using mesenchymal stem cells. Biomaterials 31: 1114–25

56. Lee D J, Steen J, Jordan J E, et al. (2009) Endothelialization of heart valve matrix using a computer-assisted pulsatile bioreactor. Tissue Eng Part A 15: 807–14

57. van der Pol U, Mathieu L, Zeiter S, et al. (2010) Augmentation of bone defect healing using a new biocomposite scaffold: An in vivo study in sheep. Acta Biomater 6(9): 3755–62

58. Beier J P, Horch R E, Hess A, et al. (2010) Axial vascularization of a large volume calcium phosphate ceramic bone substitute in the sheep AV loop model. J Tissue Eng Regen Med 4: 216–23

59. Ledet E H, Jeshuran W, Glennon J C, et al. (2009) Small intestinal submucosa for anular defect closure: long-term response in an in vivo sheep model. Spine (Phila Pa 1976) 34: 1457–63

60. Schulze-Tanzil G, Muller R D, Kohl B, et al. (2009) Differing in vitro biology of equine, ovine, porcine and human articular chondrocytes derived from the knee joint: an immunomorphological study. Histochem Cell Biol 131: 219–29

61. Kon E, Chiari C, Marcacci M, et al. (2008) Tissue engineering for total meniscal substitution: animal study in sheep model. Tissue Eng Part A 14: 1067–80

62. Hosper N A, Eggink A J, Roelofs L A, et al. (2010) Intra-uterine tissue engineering of full-thickness skin defects in a fetal sheep model. Biomaterials 31: 3910–9

63. Redwan e-R M (2009) Animal-derived pharmaceutical proteins. J Immunoassay Immunochem 30: 262–290

64. Kofler K, Ainoedhofer H, Hollwarth M E, et al. (2010) Fluorescence-activated cell sorting of PCK-26 antigen-positive cells enables selection of ovine esophageal epithelial cells with improved viability on scaffolds for esophagus tissue engineering. Pediatr Surg Int 26: 97–104

65. Starkey M P, Scase T J, Mellersh C S, et al. (2005) Dogs really are man's best friend–canine genomics has applications in veterinary and human medicine! Brief Funct Genomic Proteomic 4: 112–28

66. Kirkness E F, Bafna V, Halpern A L, et al. (2003) The dog genome: survey sequencing and comparative analysis. Science 301: 1898–903

67. Lindblad-Toh K, Wade C M, Mikkelsen T S, et al. (2005) Genome sequence, comparative analysis and haplotype structure of the domestic dog. Nature 438: 803–19

68. Horn P A, Morris J C, Neff T, et al. (2004) Stem cell gene transfer – efficacy and safety in large animal studies. Mol Ther 10: 417–31

69. Kolb H J, Gunther W, Schumm M, et al. (1997) Adoptive immunotherapy in canine chimeras. Transplantation 63: 430–6

70. Hatoya S, Torii R, Kondo Y, et al. (2006) Isolation and characterization of embryonic stem-like cells from canine blastocysts. Mol Reprod Dev 73: 298–305

71. Schneider M K, Seebach J D (2009) Xenotransplantation literature update: November-December, 2008. Xenotransplantation 16: 50–3

72. Hayes B, Fagerlie S R, Ramakrishnan A, et al. (2008) Derivation, characterization, and in vitro differentiation of canine embryonic stem cells. Stem Cells 26: 465–73

73. Lane M A (2000) Nonhuman primate models in biogerontology. Exp Gerontol 35: 533–41
74. Gaur L K (2004) Nonhuman primate models for islet transplantation in type 1 diabetes research. ILAR J 45: 324–33
75. Clarkson T B, Mehaffey M H (2009) Coronary heart disease of females: lessons learned from nonhuman primates. Am J Primatol 71: 785–93
76. Vierboom M P, Jonker M, Bontrop R E, et al. (2005) Modeling human arthritic diseases in nonhuman primates. Arthritis Res Ther 7: 145–54
77. Archer D F (2004) Role of the nonhuman primate for research related to women's health. ILAR J 45: 212–9
78. Furlan R, Cuomo C, Martino G (2009) Animal models of multiple sclerosis. Methods Mol Biol 549: 157–73
79. Kaplan J R, Manuck S B (1999) Status, stress, and atherosclerosis: the role of environment and individual behavior. Ann N Y Acad Sci 896: 145–61
80. Ham K D, Carlson C S (2004) Effects of estrogen replacement therapy on bone turnover in subchondral bone and epiphyseal metaphyseal cancellous bone of ovariectomized cynomolgus monkeys. J Bone Miner Res 19: 823–9
81. Ham K D, Loeser R F, Lindgren B R, et al. (2002) Effects of long-term estrogen replacement therapy on osteoarthritis severity in cynomolgus monkeys. Arthritis Rheum 46: 1956–64
82. Wagner J E, Kavanagh K, Ward G M, et al. (2006) Old world nonhuman primate models of type 2 diabetes mellitus. ILAR J 47: 259–71
83. Wood C E, Chen Z, Cline J M, et al. (2007) Characterization and experimental transmission of an oncogenic papillomavirus in female macaques. J Virol 81: 6339–45
84. Thomson J A, Kalishman J, Golos T G, et al. (1995) Isolation of a primate embryonic stem cell line. Proc Natl Acad Sci U S A 92: 7844–8
85. Nakatsuji N, Suemori H (2002) Embryonic stem cell lines of nonhuman primates. Sci World J 2: 1762–73
86. Wang P, Liu X M, Ma B F, et al. (2008) Isolation, characterization and gene modification of fetal neural stem/progenitor cells from cynomolgus monkey. Neuroreport 19: 419–24
87. Hermann B P, Sukhwani M, Hansel M C, et al. (2010) Spermatogonial stem cells in higher primates: are there differences from those in rodents? Reproduction 139: 479–93
88. Masuda S, Ageyama N, Shibata H, et al. (2009) Cotransplantation with MSCs improves engraftment of HSCs after autologous intra-bone marrow transplantation in nonhuman primates. Exp Hematol 37: 1250–1257
89. Williams J K, Baptista P M, Daunais J B, et al. (2008) The effects of ethanol consumption on vasculogenesis potential in nonhuman primates. Alcohol Clin Exp Res 32: 155–61
90. Parolini O, Soncini M, Evangelista M, et al. (2009) Amniotic membrane and amniotic fluid-derived cells: potential tools for regenerative medicine? Regen Med 4: 275–91
91. Rosson G D, Williams E H, Dellon A L (2009) Motor nerve regeneration across a conduit. Microsurgery 29: 107–14
92. Leschik J, Stefanovic S, Brinon B, et al. (2008) Cardiac commitment of primate embryonic stem cells. Nat Protoc 3: 1381–7
93. Contreras J L, Smyth C A, Curiel D T, et al. (2004) Nonhuman primate models in type 1 diabetes research. ILAR J 45: 334–42
94. Takahashi Y, Yamamoto M, Yamada K, et al. (2007) Skull bone regeneration in nonhuman primates by controlled release of bone morphogenetic protein-2 from a biodegradable hydrogel. Tissue Eng 13: 293–300

95. Ripamonti U, Ferretti C, Teare J, et al. (2009) Transforming growth factor-beta isoforms and the induction of bone formation: implications for reconstructive craniofacial surgery. J Craniofac Surg 20: 1544–55

96. Englesbe M J, Davies M G, Hawkins S M et al. (2004) Arterial injury repair in nonhuman primates-the role of PDGF receptor-beta. J Surg Res 119: 80–4

97. Ekser B, Rigotti P, Gridelli B et al. (2009) Xenotransplantation of solid organs in the pig-to-primate model. Transpl Immunol 21: 87–92

98. Fodor W L (2003) Tissue engineering and cell based therapies, from the bench to the clinic: the potential to replace, repair and regenerate. Reprod Biol Endocrinol 1: 102

99. Fink J S, Schumacher J M, Ellias S L, et al. (2000) Porcine xenografts in Parkinson's disease and Huntington's disease patients: preliminary results. Cell Transplant 9: 273–8

100. Schumacher J M, Ellias S A, Palmer E P, et al. (2000) Transplantation of embryonic porcine mesencephalic tissue in patients with PD. Neurology 54: 1042–50

101. Deacon T, Schumacher J, Dinsmore J, et al. (1997) Histological evidence of fetal pig neural cell survival after transplantation into a patient with Parkinson's disease. Nat Med 3: 350–3

102. Groth C G, Tibell A, Wennberg L, et al. (1999) Xenoislet transplantation: experimental and clinical aspects. J Mol Med 77: 153–4

103. Levy M F, Crippin J, Sutton S, Netto G, McCormack J, Curiel T, Goldstein R M, Newman J T, Gonwa T A, Banchereau J, Diamond L E, Byrne G, Logan J, Klintmalm G B. (2000) Liver allotransplantation after extracorporeal hepatic support with transgenic (hCD55/hCD59) porcine livers: clinical results and lack of pig-to-human transmission of the porcine endogenous retrovirus. Transplantation. 69(2): 272–80

104. Switzer W M, Michler R E, Shanmugam V, et al. (2001) Lack of cross-species transmission of porcine endogenous retrovirus infection to nonhuman primate recipients of porcine cells, tissues, or organs. Transplantation 71: 959–65

105. Dinsmore J H, Manhart C, Raineri R, et al. (2000) No evidence for infection of human cells with porcine endogenous retrovirus (PERV) after exposure to porcine fetal neuronal cells. Transplantation 70: 1382–9

106. Martin U, Steinhoff G, Kiessig V, et al. (1998) Porcine endogenous retrovirus (PERV) was not transmitted from transplanted porcine endothelial cells to baboons in vivo. Transpl Int 11: 247–51

107. Paradis K, Langford G, Long Z, et al. (1999) Search for cross-species transmission of porcine endogenous retrovirus in patients treated with living pig tissue. The XEN 111 Study Group. Science 285: 1236–41

108. Brevini T A, Antonini S, Cillo F, et al. (2007) Porcine embryonic stem cells: Facts, challenges and hopes. Theriogenology 68 Suppl 1: S206–13

109. Amano S (2002) [Transplantation of corneal endothelial cells]. Nippon Ganka Gakkai Zasshi 106: 805–35; discussion 836

110. Kalpidis C D, Ruben M P (2002) Treatment of intrabony periodontal defects with enamel matrix derivative: a literature review. J Periodontol 73: 1360–76

111. Allen J W, Bhatia S N (2002) Engineering liver therapies for the future. Tissue Eng 8: 725–37

112. Kropp B P, Badylak S, Thor K B (1995) Regenerative bladder augmentation: a review of the initial preclinical studies with porcine small intestinal submucosa. Adv Exp Med Biol 385: 229–35

113. Balazs E A, Bland P A, Denlinger J L, et al. (1991) Matrix engineering. Blood Coagul Fibrinolysis 2: 173–8

114. Vara D S, Salacinski H J, Kannan R Y, et al. (2005) Cardiovascular tissue engineering: state of the art. Pathol Biol (Paris) 53: 599–612

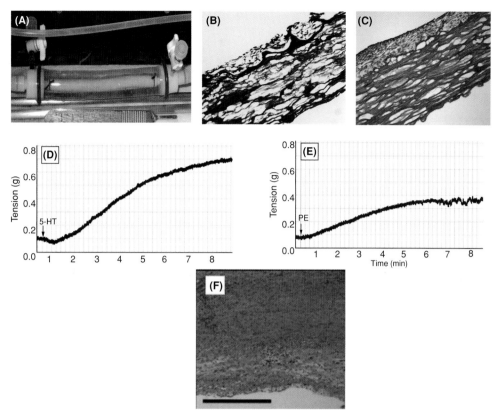

Plate 1. Illustration of the applicability of regenerative pharmacology to the development of tissue-engineered blood vessels (TEBVs). (**A**) Bioreactor flow system containing the scaffold seeded with endothelial cells (ECs) on the luminal side and with smooth muscle cells (SMCs) on the abluminal side. The bioreactor provides an external media bath, optical access, a bypass system, control over flow and pressure conditions, and the ability to maintain sterility. (**B**) Hematoxylin and eosin (H&E) stain of representative example of statically seeded SMCs on a decellularized construct after 48 hours and (**C**) after longer-term (3–4 weeks) bioreactor preconditioning. As shown, this period of bioreactor conditioning is sufficient to cause formation a substantive medial SMC layer. As noted by Yazdani et al. [10], Fura-2–based digital imaging microscopy experiments revealed no receptor mediated increases intracellular calcium levels. However, as indicated by the representative tracings shown in (**D**) and (**E**), retrieval of TEBV 4 months after implantation as a carotid artery interposition graft in sheep (Neff et al. [11]), revealed pharmacologically mediated contractile responses to 10 μM 5-Hydroxytryptamine (**D**) and 10 μM phenylephrine (**E**). *Arrows* indicate the application of agonists. (**F**) Representative H&E staining of a retrieved TEBV 4 months after implantation. Scale bar = 400 μM (Modified from Yazdani et al., 2009; Neff et al., 2011).

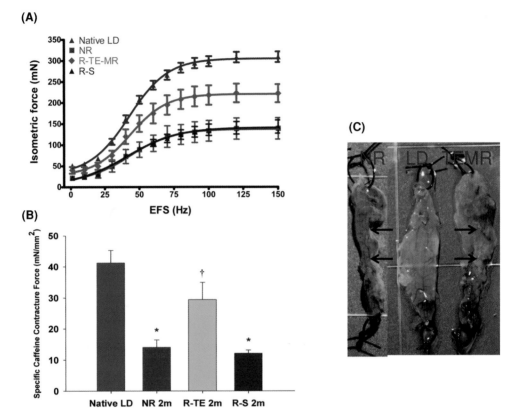

(A)

(B)

(C)

Plate 2. Morphologic assessment and functional recovery of retrieved tissues from the mouse volumetric muscle loss (VML) injury model. For these studies, bioengineered skeletal muscle implants were sutured into a surgically created VML injury by removal of approximately 50 percent of the murine latissimus dorsi (LD) muscle (see Machingal et al. [12] for details). (**A**) The mean values for the electrical field stimulation (EFS)–induced contractions observed on all retrieved tissues 2 months after injury or implantation. The sample sizes are native LD = 20, no repair (NR) (see C) = 5, repair with tissue-engineered muscle repair implantation (R-TE-MR) = 5, and R-S (repaired with a scaffold alone – no cells) = 5. The isometric absolute force (mN) is displayed as a function of stimulation frequency. Additionally, in (**B**) after force-frequency testing contralateral native LD muscles ($n = 6$), NR ($n = 4$), R-TE-MR ($n = 3$), or R-S ($n = 4$) at the 2-month time point were subjected to twitch contractions at 0.2 Hz in the presence of a maximally stimulating concentration of caffeine (50 mM). The *asterisk* denotes that group means are significantly different from that of control ($p < .05$). Values are means ± standard error of the mean. *Dagger* indicates that the group mean is significantly different from that of all other groups ($P < .05$). (**C**) shows representative examples of the gross morphology of retrieved LD tissues for an NR, native LD, and TEMR animal. *Arrows* indicate the original site of the surgical defect. Morphologic examination of tissue demonstrates robust tissue formation and remodeling of the TEMR construct but little or no tissue formation in the NR group. (Modified from Machingal et al. [12].)

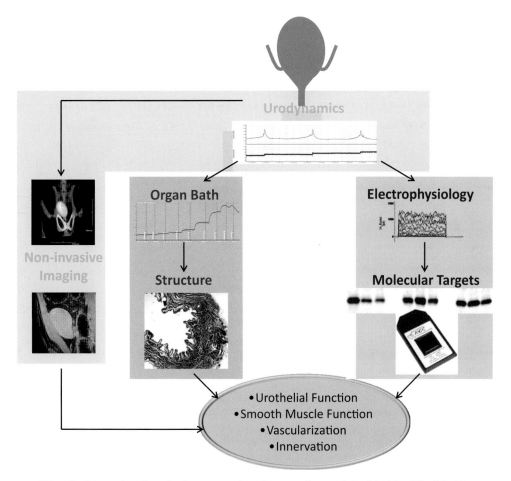

Plate 3. Dissecting (passive) regenerative pharmacology of the bladder. The bladder can be used as a model system that integrates multidisciplinary studies to evaluate organ regeneration (i.e., function and structure) on the whole organ (*green text*), tissue (*red text*), and cellular (*blue text*) levels. In vivo urodynamic studies can be used to examine overall bladder function. After euthanasia, bladder tissue can be cut into strips and stimulated to contract in an organ bath system (pharmacological studies), or sliced into sections for structural analysis (histological studies). Additionally, both gene and protein levels can be evaluated (molecular studies) and patch clamp methods can be used (electrophysiological studies) to study regenerated tissue. Noninvasive CT and MR imaging can be used longitudinally to examine organ morphology during regeneration, and possibly provide information on aspects of tissue phenotype gained via other methods. The information obtained from these studies can be used to design therapeutic interventions (see Fig. 2-2).

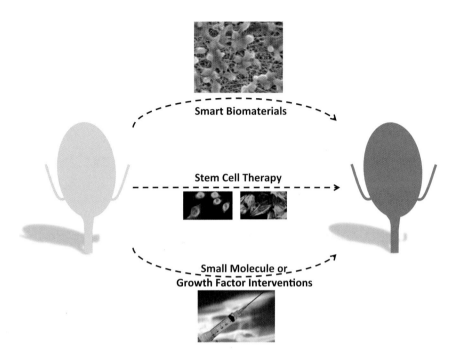

Plate 4. Directing (active) regenerative pharmacology of the bladder. Dissecting the process of bladder regeneration (Fig. 2-1) can identify specific processes (e.g., cell proliferation, differentiation, angiogenesis, innervation, and stem cell migration) that can be manipulated pharmacologically to direct tissue engineering and regenerative medicine strategies for the bladder. (*Top*) Tissue-engineered constructs currently used for bladder augmentation techniques can be altered to include, for example, different cell types and/or controlled oxygen delivery to enhance regeneration. (*Middle*) Supplementation of stem cells may modulate different aspects of bladder regeneration in a paracrine fashion. (*Bottom*) Pharmacological manipulation with small molecules or growth factors may be used to target specific signaling cascades involved in bladder regeneration. The ultimate goal with any of these interventions is to maximize bladder regeneration to restore normal bladder function.

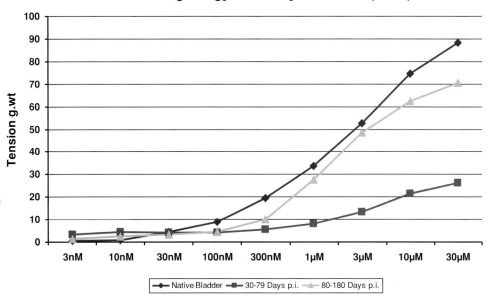

Pharmacologic Log[Carbachol] Stimulation (Mean)

Plate 5. Carbachol stimulation of regenerated versus native bladder tissue in large mammals. Chronopharmacological evaluation of bladder tissues retrieved from canines at necropsy demonstrates that the receptor–ligand pathway is restored by 6 months after initiating the regenerative process (compare the *green line* with the *red line*). The lower concentrations represent physiological and pharmacological conditions.

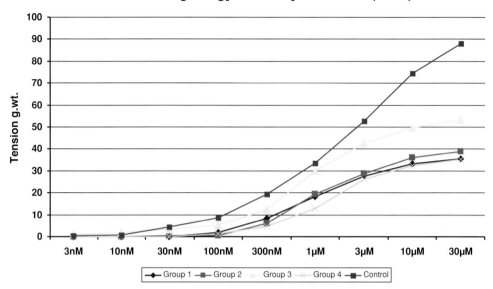

Pharmacologic Log[Carbachol] Stimulation (Mean)

Plate 6. Influence of cell number on carbachol stimulation of regenerated versus native bladder in large mammals. The regenerative process is primed by including more cells in the cell–biomaterial scaffold regenerative template (i.e., construct). Force generated by the regenerated bladder tissue retrieved from group 3 dogs that received a higher number of cells than groups 1 and 3 is most similar to that of native canine bladder tissue at the lower agonist concentrations that are closer to physiological and pharmacological conditions. At higher carbachol concentrations, the force generated by neo-tissues retrieved from group 3 dogs was also greater than that generated by neo-tissues from constructs having fewer cells and approached the response seen from native tissue.

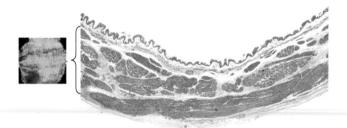

Plate 7. Histologic evaluation of regenerated bladder demonstrates a full-thickness multilayer structure. When stimulated with the calcium ionophore (A23187), the detrusor muscle mobilizes calcium as a syncytial tissue as would be observed in a native bladder detrusor muscle.

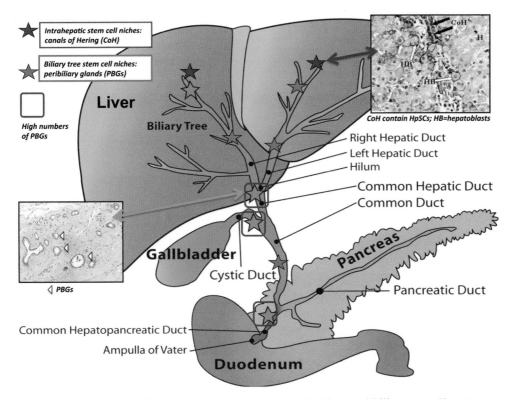

Plate 8. Schematic diagram of stem cell niches in the liver and biliary tree. *Hepatic stem cells* (HpSCs) are found within the liver in canals of Hering (CoH). *Inset top right* shows immunohistochemical staining (*brown*) for CD326 (EpCAM). HpSCs are small, strongly stained cells within CoH. *Hepatoblasts* (HBs), progenitors derived from HpSCs, are larger and characteristically show distinct staining of the cell membrane. *Inset left*, hematoxylin and eosin staining shows the location of *biliary tree stem cells in peribiliary glands* (PBGs). The pancreas contains committed progenitors but appears to lack stem cells capable of extended self-renewal.

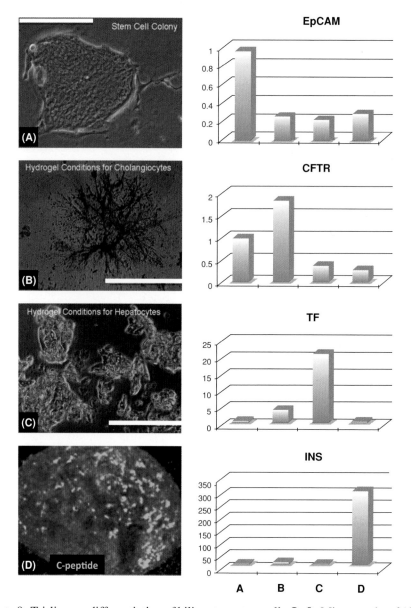

Plate 9. Tri-lineage differentiation of biliary tree stem cells. **Left**. Micrographs of (**A**) *undifferentiated biliary tree stem cells* expanded in Kubota's medium on tissue-culture plastic (bar = 0.2 mm) and (**B–D**) differentiation in three-dimensional hydrogels with appropriate growth factors and collagen types for specific fates: (**B**) *cholangiocyte lineage* showing branching ductules (bar = 1.0 mm), (**C**) *hepatocyte lineage* showing large cells with distinct bile canaliculi (bar = 0.2 mm), and (**D**) *endocrine pancreatic lineage* showing an islet-like cell cluster with positive immunofluorescent staining for insulin C-peptide. **Right**. Relative expression of representative lineage-specific transcripts assessed by quantitative polymerase chain reaction. Values are normalized to 1.0 in the undifferentiated stem cells (**A**). Differentiation conditions **B**, **C**, and **D** are as in the micrographs. CFTR = cystic fibrosis transmembrane conductance regulator, a cholangiocyte marker (much greater upregulation is observed with complete tissue-specific matrix in the hydrogel); EpCAM = CD326, expressed in stem cells, downregulated under all three differentiation conditions.; INS = proinsulin, a pancreatic β-cell marker; TR = transferrin, a hepatocyte marker. Many additional lineage markers showed comparably specific expression patterns under these differentiation conditions. (Adapted from Cardinale et al. 2011.)

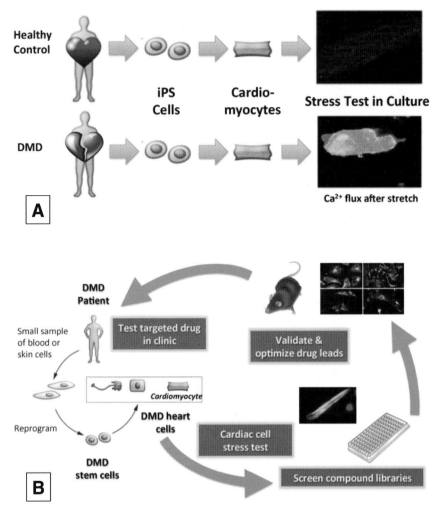

Plate 10. Disease-in-a-dish strategy to discover drugs to treat cardiomyopathy associated with Duchenne muscular dystrophy (DMD). (**A**) Screening assays will be developed using cardiomyocytes derived from DMD patient-specific induced pluripotent stem (iPS) cells. Dystrophin deficiency makes membranes of DMD cardiomyocytes more sensitive to mechanical stress. This can be detected using assays discussed in text, such as potentiation of Ca^{2+} flux, illustrated here. "Healthy control" will be syngeneic iPS cells in which the DMD mutation is corrected by introduction of a functional mini-dystrophin transgene. (**B**) Schematic of pathway from generation of DMD patient-specific iPS cells through drug discovery and preclinical development to clinical testing in DMD subjects.

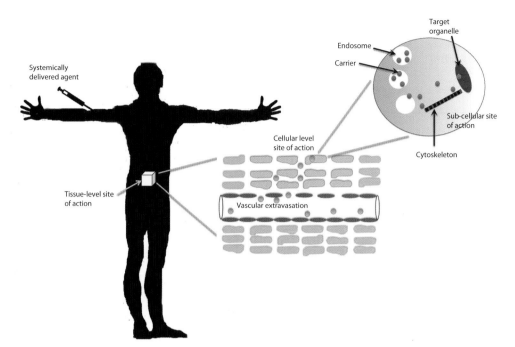

Plate 11. Schematic highlighting the hurdles to systemic delivery of therapeutic agents with micro- or nano-scale particulate carriers. These carriers are often delivered intravenously. They reach all areas of the body, including the intended tissue-level site of action, via the bloodstream. To reach the tissue, the carriers must extravasate from the vasculature. In tumors, this occurs by the enhanced permeation retention effect or "leaky vasculature." Vascular disruption may be required to allow extravasation to occur, and nanocarriers much more readily extravasate than microcarriers. Ideally, the carriers will localize to specific cells to which the therapeutic is being delivered (*gray cells*) while sparing off-target cells (*green cells*). Several mechanisms exist to achieve cellular uptake, including the use of targeting ligands. After cellular uptake, the carriers or their payload (or both) must reach the subcellular site of action. This often requires achieving escape from the endosome, after which the carrier may traffic to the target organelle (e.g., the nucleus) via actin or other cytoskeletal components.

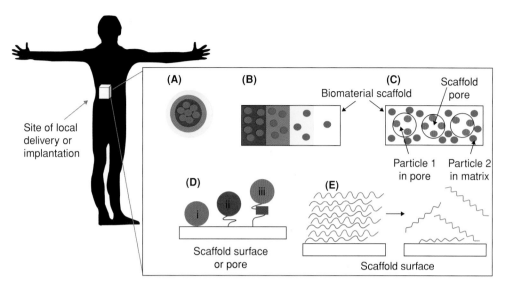

Plate 12. Micro- and nanoparticles may be used to achieve spatiotemporal control over delivery of therapeutic agents when delivered locally. (**A**) When delivered alone, the release profile may establish a gradient because of diffusional control over movement of the therapeutic agent. (**B**) When incorporated into a biomaterial scaffold, a similar gradient profile may be established. (**C**) By controlling the spatial location of the particulate carrier, control over the timing of release of single or multiple agents may be controlled. (**D**) Nanoscale carriers may be attached to the surface of biomaterials by adsorption (i) or covalent cross-linking (ii). Enzymatic cleavage sites may also be incorporated into tethers (iii) used to achieve covalent cross-linking to allow cell-mediated release. (**E**) Layer-by-layer release of therapeutic agents allows for temporal control as the layers of the system sequentially degrade, slowly releasing the contents of the subsequent layer.

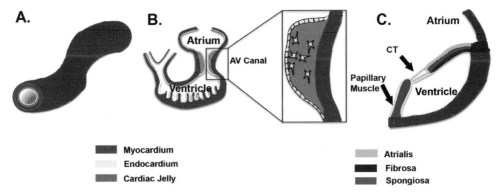

■ Myocardium	■ Atrialis
■ Endocardium	■ Fibrosa
■ Cardiac Jelly	■ Spongiosa

Plate 13. Early development of the atrioventricular (AV) valves. (**A**) The early heart tube consists of myocardium (*red*) and endocardium (*yellow*) with a layer of extracellular matrix known as the cardiac jelly (*blue*) between them. (**B**) In the AV canal region of the developing heart, the cardiac jelly expands to form padlike structures that eventually fuse and are filled by migrating stellate-shaped mesenchyme produced as the result of epithelial-to-mesenchymal transformation. (**C**) In the mature heart, this pad is sculpted as a result of fluid dynamics coupled with cellular reprogramming to produce a trilaminar structure. The atrialis (*green*) consists of primarily of elastin fibers, the spongiosa (*blue*) contains glycosaminoglycans, and the fibrosa (*purple*) is mostly collagen type I. This trilaminar structure is maintained in both the AV and semilunar valves. CT = chordae tendinae.

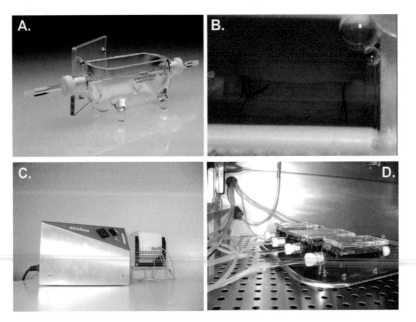

Plate 14. Fluid flow bioreactor system. (**A**) The glass bioreactor. (**B**) The collagen tube scaffold attached to the bioreactor. (**C**) The positive displacement pump. (**D**) Fluid flow bioreactor systems inside an incubator.

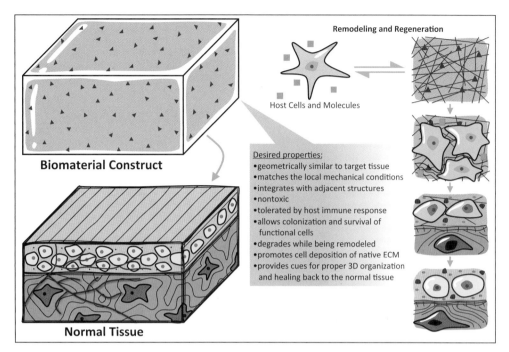

Plate 15. An ideal biomaterial construct for tissue engineering incorporates the physical features of the biomaterial with active biological factors. The in vivo regeneration process, dictated by the material and host interplay, replaces the relatively simple temporary structure with the complex normal tissue composed of organized cell populations restricted to their respective extracellular matrices. 3D = three-dimensional.

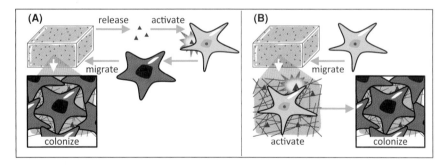

Plate 16. (**A**) Active factors incorporated within the biomaterial can be released into the surrounding tissues and subsequently activate target cells to migrate and colonize the scaffold. (**B**) Alternatively, motile target cells that invade the functionalized biomaterial can be induced to attach, differentiate, and populate the construct.

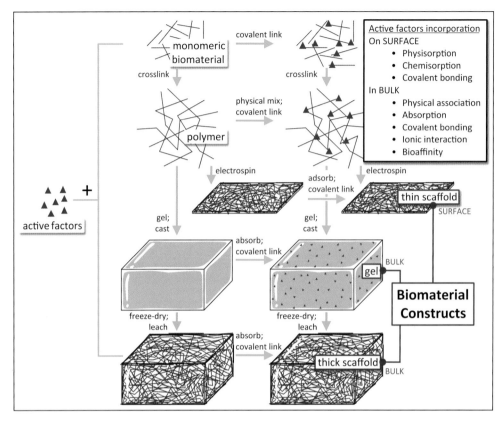

Plate 17. Bioactive pharmacological substances can be incorporated at various stages of the biomaterial construct synthesis. They can be added to the monomeric units, unassembled polymers, and final products after electrospinning, gelation, or scaffold formation.

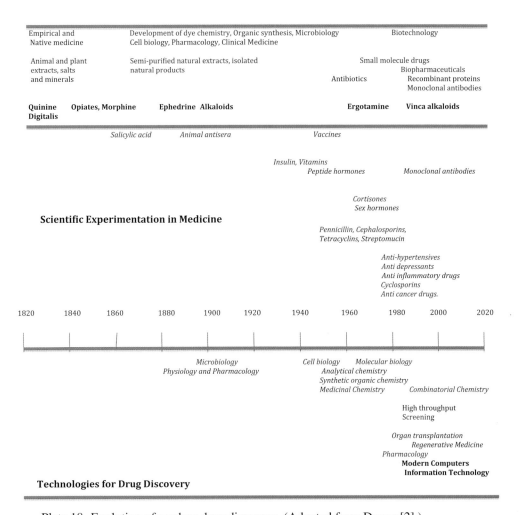

Plate 18. Evolution of modern drug discovery. (Adapted from Drews [2].)

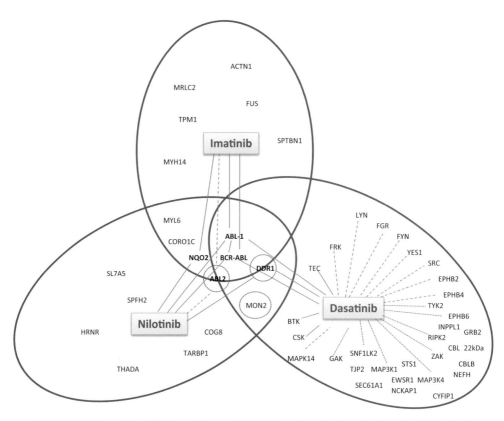

Plate 19. Interaction of kinase drugs with their molecular targets in cells. Chemical modulation of cellular function. *Solid lines* denote target–drug interactions that are well established, and the *dotted lines* represent potential or probable interactions. No connections indicate suspected interactions yet to be confirmed. (Reproduced with permission from Royal Society of Chemistry [13].)

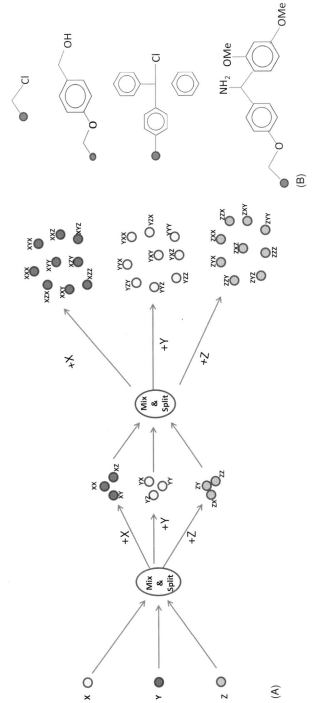

Plate 20. Basic combinatorial chemistry design. (**A**) Mix and split solid phase synthesis to synthesize trimeric molecules with three building blocks: X, Y, and Z. Solid phase methods allow to wash away excess reagents and unwanted by-products at every step. (**B**) Types of commercial resins used for solid phase synthesis. (Reproduced with permission from Drews [14]).

Microtiter plate types

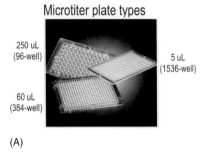

250 uL
(96-well)

5 uL
(1536-well)

60 uL
(384-well)

(A)

Plate 21. (**A**) Microtiter plate types used in high-throughput screening (HTS) and lead optimization studies. Maximum reaction volume capacities are shown for each well type.

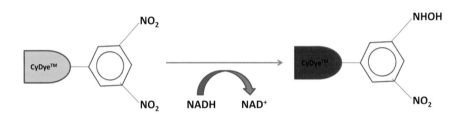

A non-fluorescent cell-permeable substrate is converted to fluorescent product in the cell by nitroreductase enzyme co-expressed with a gene of interest. This is a reporter system in which cells are intact for the readout while having enzymatic amplification for high sensitivity.

Plate 22. Reporter systems: chemiluminescence. (From [24]).

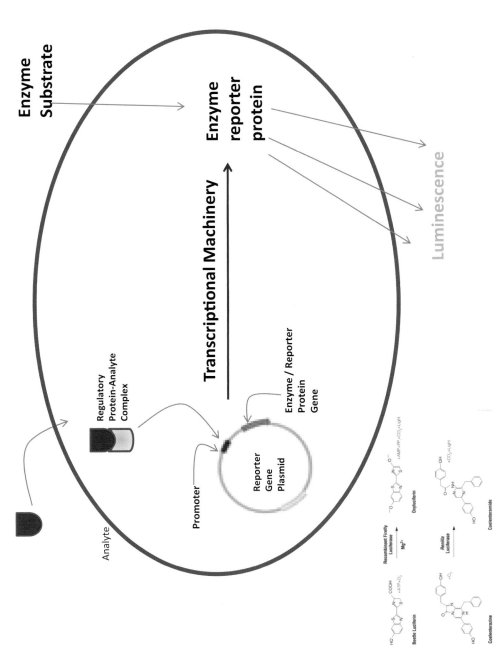

Plate 23. Luciferase reporter system for cell-based assays. A nonfluorescent cell-permeable substrate is converted to fluorescent product in the cell by nitroreductase enzyme coexpressed with a gene of interest. This is a reporter system in which cells are intact for the readout while having enzymatic amplification for high sensitivity. (Adapted from Amersham Biosciences.)

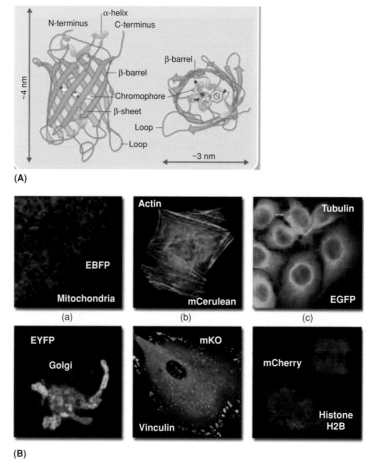

(A)

(B)

Plate 24. (**A**) β-Barrel structure of green fluorescent protein (GFP). (Adapted with permission from D. Piston, 2011.) (**B**) Subcellular localization of fluorescent proteins. EBFP = engineered blue fluorescent protein; EGFP = engineered green fluorescent protein; EYFP = engineered yellow fluorescent protein.

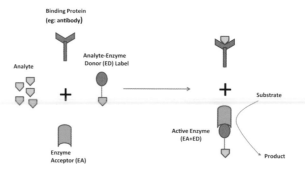

Plate 25. Enzyme complementation assay for a second messenger. EA = enzyme acceptor; ED = enzyme donor. (Adapted from DiscoveRx Inc: http://www.discoverx.com/technology/technology-hithunter.php.)

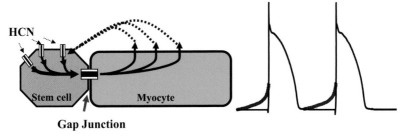

Gap Junction

Plate 26. A model of the two-cell pacing syncytium composed of a human bone marrow mesenchymal stem cell (hMSC) and a ventricular myocyte. HCN = hyperpolarization-activated cyclic nucleotide-gated (HCN) channel.

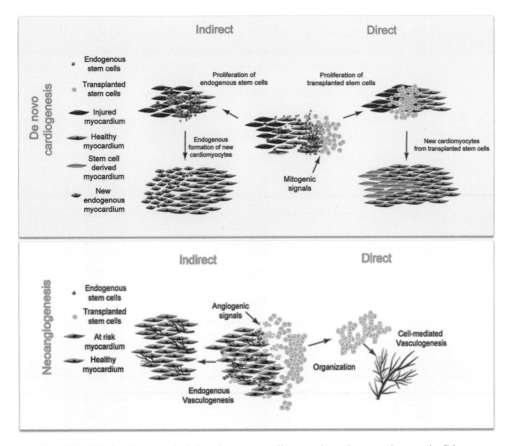

Plate 27. Mechanisms underlying de novo cardiogenesis and neoangiogenesis. Direct influence denotes regeneration of target organ following stem cell differentiation and engraftment. Indirect indicates a reparative paracrine influence of transplanted stem cells on resident stem cells.

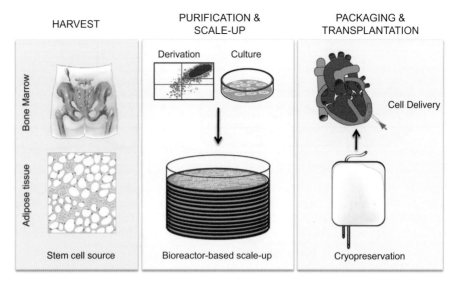

HARVEST PURIFICATION & SCALE-UP PACKAGING & TRANSPLANTATION

Plate 28. Critical steps in clinical application of stem cell therapy. GMP-grade manufacturing of cell biotherapeutics involves a three-step approach: (1) harvest of stem cells from sources such as adipose tissue and bone marrow; (2) derivation, purification, and scale-up of the stem cell product; and (3) packaging, storage (e.g. cryopreservation), and delivery into the diseased organ.

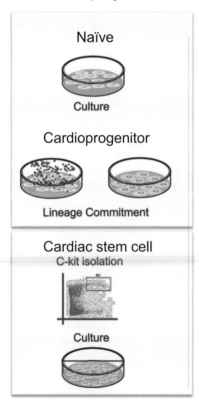

Plate 29. Organ specific stem cells: A new paradigm in regeneration. Organ specification can be achieved either by ex vivo conditioning of patient-derived stem cells, or derivation and purification of cells from the organ of interest.

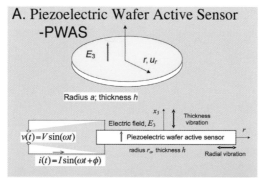

A. Piezoelectric Wafer Active Sensor -PWAS

E_3 r, u_r

Radius *a*; thickness *h*

x_3 Thickness vibration

Electric field, E_3

$v(t) = V\sin(\omega t)$ Piezoelectric wafer active sensor

radius r_a, thickness *h*   Radial vibration

$i(t) = I\sin(\omega t + \phi)$

B. Implantation of PWAS DEVICE

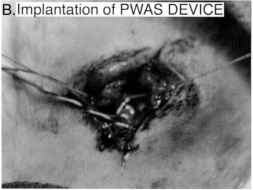

C. PWAS Response to αCT1 4-Weeks Following Implantation

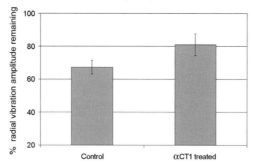

% radial vibration amplitude remaining

Control   αCT1 treated

Plate 30. Mechanical testing of αCT1-treated contraction capsules around silicone implants. (**A**) Principal modes of vibration of a circular piezoelectric wafer under oscillatory voltage excitation. (**B**) Subdermal or intramuscular implantation of wired piezoelectric wafer active sensor (PWAS) device in vivo in a rat. (**C**) αCT1 reduces dampening of the PWAS amplitude indicative of a less contracted capsule. (PWAS data obtained in collaboration with Victor Giurgiutiu PhD USC – Mechanical Engineering.)

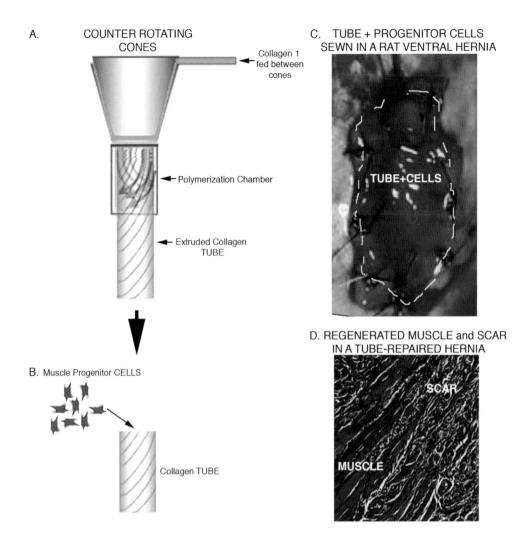

A. COUNTER ROTATING CONES

Collagen 1 fed between cones

Polymerization Chamber

Extruded Collagen TUBE

B. Muscle Progenitor CELLS

Collagen TUBE

C. TUBE + PROGENITOR CELLS SEWN IN A RAT VENTRAL HERNIA

TUBE+CELLS

D. REGENERATED MUSCLE and SCAR IN A TUBE-REPAIRED HERNIA

SCAR

MUSCLE

Plate 31. Tissue-engineered device for hernia repair. (**A**) Schema for device generating collagen tubes. (**B**) Skeletal muscle progenitor cells (satellite cells) are added to the collagen tube generating the tissue-engineered device. (**C**) The collagen tube with added muscle progenitor cells sewn into a ventral hernia in a rat. (**D**) Histologic section of a repaired ventral hernia 4 weeks after sewing in the tissue-engineered device. The device mediated a partial repair of the muscle defect. However, it did so imperfectly because the repair exhibited a mixture of regenerated muscle and scar tissue. Pharmacological approaches such as αCT1 may further decrease fibrosis, increasing the proportion of muscle to scar in the repaired hernia.

Section III

Future Applications of Regenerative Pharmacology

11

Gap Junction–Mediated Therapies to Eliminate Cardiac Arrhythmias

PETER R. BRINK, VIRGINIJUS VALIUNAS, AND IRA S. COHEN

Cardiac rhythm is initiated in the sinoatrial (SA) node cells, where action potential propagation to the atrium is accomplished by intercellular communication via gap junctions. Gap junction–mediated communication from the atrium to the atrioventricular (AV) node allows subsequent spread of the cardiac impulse rapidly throughout the ventricles via Purkinje fibers. Of clinical importance is the fact that reentrant cardiac arrhythmias dependent on abnormal conduction can arise in any of these myocardial tissue types. Arrhythmias can arise as a result of local ischemia or as a result of channelopathies such as those that occur with mutations of select K^+ or Na^+ channels resulting in slow conduction.

The essential role of gap junction channels in allowing current flow from cell to cell represents a major factor in normal and abnormal conduction. The central tenet of the following discussion is to first review the role of gap junction mediated communication as it relates to action potential conduction in the heart and to further introduce two potentially useful approaches to reduce or eliminate arrhythmias. The first is alteration of endogenous expression of connexins, and the second is a cellular delivery system able to deliver gene products to myocytes that in turn are able to affect cardiac pacing and potentially be a tool for curing cardiac arrhythmias.

Junctions Formed by Connexins

Gap junction channels in vertebrates are formed from subunit proteins called connexins. Each gap junction channel is composed of two hemichannels, each of which contains six connexins. When two cells are in close apposition, hemichannels from each cell can link together via the extracellular loops of the component connexins to form gap junction channels. This composite channel represents a unique intercellular pathway because it is the only form of intercellular communication that excludes the extracellular space. For reasons that are not completely understood but have been attributed to lipid membrane domains, including lipid rafts, gap junction channels tend

Table 11-1. *Connexin distribution in the heart*

Tissue	Connexins
Ventricle	Cx43
Purkinje cells	Cx40 > Cx43
Atrium	Cx40 > Cx43
AV node	Cx45 = Cx31.9?
SA node	Cx45 > Cx40 > Cx43

AV = atrioventricular; SA = sinoatrial.
Data from Van Veen et al., 2001; Boyett et al., 2006.

to aggregate and form plaques containing tens to thousands of channels (Locke et al., 2005). The major connexin types expressed within the human heart are connexin 43 (Cx43), Cx40, and Cx45 (Severs et al., 2006; Van Veen et al., 2001). The gap junction channels formed by these connexins participate in the generation of the local circuit currents necessary for action potential propagation. Table 11-1 illustrates the type of myocardium and the connexins expressed.

Recently, mouse Cx30.2 was shown to be expressed in the AV node of mice (Bukauskas et al., 2006) and Belluardo et al. (2001) have shown human Cx31.9 to be its ortholog. Cx31.9 has also been shown to form functional gap junction channels in vitro, and White et al. (2002) demonstrated that it is expressed in human heart. However, its exact distribution is not known in the human heart.

In general, coexpression of two or more connexins within a cell can give rise to a mixed gap junction channel such that the 12 subunits are not all the same. These channels are referred to as heteromeric. The two major cardiac connexins, Cx43 and Cx40, have been shown to form heteromeric channels (Brink et al., 1997; Valiunas et al., 2002). There are no data illustrating whether Cx31.9 is able to mix and form heteromeric channels with Cx43 or Cx40 in vivo, although the data for Cx30.2 in the mouse AV node suggest that it forms heteromers with Cx40 in vivo, resulting in reduced conductance, which could contribute to slow conduction velocity within the AV node.

Gap Junction Channel Permeability

Early studies on gap junction channels composed of connexins generated a consensus view that they were not permeable to molecules with molecular weights greater than 1.5 kD (Simpson et al., 1977; Schwarzmann et al., 1981) or with minor diameters greater than 1.2 to 1.3 nm (Neijssen et al., 2005). Recent publications show the passage of rod-shaped oligonucleotides and siRNA with minor diameters of 1.2 nm or less but with major diameters of 3 to 8 nm (Valiunas et al., 2005) and weights up to 4–5 kD is possible. This has redefined the limits of gap junction channel permeability. More importantly, the demonstration of the ability of siRNA to traverse gap junction channels (Valiunas et al., 2005) adds yet another dimension to the role gap junction channels play in coordinated tissue functions. Hence, besides allowing the movement of monovalent ions and second messengers and metabolites, gap junctions are also able to facilitate gene silencing. Whether this new-found ability of gap junctions will be a tool for combating arrhythmias remains to be seen.

Interestingly, not all connexins have the same biophysical properties. Most notable are single channel conductance and the selectivity or permselectivity of gap junction channels (Valiunas et al., 2002; Goldberg et al., 2004; Brink et al., 1996; Ek-Vitorin et al., 2005; Brink et al., 2006). For example, Cx43 single channel conductance measured in Cs or K salt is approximately 90 pS, and that of Cx40 is 140 pS. In Cs or K solutions using aspartate as the major anion, the conductances are 60 and 125 pS, respectively (Table 11-1).

The selectivity or permselectivity properties of gap junction channels also differ. The permeability ratio for Lucifer yellow (LY) relative to K^+ is 1/40 for Cx43 and 1/400 for Cx40 (Brink et al., 1997; Valiunas et al., 2002). In a recent study, Ek-Virton et al. (2005) found that LY permeability to Cx43 was less than that for cations. Ek-Virton et al. (2005) also showed that phosphorylation state can affect the permeability of cationic species dramatically. In fact, the data presented by Ek-Vitron et al. (2005) suggest that small cationic probes with minor diameters of 0.5 nm can attain permeabilities similar to that of K^+ when Cx43 is phosphorylated.

A number of studies have compared the relative transfer rate of endogenous solutes such as nucleotides and second messengers for a number of connexins (Goldberg et al., 2004; Valiunas et al., 2002; Kanaporis et al., 2008). As was the case for the exogenous probe LY, endogenous probe permeability is highly dependent on the connexin type. A number of publications have illustrated that the various connexins have different permeabilities to a variety of probes (Goldberg et al., 2004; Niessen et al., 2000). Other connexin types that have not been studied as completely as Cx43 or Cx40 are Cx37, found most abundantly in endothelium (Beyer, 1993) and Cx45, found in select regions of the heart and vascular wall (Van Veen et al., 2001). Table 11-2 lists the unitary conductances and permeability ratios for LY and K^+ when known.

The list demonstrates the diversity of electrical conductances ranging from 400 pS for Cx37 to 27 pS for Cx45. Interestingly, although Cx45 has a smaller electrical conductance than Cx43 or Cx40, it is more permeable to LY than Cx40. These data point to the diversity of properties in the multigene family of connexins. The varied permeabilities and electrical conductances of homotypic gap junction channels are also apparent with regard to the cell–cell transfer of oligonucleotides and siRNA (Valiunas et al., 2005; Kanaporis et al., 2008).

Table 11-2. *Homotypic channel conductances and permeability*

Connexin	Unitary conductance (pS)	LY/K$^+$*
Cx37	400	–
Cx31.9	15	–
Cx32	60	–
Cx40	125	1/400
Cx43	60	1/40
Cx45	27	1/100

*Ratio of Lucifer yellow to K$^+$ flux per channel.
Data from Valiunas et al., 2002; Bukauskus et al., 2006;
Oh et al., 1999.

Gap Junctions and the Heart: Action Potential Propagation

Barr and Berger (1965) and Weidmann (1970) established that currents associated with action potential propagation move from myocyte to myocyte via gap junctions and that reduction in gap junction–mediated communication results in propagation failure. Numerous publications have verified these seminal observations (Wilders et al., 1996; Cole et al., 1988; de Groot et al., 2003; Beauchamp et al., 2006; Poelzing and Rosenbaum, 2004).

An essential component for cardiac action potential propagation is longitudinal resistance, where it can be demonstrated that conduction velocity is inversely proportional to the square root of the longitudinal resistance. Longitudinal resistance is composed of both cytoplasmic resistance and junctional membrane resistance such that Ri = Rcyto + Rj. For a typical myocyte, the longitudinal resistance contributed by the cytoplasm is about 1 MΩ or 1000 nS, and the junctional resistance at the intercalated disc is about 2 MΩ or 500 nS, making junctional resistance at the intercalated disc the dominant determinant of longitudinal resistance. De Groot et al. (2003) and Cole et al. (1988) have shown that reducing junctional conductance slows propagation and can be a major determinant in conduction failure. Optical mapping of perfused ventricular wedge preparations (Poelzing and Rosenbaum, 2004) also demonstrates the critical role of gap junctions in conduction.

Longitudinal Resistance and Reentrant Arrhythmias

Reentrant rhythms have long been associated with abnormalities of conduction (Janse and Wit, 1989). Whether a reentrant pathway is anatomically defined (e.g., in association with a scar (Janse and Wit, 1989)) or whether it is functional (circular reentry (Janse and Wit, 1989)), a critical contributor to the conducting properties in the heart in general and in the reentrant circuit is the gap junctions and their component connexins. Studies of cardiac failure and reentrant ventricular arrhythmias have shown reduced expression and abundance of Cx43 such that the length constant is significantly reduced relative to wild type (Poelzing and Rosenbaum, 2004; Gutstein et al., 2001).

Modulating gap junctions as an antiarrhythmic strategy initially was conceived to bring about a block of conduction. Regrettably, the gap junctional blockers used to date have not been channel specific or isoform specific, and disrupting coupling between cells has been found to cause potentially fatal arrhythmias (Dhein, 2002). For example, eliminating conduction by reduced gap junctional conductance in reentrant circuits can create new reentrant circuits when gap junction conductance is reduced in surrounding normal myocytes. On the positive side, antiarrhythmic peptides have been used to increase junctional conductance. One such peptide, rotigaptide, appears to target Cx43 specifically (Dhein et al., 2003) and is purportedly antiarrhythmic.

Other recent studies have shown the importance of connexins and hence gap junctions in arrhythmias. For example, overexpression of Cx45 results in ventricular tachycardia in mice (Betsuyaku et al., 2006, 2004), and mutations of Cx40 are associated with atrial fibrillation in humans (Gollob et al., 2006). The connexin mCx30.2 (the ortholog of h31.9) has been shown to slow conduction in the murine AV node (Kreuzberg et al., 2005). Studies of the epicardial border zone of healing canine myocardial infarcts have demonstrated that altered connexin distribution and density in regions important to the generation of reentrant ventricular tachycardia (Peters et al., 1997).

Ischemia and pH Dependence of Cardiac Gap Junction Channels

One feature of ischemia that has been illustrated in vitro is the acidification of myocytes (Duffy et al., 2004; Cascia et al., 2005). A recent study by Schroeder et al. (2010) has shown that ischemia in rat hearts results in intracellular pH declining 0.5 pH units over a 20-minute period. The linkage between ischemia and connexins arises because gap junction channels are pH sensitive (Morley et al., 1997). Acidification of the cytoplasm causes gap junction channels to close. There is one notable exception, Cx32 (Morley et al., 1997), which is the least pH-sensitive connexin thus far documented. In addition, Cx32 does not readily form heteromeric channels with Cx43 (Das Sarma et al., 2001). Thus, once they are transfected into cardiac myocytes, Cx32-derived gap junctions represent an independent population of channels acting without influence from interactions with endogenous connexins. The notion of Cx32 functioning within the heart is not novel. In fact, Plum et al. (2000) generated a mouse in which Cx43 was replaced with Cx32. The latter rescued the Cx43-deficient mice that would otherwise have died at birth. Whether this phenotype would be more or less susceptible to ischemia remains to be determined.

Novel Therapies for Cardiac Arrhythmias

Overexpression of Connexins

Among the ways to upregulate connexin expression are stress in the form of mildly elevated temperatures (VanSlyke and Musil, 2005), increasing expression of adhesion molecules such as α- and β-catenins and cadherin (Jongen et al., 1991; Prowse et al., 1997; Wei et al., 2005), and chemical stimulation with 4-phenylbutyrate (4PB) (Asklund et al., 2004) or the synthetic antiarrhythmic peptide zp123 (Axelsen et al., 2006; Eloff et al., 2003). 4PB is a Food and Drug Administration–approved drug that can be administered orally and that is being tested for effectiveness in spinal muscular atrophy (Wirth et al., 2006) and cystic fibrosis (Singh et al., 2006).

In cells that already make sufficient amounts of catenins and cadherins, connexin overexpression is not as effective as it is with cells that are deficient in catenin or cadherin expression. Human bone marrow mesenchymal stem cells (hMSCs) make both α- and β-catenins and express both E and N-cadherins. Cardiac myocytes express catenins and N-cadherins as well. Interestingly, if N-cadherin is overexpressed in cardiac myocytes, then cardiomyopathies occur (Ferriera-Cornwall et al., 2002; Li et al., 2006). Thus, the use of adhesion molecules as a tool to promote and increase the number of functional gap junction channels presents some potential hazards. Another approach is pharmacological stimulation of connexin synthesis and function. The chemical chaperone (4PB) inhibits histone deacetylase, an enzyme associated with inactivation of gene transcription (Asklund et al., 2004; Perlmutter, 2002; Iwasaki et al., 2006). 4PB concentrations in the mM range increase Cx43 production two- to fivefold during exposure times of hours to days (Asklund et al., 2004; Wirth et al., 2006; Permutter, 2002). Not only is Cx43 production elevated, but enhanced dye transfer has also been observed (Asklund et al., 2004). The use of 4PB as an antiarrhythmic drug has yet to be tested in animal models. The drawback in using drugs such as 4PB or rotogaptide to affect Cx43 or other connexin expression in vivo is a lack of specificity.

Viral delivery of connexins is yet another approach that has potential in the treatment of arrhythmias. There have been no published studies using viral delivery of Cx43 to affect arrhythmias, but there studies have targeted cancer cells using in vitro approaches (Mao et al., 2000; Hattori et al., 2007) that demonstrate that upregulation reduces tumor cell growth rate. Unfortunately, the viral delivery also presents the hazard of global delivery to a tissue or organ.

Stem Cells: Their Use as a Tool for Remedying Cardiac Arrhythmias

Adult mesenchymal stem cells represent an attractive cell type for cell-based therapy for two reasons. First, these cells can be used as vehicles to deliver gene products or small molecules because they are either autologous if derived from the same person

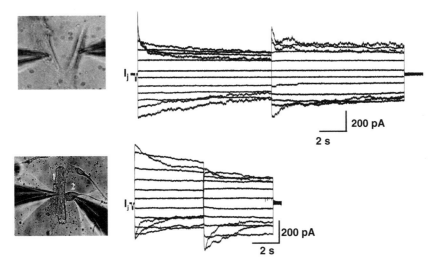

Figure 11-1. Junctional conductance between human bone marrow mesenchymal stem cells (hMSCs) is shown in the *upper panel*. hMSC to ventricular myocyte coupling is shown in the *lower panel*.

for whom one is creating a therapy or allogenic because of their immune privileged status. Second, they readily form gap junctions with themselves and other cell types in vitro and most importantly in vivo (Valiunas et al., 2004, 2009; Potapova et al., 2004).

To illustrate the utility of stem cells as delivery vehicles, it is necessary to determine their ability to form gap junctions and to demonstrate their ability to be engineered and express a gene product that can subsequently be delivered to a target cell. For the latter, our gene of choice has been the *HCN2* pacing gene because it has easily demonstrated signature currents as revealed with whole-cell patch clamp (Valiunas et al., 2009).

Human Bone Marrow Mesenchymal Stem Cells Express Connexins and Can Form Functional Gap Junctions

Human bone marrow mesenchymal stem cells form gap junctions composed of Cx43 and Cx40 (Valiunas et al., 2004). In vitro measurements of junctional conductance between hMSCs range from single channel or multichannel activity to macroscopic conductances of 10 to 20 nS (Valiunas et al., 2004, 2005). Heterologous coupling between an hMSCs and cardiac myocytes also manifests macroscopic junctional conductances in the 10 nS range (Valiunas et al., 2004, 2009). Figure 11-1 illustrates an hMSC cell pair (**A**) and a heterologous hMSC–ventricular myocyte cell pair (**B**). In both cases, the cell pairs are coupled (~10 nS). Furthermore, because hMSCs form gap junctions composed of Cx43, a variety of small solutes, including cyclic adenosine monophosphate (cAMP) (Kanaporis et al., 2008) and siRNA molecules can be delivered to any cell with which a stem cell can form Cx43-based gap junctions (Valiunas et al., 2005).

Delivery of *HCN2*-Mediated Current from Human Bone Marrow Mesenchymal Stem Cells Coupled by Gap Junctions to Myocytes

The mammalian heart beats about 3 billion times in a normal lifetime. This spontaneous rhythm is myogenic in origin (Noble, 1979). Virtually all cardiac regions retain the capacity for spontaneous activity (Yu et al., 1993), although the primary pacemaker is the SA node. It is primary because it generates the highest spontaneous rate. Because all myocytes in the heart are connected to each other by gap junctions, the region that generates the highest rate drives all others. There is little doubt that the pacemaker current I_f (whose α subunit is encoded by members of the *HCN* gene family) is the major contributor. I_f is an inward current activated by hyperpolarization, and this inward current drives the membrane toward threshold for initiating the next action potential. The family *HCN* consists of four members, *HCN1* to *HCN4*; three of these (*HCN1*, *HCN2*, and *HCN4*) are expressed in the mammalian heart (Shi et al., 1999). The genes are expressed in a region-specific manner, with *HCN4* being the predominant isoform expressed in the sinus node (80%) and *HCN2* being the dominant form expressed in ventricle (>80%) (Shi et al., 1999). Mutations in *HCN4* lead to disorders of rhythm in affected patients (Schulze-Bahr et al., 2003). We also know that expression of *HCN2* is important for in vitro cardiac models to pace because a dominant negative construct of *HCN2* significantly reduces beating in rat neonatal ventricular myocytes (Er et al., 2003). Structurally, the hyperpolarization-activated cyclic nucleotide-gated (HCN) channel proteins are similar to K^+ channels containing six membrane-spanning regions (S1–S6). The S4 region is highly charged and contributes to the voltage dependence of channel open probability. The pore is between S5 and S6. The HCN channels are selective to Na^+ and K^+. The carboxy terminus contains a cAMP binding site. When cAMP is bound, the channel opens at less negative potentials.

Adult Mesenchymal Stem Cells Can Heterologously Express *HCN2* Channels and Form a Pacemaker Unit When Coupled to a Ventricular Myocyte

HCN2 expression in hMSCs is possible and, in fact, stable transfection is possible, and robust channel activity has also been demonstrated (Potapova et al., 2004; Valiunas et al., 2009). Genetic engineering of the hMSCs along with their expression of connexins and their consequent gap junctional coupling to target cells such as cardiac myocytes make hMSCs an ideal cellular delivery system (Potapova et al., 2004). Two

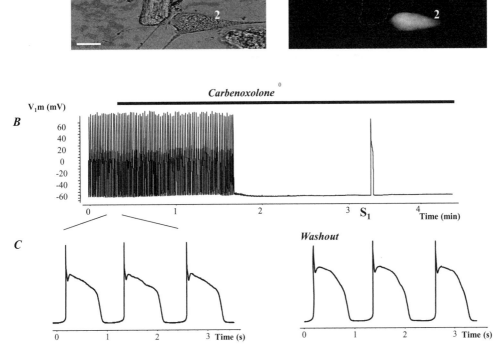

Figure 11-2. (**A**) Imaging of a ventricular myocyte–human bone marrow mesenchymal stem cell (hMSC) pair. (**B**) hMSCs expressing *HCN2* drive the pacing of the myocyte–hMSC cell pair. Carbenoxolone blocks pacing. S1 is an electrical stimulus to show that carbenoxolone does not affect the action potential. (**C**) Examples of action potentials before carbenoxolone and after.

questions can now be addressed. First, can a cell pair consisting of an hMSC that expresses *HCN2* when coupled to a ventricular myocyte act as a pacemaker and generate a constant pacing rate? Second, can *HCN2*-expressing cells be focally delivered to the heart and pace the heart? The answer to both of these questions is yes. Figure 11-2 illustrates data taken from a cell pair consisting of an hMSC coupled to a canine ventricular myocyte. In current clamp mode, a regularly generated action potential is observed in the myocyte at a rate of approximately 1 Hz. Carbenoxolone, a gap junction channel inhibitor, eliminates pacing. A stimulus applied directly to the myocyte under this condition generates an action potential. This indicates that the carbenoxolone does not affect the ability of the myocyte to generate an action potential but does illustrate the necessity of the *HCN2*-expressing hMSCs to be coupled to the myocyte to induce pacing. Expanded tracings before carbenoxolone and after washout are also shown. In both cases, a phase 4–like depolarization precedes the upstroke of the action

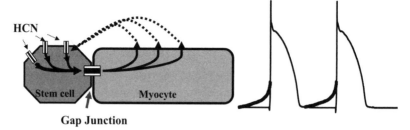

Figure 11-3. A model of the two-cell pacing syncytium composed of a human bone marrow mesenchymal stem cell (hMSC) and a ventricular myocyte. HCN = hyperpolarization-activated cyclic nucleotide-gated (HCN) channel. (See color plate 26.)

potential. Figure 11-3 illustrates the functional interactions between the hMSC and myocyte mediated by gap junctions. Clearly, the in vitro data support the notion that an hMSC can form a functional two-cell pacemaker syncytium.

Can *HCN2*-expressing cells be delivered the heart and act as a pacemaker? In fact, Potapova et al. (2004) did just that. Approximately 1 million cells were focally delivered (via catheter) to the left ventricular myocardium. In some animals, the hMSCs contained no *HCN2*, but in others, the hMSCs were expressing *HCN2*.

After 3 to 12 days, vagal stimulation was used to inhibit the SA node. In control animals, the pacing rate was 45 beats/min, but in animals with hMSCs expressing *HCN2*, the pacing rate was 60 beats/min. Histologic analysis demonstrated that the site of injection contained hMSCs and further mapping revealed the injection site to be the source of pacemaker activity. Additional studies by Plotnikov et al. (2007) have shown consistent pacing rates generated by delivered *HCN2*-expressing cells up to 16 weeks after injection as long as 700,000 or more cells were delivered.

A concern when considering this type of approach is effectiveness over time. Do the cells wander, or do they remain at a site of injection? Rosen et al. (2007) addressed the question by labeling hMSCs with quantum dots. Labeled cells were injected and histologic sections made to reconstruct the injection site 1 hour and 24 hours after injection. The data indicated that over the time frame used, little cell wandering occurred. What about longer times? Will cell migrate away from an injection site with time or remain? Conversely, can hMSCs be delivered systemically and home to specific sites? Both wandering and homing remain as unanswered questions that need answers before cellular-based delivery becomes truly viable.

Conclusions

Gap junction–mediated conductance is essential to normal action potential conduction in the heart, and evidence strongly suggests dysfunction as a major causative component of many cardiac arrhythmias. The therapeutic approaches available for affecting junction conductance to alleviate arrhythmias have some promise in the form 4PB and rotigaptide, but the effects of these agents on the heart will be global. A similar problem is presented if viral delivery is used. Another very promising approach is the engineering of adult stem cells to produce specific gene products and using those cells to delivery that product to target cells in the body. This approach can be used for focal delivery of cells without global consequence or systemically if delivery cells can home to sites of interest. One example of focal delivery is *HCN2*-expressing cells that are able to couple to ventricular myocytes and pace the heart. This observation represents proof of principle for such cell-based therapy (Potapova et al., 2004). A related aspect of cellular delivery mediated by gap junction channels is the delivery siRNA able to silence appropriate genes such as those required for excitability to combat arrhythmias. At present, this is a very exciting idea still in its infancy.

The primary question from a therapeutics perspective becomes: which gene products are antiarrhythmic and which are proarrhythmic? Or can the same gene product be both antiarrhythmic or proarrhythmic depending on our ability to target delivery to specific locations?

Acknowledgments

Supported by NIH grants 88180 and 088181.

References

Asklund, T., I.B. Appelskog, O. Ammerpohl, T.J. Ekstrom, and P.M. Almqvist. Histone Deacetylase Inhibitor 4-phenylbutyrate Modulates Glial Fibrillary Acidic Protein and Connexin 43 Expression, and Enhances Gap-junction Communication, in Human Glioblastoma Cells. Eur. J. Cancer 40: 1073–1081, 2004.

Axelsen, L.N., M. Stahlhut, S. Mohammed, B.D. Larsen, M. Nielsen, N. Holstein-Rathlou, S. Andersen, O.N. Jensen, J.K. Hennan, and A.L. Kjolbye. Identification of Ischemia-regulated Phosphorylation Sites in Connexin43: A Possible Target for the Antiarrhythmic Peptide Analogue Rotigaptide (ZP123). J. Mole. Cell. Cardiol. 40: 790–798, 2006.

Barr, L., M. Dewey, and Berger, W. Propagation of Action Potentials and the Structure of the Nexus in Cardiac Muscle. J. Gen. Physiol. 48: 797–823, 1965.

Beauchamp, P. K. Yamada, A Baertschi, K. Green, E. Kanter, J. Saffitz, and A. Kleber. Relative contributions of connexins 40 and 43 to atrial impulse propagation in synthetic strands of neonatal and fetal murine cardiomyocytes. Circ. Res. 99: 1216–1224, 2006.

Belluardo, N., T.W. White, M. Srinivas, A. Trovato-Salinaro, H. Ripps, G. Mudo, R. Bruzzone, and D.F. Condorelli. Identification and functional expression of HCx31.9. Cell Comm. Adhesion, 8(4–6): 173–178, 2001.

Betsuyaku, T., S. Kanno, D.L. Lerner, R.B. Schuessler, J.E. Saffitz, and K.A. Yamada. Spontaneous and inducible ventricular arrhythmias after myocardial infarction in mice. Cardiovasc. Pathol. 13: 156–164, 2004.

Betsuyaku, T., N.S. Nnebe, R. Sundset, S. Patibandla, C.M. Drueger, and K.A. Yamada Overexpression of cardiac Connexin45 increases susceptibility to ventricular tachyarrhythmias in vivo. Am. J. Physiol. Heart Circ. Physiol. 290: H163–171, 2006.

Beyer, E.C. Gap junctions. Int Rev Cytol. 137C: 1–37, 1993.

Boyett, M., S. Inada, S. Yoo, J. Li, J. Liu, J. Tellez, I. Greener, H. Honjo, R. Billeter, M. Lei, H. Zhang, I. Efimov, and H. Dorzynski Connexins in the SA and AV nodes. Adv. Cardiol. 42:175–197, 2006.

Brink, P.R., V. Valiunas, H.Z. Wang, W. Zhao, K. Davies, and G.J. Christ. Experimental diabetes alters connexin43 derived gap junction permeability in short-term cultures of rat corporeal vascular smooth muscle cells. J. Urol. 175(1): 381–386, 2006.

Brink, P.R., K. Cronin, K. Banach, E. Peterson, E. Westphale, K.H. Seul, S.V. Ramanan, and E.C. Beyer. Evidence of heteromeric gap junction channels Formed from rat connexin43 and human connexin37. Am. J. Physiol. 273: C1386–C1396, 1997.

Brink, P.R., S.V. Ramanan, and G.J. Christ. Human connexin43 gap junction channel gating: evidence for mode shifts and/or heterogeneity. Am. J. Physiol. 271: C321–C331, 1996.

Bukauskas, F.F., M.M. Kreuzberg, M. Rackauskas, A. Bukauskiene, M.V.L. Bennett, V.K. Verselis, and K. Willecke. Properties of mouse connexin 30.2 and human connexin 31.9 hemichannels: implications for atrioventricular conduction in the heart. PNAS. 103(25): 9726–9731, 2006.

Cascia, W.E., H. Yang, B.J. Muller-Borer, and T.A. Johnson. Ischemia-induced Arrhythmia: the role of connexins, gap junctions, and attendant changes in impulse propagation. J. Electrocardiol. 38: 55–59, 2005.

Cole, W.C., J.B. Picone, and N. Sperelakis. Gap junction uncoupling and discontinuous propagation in the heart. a comparison of experimental data with computer simulations. Biophys. J. 53(5): 809–818, 1988.

Das Sarma, J., R.A. Meyer, F. Wang, V. Abraham, C.W. Lo, and M. Koval. Multimeric connexin interactions prior to the trans-golgi network. J. Cell Sci. 114: 4013–4024, 2001.

de Groot, J.R., T. Veenstra, A.O. Verkerk, R. Wilders, J.P. Smits, F.J. Wilms-Schopman, R.F Wiegerinck, J. Bourier, C.N. Belterman, R. Coronel, and E.E. Verheijck. Conduction slowing by the gap junctional uncoupler carbenoxolone. Cardiovasc. Res. 60(2): 288–297, 2003.

Dhein, S. Peptides acting at gap junctions. Peptides. 23: 1701–1709, 2002.

Dhein, S., B.D. Larsen, J.S. Petersen, and F.W. Mohr. Effects of the new antiarrhythmic peptide ZP123 on epicardial activation and repolarization pattern. Cell Commun. Adhes. 10: 371–378, 2003.

Duffy, H.S., A.W. Ashton, P. O'Donnell, W. Coombs, S.M. Taffet, M. Delmar, and D. C. Spray. Regulation of connexin43 protein complexes by intracellular acidification. Circ. Res. 94: 215–222, 2004.

Eloff, B.C., E. Gilat, X. Wan, and D.S. Rosenbaum. Pharmacological modulation of cardiac gap junctions to enhance cardiac conduction. Circulation. 108: 3157–3163, 2003.

Ek-Vitorin, J.F. and J.M. Burt. Quantification of gap junction selectivity. Am. J. Physiol. Cell Physiol. 289(6): C1535–C1546, 2005.

Er, F., R. Larbig, A. Ludwing, M. Bie, F. Hofmann, D. J. Beuckelmann, and U.C. Hoppe. Dominant-negative suppression of HCN channels markedly reduces the native pacemaker current if and undermines spontaneous beating of neonatal cardiomyocytes. Circulation. 107(3): 485–489, 2003.

Ferriera-Cornwall, M., L. Yang, N. Narula, J. Lenxon, M. Lieberman, and G. Radice. Remodeling the intercalated disc leads to cardiomyopathy in mice misexpressing cadherins in the heart. J. Cell Sci. 115: 1623–1634, 2002.

Goldberg, G., Valiunas, V., and Brink, P.R. Selectivity permeability of gap junction channels. Biochem. Biophysics Acta. 662: 96–101, 2004.

Gollob, M.H., D.L. Jones, A.D. Krahn, L. Danis, X. Gong, Q. Shao, X. Liu, J.P. Veinot, A. Tang, A. Stewart, F. Tesson, G. Klein, R. Yee, A. Skanes, G. Guiraudon, L. Ebihara, and D. Bai. Somatic mutations in the connexin 40 gene (GJA5) in atrial fibrillation. N. Engl. Med. 354: 25, 2006.

Gutstein, D.E., G.E. Morley, D. Vaidya, F. Liu, F.L. Chen, H. Stuhlmann, and G.I. Fishman. Heterogeneous expression of gap junction channels in the heart leads to conduction defects and ventricular dysfunction. Circulation. 104: 1194–1199, 2001.

Hattori, Y., M. Fukushima, and Y. Maitani. Non-viral delivery of connexin 43 gene with histone deacetylase inhibitor to human nasopharyngeal tumor cells enhances gene expression and inhibits in vivo tumor growth. Int. J. Oncol. 30: 1427–1439, 2007.

Hodgkin, A.L. and A.F. Huxley. A quantitative description of membrane current and its application to conduction and excitation in nerve. J. Physiol. 117:500–544, 1952.

Janse, M. and A. Wit. Electrophysiological mechanisms of ventricular arrhythmias resulting from myocardial ischemia and infarction. Phys. Rev. 69: 1049–1169 1989.

Jongen, W.M., D.J. Fitzgerald, M. Asamoto, C. Piccoli, T.J. Slaga, D. Gros, M. Takeichi, and H. Yamasaki. Regulation of connexin 43-mediated gap junctional intercellular communication by Ca2+ in mouse epidermal cells is controlled by E cadherin. J. Cell Biol. 114(3): 545–555, 1991.

Kanaporis, G, G. Mese, L. Valiuniene, T.W. White, P.R. Brink, and V. Valiunas. Gap junction channels exhibit connexin-specific permeability to cyclic nucleotides. J. Gen. Physiol. 131: 293–305, 2008.

Kreuzberg, M.M., G. Sohl, J. Kim, V.K. Verselis, K. Willecke, and F.F. Bukauskas. Functional properties of mouse connexin30.2 expressed in the conduction system of the heart. Circ. Res. 96: 1169–1177, 2005.

Li, J., V.V. Patel and G.L. Radice. Dysregulation of cell adhesion proteins and cardiac arrhythmogenesis. Clin. Med. Res. 4(1): 42–52, 2006.

Locke, D., J. Liu, and A.L. Harris. Lipid rafts prepared by different methods contain different connexin channels, but gap junctions are not lipid rafts. Biochemistry 44(39): 13027–13042, 2005.

Mao, A., J. Bechberger, D. Lidington, J. Galipeau, D. Larid, and C. Naus. Neuronal differentiation and growth control of Neuro-2a cells after retroviral gene delivery of Connexin43. J. Biol. Chem. 275: 34407–34417, 2000.

Morley, G.E., J.F. Ek-Vitorin, S.M. Taffet, and M. Delmar. Structure of Connexin43 and its regulation by pHi. J. Cardiovasc. Electrophysiol. 8: 939–951, 1997.

Niessen, H., Harz, H., Bedner, P., Kramer, K., and Willecke, K. Selective permeability of different connexin channels to the second messenger IP3. J. Cell Sci. 113: 1365–1372, 2000.

Noble, D. The Initiation of the Heartbeat. 2nd ed. Clarendon Press, Oxford, 1979.

Oh, S., J.B. Rubin, M.V. Bennett, V.K. Verselis, and T.A. Bargiello. Molecular determinants of electrical rectification of single channel conductance in gap junctions formed by connexins 26 and 32. J. Gen. Physiol. 114: 339–364, 1999.

Perlmutter, D.H. Chemical chaperones: a pharmacological strategy for disorders of protein folding and trafficking. Pediatr. Res. 52: 832–836, 2002.

Peters, N.S., J. Coromilas, N.J. Severs, and A.L. Wit. Disturbed connexin43 gap junction distribution correlates with the location of reentrant circuits in the epicardial border zone of healing canine infarcts that cause ventricular tachycardia. Circulation. 95(4): 988–996, 1997.

Plotnikov, A.N., I. Shlapakova, M.J. Szabolcs, P. Danilo, Jr, B.H. Lorell, I.A. Potapova, Z. Lu, A.B. Rosen, R.T. Mathias, P.R. Brink, R.B. Robinson, I.S. Cohen, and M.R. Rosen. Xenografted adult human mesenchymal stem cells provide a platform for sustained biological pacemaker function in canine heart. Circulation. 116: 706–713. 2007.

Plum A., G. Hallas, T. Magin, F. Dombrowski, A. Hagendorff, B. Schumacher, C. Wolpert, J. Kim, W.H. Lamers, M. Evert, P. Meda, O. Traub, and K. Willecke. Unique and shared functions of different connexins in mice. Curr. Biol. 10(18): 1083–1091, 2000.

Poelzing, S. and D.S. Rosenbaum. Altered connexin43 expression produces arrhythmia substrate in heart failure. Am. J. Physio. Heart Circ. Physiol., 287: H1762–H1770, 2004.

Potapova, I., A. Plotnikov, Z. Lu, P. Danilo, Jr., W. Valiunas, J. Qu, S. Doronin, J. Zuckerman, I.N. Shlapakova, J. Gao, Z. Pan, A.J. Herron, R.B. Robinson, P.R. Brink, M.R. Rosen, and I.S. Cohen. Human mesenchymal stem cells as a gene delivery system to create cardiac pacemakers. Circ Res. 94: 952–959, 2004.

Prowse, D.M., G.P. Cadwallader, and J.D. Pitts. E-cadherin expression can alter the specificity of gap junction formation. Cell Biol. Int. 21(12): 833–843, 1997.

Rosen, A.B., D.J. Kelly, A.J. Schuldt, J. Lu, I.A. Potapova, S.V. Doronin, K.J. Robichaud, R.B. Robinson, M.R. Rosen, P.R. Brink, G.R. Gaudette, and I.S. Cohen. Finding fluorescent needles in the cardiac haystack: tracking human mesenchymal stem cells labeled with quantum dots for quantitative in vivo three-dimensional fluorescence analysis. Stem Cells. 25(8):2128–2138, 2007.

Schroeder, M., P. Swietach, H. Atherton, F. Callagher, P. Lee, G. Radd, K. Clarke, and D. Tyler. Measuring intracellular pH in the heart using hyperpolarized carbon dioxide and bicarbonate: a C13 and P31 magnetic resonance spectroscopy study Cardiovasc. Res 86: 82–91, 2010.

Schulze-Bahr, E., A. Neu, P. Friederich, B. Kaupp, G. Breithardt, O. Pongs, and D. Isbrandt. Pacemaker channel dysfunction in a patient with sinus node disease. J. Clin. Invest. 111: 1537–1545, 2003.

Schwarzmann, G., H. Wiegarndt, B. Rose, A. Zimmerman, D. Ben-Haim, and W. Loewenstein. Diameter of the cell to cell junctional membrane channels as probed with neutral molecules. Science. 213: 551–553, 1981.

Severs, N.J., E. Dupont, N. Thomas, R. Kaba, S. Rothery, R. Jain, K. Sharpey, and C.H. Fry. Alterations in cardiac connexin expression in cardiomyopathies. Adv. Cardiol. 42: 228–242, 2006.

Shi, W., R. Wymore, H. Yu, J. Wu, R.T. Wymore, Z. Pan, R.B. Robinson, J.E. Dixon, , D. McKinnon, and I.S. Cohen. Distribution and prevalence of hyperpolarization-activated cation channel HCN0 mRNA expression in cardiac tissues. Circ. Res. 85: E1–E6, 1999.

Simpson, I., B. Rose, and W.R. Loewenstein. Size limit of molecules permeating the junctional membrane channels. Science. 195: 294–296, 1977.

Singh, O.V., N. Vij, P.J., Mogayzel, Jr., C. Jozwik, H.B. Pollard, and P.L. Zeitlin. Pharmacoproteomics of 4-phenylbutyrate-treated IB3–1 cystic fibrosis bronchial. J. Proteome Res. 5(3): 562–571, 2006.

Valiunas, V., E.C. Beyer, and P.R. Brink. Gap junction channels show a quantitative difference in selectivity. Circ. Res. 91(2):104–111, 2002.

Valiunas, R., S. Doronin, L. Valiuniene, I. Potapova, J. Zuckerman, B. Walcott, R.B. Robinson, M.R. Rosen, P.R. Brink, and I.S. Cohen. Human mesenchymal stem cells make cardiac connexins and form functional gap junctions. J. Physiol: 555: 617–626, 2004.

Valiunas, V., G. Kanaporis, L. Valiuniene, C. Gordon, H. Wang, L. Li, R.B. Robinson, M.R. Rosen, I.S. Cohen, and P.R. Brink. Coupling an HCN2 expressing cell to a myocyte creates a two cell pacing unit. J. Physiol. 587: 5211–5226, 2009.

Valiunas, V., Y. Polosina, H. Miller, I. Potapova, L. Valiuniene, S. Doronin, R.T. Mathias, R.B. Robinson, M.R. Rosen, I.S. Cohen, and P.R. Brink. Connexin-specific cell-to-cell transfer of short interfering RNA by gap junctions. J. Physiol. 568: 459–468, 2005.

VanSlyke, J.K. and L.S. Musil. Cytosolic stress reduces degradation of connexin43 internalized from the cell surface and enhances gap junction formation and function. Mol. Biol. Cell. 16: 5247–5257, 2005.

Van Veen, T.A.B., H.W.M. van Rijen, and T. Opthof. Cardiac gap junction channels: modulation of expression and channel properties. Cardiovasc. Res. 51: 217–229, 2001.

Wei, C.J., R. Francis, X. Xu, and C.W. Lo. Connexin43 associated with an N-cadherin-containing multiprotein complex is required for gap junction formation in NIH3T3 cells. J. Biol. Chem. 280(20): 19925–19936, 2005.

Weidman, S. Electrical constants of trabecular muscle from mammalian heart. J. Physiol. 210: 1041–1054, 1970.

Wilders, R., E.E. Verheijck, R. Kumar, W.N. Goolsby, A.C. van Ginneken, R.W. Joyner, and H.J. Jongsma. Model clamp and its application to synchronization of rabbit sinoatrial node cells. Am. J. Physiol. 271: H2168–H2182, 1996.

White, T.W., M. Srinivas, H. Ripps, A. Trovato-Salinaro, D.F. Condorelli, and R. Bruzzone. Virtual cloning, functional expression, and gating analysis of human Connexin31.9. Am. J. Physiol. Cell Physiol. 283(3): C960–C967, 2002.

Wirth, B., L. Brichta, and E. Hahnen. Spinal muscular atrophy: from gene to therapy. Semin. Pediatr. Neurol. 13(2): 121–131, 2006.

Yu, H., F., Chang, and I.S. Cohen. Pacemaker current exists in ventricular myocytes. Circ. Res. 72: 323–336, 1993.

12

Regenerative Cardiac Pharmacology: Translating Stem Cell Biology into Therapeutic Solutions

ATTA BEHFAR AND ANDRE TERZIC

Introduction

Heart Disease: An Epidemic

Ischemic heart disease accounts for 20 million of global deaths annually.[1] Advanced ischemic cardiomyopathy manifests as an overt congestive heart failure syndrome, the largest cause of repeat hospitalizations and mortality in the developed world. At present, more than 5 million Americans and 20 million patients worldwide have heart failure with 550,000 new cases recorded each year in the United States alone.[2] Symptomatic heart failure has a poor prognosis and carries a 5-year mortality rate exceeding 50 percent. Despite aggressive medical management and increased access to interventional therapies, the malignant nature of heart failure imposes an annual cost of more than $80 billion in the United States, warranting new therapeutic solutions.[3]

Revascularization at the time of infarction has reduced acute mortality but has paradoxically caused an epidemic of chronic heart failure because of massive myocardial damage in the surviving patient population.[4] Current clinical management is focused at symptomatic palliation yet lacks the capacity to salvage the infarcted myocardium. Life-extending measures – such as left ventricular assist devices or organ replacement – are ultimately the only therapeutic options.[5] However, only a limited number of patients can benefit from such complex interventions. Accordingly, there is a large and immediate need for the development and implementation of effective repair strategies accessible to a broad patient population.

The Stem Cell Paradigm

The stem cell regenerative paradigm challenges the notion of the heart as an organ incapable of repair.[6,7] In male recipients of female donor hearts, myocardial tissue harbors Y chromosome–positive cells, indicating that circulating progenitors have cardiac homing capacity.[8] In fact, quantitative monitoring of innate cardiomyogenesis has recently established a significant growth reserve of the adult human heart capable of replacing myocyte and nonmyocyte compartments during lifespan.[9,10] Although the process of rejuvenation may be sufficient to respond to homeostatic demand, in the context of severe destruction associated with ischemic injury, the endogenous regenerative potential is largely insufficient to rescue the progressively deteriorating failing heart.[11] This limitation mandates alternative approaches that would boost the innate repair capacity.

The recognition that stem cells can differentiate into specified cell phenotypes that produce beneficial outcome when transplanted into diseased heart, often beyond that achieved with current standards of care, has introduced a novel paradigm in cardiovascular pharmacology.[12–15] Initially hypothesized to directly replace nonviable myocardium through de novo cardiogenesis, evaluation of stem cell–based regeneration has implicated a therapeutic mode of action that cannot be explained by direct replacement alone.[16,17] Accordingly, recent iterations of the regenerative pharmacology paradigm move beyond the notion that transplanted cells serve per se as myocardial building blocks to a model that imposes, at the molecular level, a repair process within the myocardial microenvironment. Such indirect stem cell–driven paracrine signaling could modulate inflammation, ischemic tolerance, endogenous healing, and inotropy to promote regeneration. To this end, repair models have been amended to include augmentation of endogenous capacity for neoangiogenesis, myocardial cytoprotection, and activation of reparative resident cardiac stem cells as potential mechanisms of stem cell benefit (Fig. 12-1).[6,12,18–21]

Initial Clinical Experience

To date, more than 3,000 patients have been enrolled and treated in clinical trials evaluating adult stem cell therapy in heart disease.[22,23] Initial studies with skeletal muscle–derived myoblasts and circulating progenitor cells have progressed to the use of bone marrow–derived stem cells tested in patients presenting with acute myocardial infarction or heart failure in the setting of ischemic heart disease.[24–26] Collectively, these studies indicate that stem cell transplantation is associated with limited benefit on function. However, evidence implies induction of cardioprotective and vasculogenic factors as potential mechanisms of repair.[27,28] Paracrine secretion, transdifferentiation or myocardial fusion, along with activation of the cardiac stem cell niche are proposed as regenerative components working in concert to achieve augmentation of cardiomyocyte content after stem cell transplantation.[29] It is still uncertain, however, whether implanted stem cells reliably contribute to long-term regeneration because clinical trials show various degrees of efficacy on follow-up.[17,30] Although cell-based therapies have in principle demonstrated safety and feasibility, meta-analyses have yielded rather modest signals of improved cardiac performance.[31] Variability noted between trials and within patient-treated populations has resulted in concerns

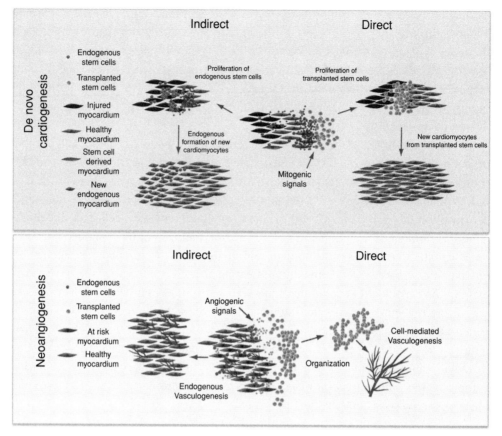

Figure 12-1. Mechanisms underlying de novo cardiogenesis and neoangiogenesis. Direct influence denotes regeneration of target organ following stem cell differentiation and engraftment. Indirect indicates a reparative paracrine influence of transplanted stem cells on resident stem cells. (See color plate 27.)

for potential of divergent outcome after cell delivery with unpredictable efficacy on follow-up.[30]

To ensure translational benefit, there has been a call for strategies that would enhance the cellular repair capacity. Here, two most recent approaches implemented from preclinical proof-of-principle to clinical trials are highlighted as novel therapeutic paradigms. The first uses the myocardium as the tissue source to recruit progenitor cells, and the second induces lineage specification of adult stem cells through exposure to natural cardiogenic cues to uniformly recruit cardiogenic progenitors for enhanced outcome.

En Route to Translation

With demonstrated safety and feasibility of stem cell–based therapy and initial delineation of putative modes of action, current emphasis is placed on optimizing regenerative cell-based products for cardiovascular applications. Beyond the establishment of proof of principle and validation through preclinical testing, realization of first-in-human studies leading to pivotal clinical trials of next-generation products mandates robust scale-up and quality control to ensure proper culture, cryostorage, transport, and cell handling before optimal delivery.[32]

Scale-Up Production

Stem cell production scaled up to yield a clinically viable biologic requires utilization of a fixed and humanized process aligned with the standards imposed by good manufacturing practice (GMP) guidelines.[33] To date, fetal bovine serum (FBS) has been used as the standard adjuvant in clinical derivation.[34] Although the risk of zoonoses associated with FBS culture is small, scrutiny in stem cell banks for prions and zoonotic pathogens remains high.[35,36] In fact, recent reports have raised the concern for potential immunogenic reactions at the time of transplantation caused by xenogenic proteins transmitted from FBS.[37] Specific cases have documented the risk for anaphylactoid response, with reported diffuse urticaria and production of antibodies against FBS proteins after repeated stem cell treatment cycles.[37–40] In addition, lot-to-lot variability seen with FBS use creates an inherent heterogeneity in the derivation and propagation of stem cell products. As such, the use of FBS may impede adherence to regulatory requirements, hampering development of clinically applicable cell-based products.[34,41] Accordingly, to ensure pathogen-free generation of master cell banks devoid of growth and phenotype variability and to address the potential immune response to bovine protein after repeat therapy, humanization of clinical-grade cultures has come into focus.[35,37–40,42–46]

To this end, testing of humanized substitutes allowing expedited therapeutic translation is increasingly considered.[34,41,47,48] Such substitutes should mimic naturally occurring microenvironments to optimally support stem cell proliferation while maintaining cellular phenotype, multipotency, and chromosomal stability. Platelets provide a unique opportunity for stem cell culture because they naturally contain intracellular granules abundant in potent reparative and mitogenic substances.[49] At the time of tissue injury, platelet-derived bioactive factors are released into the clot and influence tissue regeneration by triggering stromal cell proliferation, migration, and differentiation. Moreover, stem cell proliferation and chemotaxis in tissue restoration are a direct response to signals after injury.[50] Compared with standard FBS, GMP-adherent pooled human platelet lysate (GMP-hPL) provides an adjuvant for accelerated expansion, maintenance of phenotype stability, and absence of clonal chromosomal aberrancy in adult stem cell cultures. Proteomic dissection of this nonzoonotic milieu has recently resolved signals that clustered within nonstochastic pathways of tissue repair and cell proliferation, identifying the molecular substrate underlying human platelet lysate support of efficient and safe adult stem cell procurement (Fig. 12.2).

HARVEST PURIFICATION & SCALE-UP PACKAGING & TRANSPLANTATION

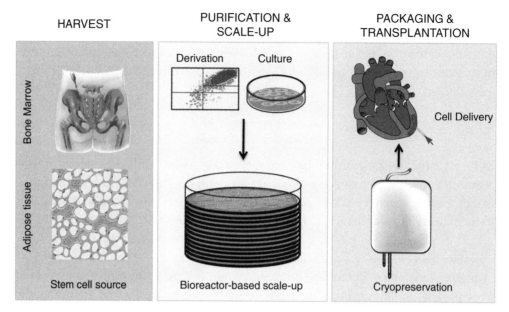

Figure 12-2. Critical steps in clinical application of stem cell therapy. GMP-grade manufacturing of cell biotherapeutics involves a three-step approach: (1) harvest of stem cells from sources such as adipose tissue and bone marrow; (2) derivation, purification, and scale-up of the stem cell product; and (3) packaging, storage (e.g. cryopreservation), and delivery into the diseased organ. (See color plate 28.)

Quality Control

Beyond scale-up production, consensus with regard to tissue source and harvest, industrialization of derivation, clinical-grade culture, packaging, and transport continues to be a focus for optimization.[29] Furthermore, to date, cells have been transplanted without a robust correlation between cellular phenotype and reparative action requiring the establishment of adequate biomarkers to predict outcome.[12,51,52] Cell-based medicinal products involve cell samples of limited amounts, mostly to be used in a patient-specific manner. This raises specific issues pertaining to quality-control testing designed for each product under examination. The manufacture of cell-based medicinal products is carefully designed and validated to ensure product consistency and traceability. Control and management of manufacturing and quality-control testing are carried out according to GMP requirements. Screens for purity, potency, infectious contamination, and karyotype stability have become necessary elements (i.e., release criteria) in compliance with standard operating practices for production and banking of cells. Accordingly, the U.S. Food and Drug Administration and the European Medicine Agency impose regulatory guidelines for risk assessment, quality of manufacturing, preclinical and clinical development, and postmarketing surveillance of stem cell biologics for translation from bench to bedside to populations. Such adherence allows prospective evaluation of clinical trial outcomes and provides an approach to identify process-based or phenotypic criteria that ultimately correspond to repair.[33,53]

Modes of Delivery

Efficient delivery and bioavailability of stem cell biologics are necessary to achieve or assess therapeutic benefit. To date, this pivotal issue remains one of the most complex components of translation because no approved method currently exists to either deliver stem cells to the myocardium or track cell homing after transplantation.[54] Four routes are commonly considered: peripheral intravenous (IV) injection, percutaneous intracoronary delivery, percutaneous endocardial transplantation, and epicardial injection during cardiothoracic surgery.[55]

Peripheral IV delivery provides the smallest degree of myocardial homing and would be applicable if the mode of action solely relied on paracrine secretion into the circulation. Although limited in efficiency, if optimized, this approach would be an attractive option because of the broad applicability in clinical practice. Recent preclinical studies have provided proof of concept by demonstrating benefit without need for homing because of the bioavailability of secreted anti-inflammatory proteins from the peripheral circulation.[56] Alternatively, intracoronary delivery is limited to facilities with a track record of catheter-based interventions and has been used by most of the clinical trials.[57–61] Endocardial transplantation has been used in the treatment of subacute to chronic postinfarction settings,[62–64] with execution of this approach limited to centers of excellence capable of coupling cell transplantation with advanced imaging techniques to guide site-specific delivery of stem cells.[65,66] Epicardial transplantation is limited to individuals who have a primary indication for heart surgery. Because different delivery techniques are applicable to certain clinical conditions, mode of action, and stem cell of interest, the specific patient population will likely dictate the method of transplantation that is utilized.

Cardiac Stem Cells

Traditionally, the heart was considered a postmitotic organ composed of a predetermined number of myocytes established at birth.[67] However, significant strides have been made in the identification, isolation, and evaluation of progenitor cells residing within the myocardium. Unlike extracardiac stem cells isolated from tissues such as bone marrow or adipose tissue, stem cells intrinsic to the heart itself mediate cardiogenesis and angiogenesis via direct and indirect mechanisms.[68] Resident cardiac stem cells demonstrate multipotency both in vitro and in vivo through differentiation into cardiomyocytes, vascular smooth muscle, and endothelial cells. Recognition that

Cardiopoiesis *versus*
Resident progenitors

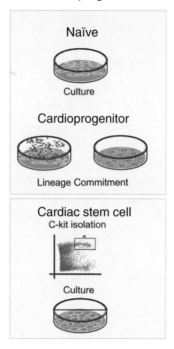

Figure 12-3. Organ specific stem cells: A new paradigm in regeneration. Organ specification can be achieved either by ex vivo conditioning of patient-derived stem cells,
or derivation and purification of cells from the organ of interest. (See color plate 29.)

cardiac stem cells can, within the heart, germinate into mature cardiovascular lineages
provides evidence that the myocardium is self-renewing.[6,69] Resident stem cell pools,
stored in niches, control the cardiac cell turnover and contribute to the replenishment
of old or dying cells within the myocardium. Delineation of resident cardiac stem cell
function in health and disease is an important line of investigation with the prospect
of delineating molecular targets for prevention of or protection from ischemic cardiomyopathy along with measures that could ultimately be used in clinical practice
(Fig. 12.3).[70]

Cell Phenotype and Isolation

Cardiac stem cells isolated from the myocardium have created significant interest
as a potential source for regenerative stem cell products. For the human heart, C-
kit–positive populations are successfully isolated from the adult myocardium with a
demonstrated capacity for myocardial transdifferentiation.[69,71] C-kit or CD117 is a
cytokine receptor that binds stem cell factor, a stem cell–specific mitogenic agent.
Islet-1 (Isl-1) is an additional marker identified in embryonic and neonatal hearts as

having the capacity for ex vivo cardiogenesis, but their isolation from adult hearts has yet to be shown.[72,73]

Two distinct methods have been used to isolate resident cardiac stem cells. The first approach digests the myocardium with protracted in vitro culture of derived cardiac fibroblasts and yields recruitment of the cardiac stem cell population within cardiospheres. These spherical structures contain resident cardiac progenitors, including C-kit[+] cells whose growth in clusters is thought to be required, serving as a niche for maintenance of "stemness."[69,74,75] The second method digests the myocardium to derive a mononuclear phase, and from this phase, C-kit[+] cells are sorted out using an antibody-based technique such as flow assisted cell sorting (FACS). When isolated in this fashion, cardiac stem cells have the capacity to proliferate as a monolayer yielding, unlike the cell cluster approach, a homogeneous population of cardiac stem cells.

Clinical Translation

Clinical evaluation of resident cardiac stem cells is currently underway in the CADUCEUS (CArdiosphere-Derived aUtologous stem CElls to reverse ventricUlar dysfunction) and SCIPIO (Cardiac Stem Cell Infusion in Patients With Ischemic CardiOmyopathy) trials.[21,76–78] Whereas the CADUCEUS study uses the cell cluster or cardiosphere approach for derivation and propagation, the SCIPO trial implements an antibody-based method to derive a homogenous C-kit[+] population. CADUCEUS focuses on individuals with either acute myocardial infarction or chronic ischemic cardiomyopathy, with harvest of the patient's own myocardial tissue to yield an autologous therapeutic delivered via coronary arteries. The SCIPIO study uses right atrial tissue obtained during coronary artery bypass grafting for autologous intracoronary transplantation of derived C-kit[+] human cardiac stem cells. Both studies are first-in-human trials powered to assess safety and feasibility.

Engineering Lineage Specification

Because adult stem cells can achieve lineage specification in vivo, it has been postulated that highly plastic cells, such as mesenchymal stem cells (MSCs), could be guided toward a similar fate ex vivo.[79,80] This notion is supported by early evidence of adult stem cell multipotency with demonstration that MSCs demonstrate multilineage specification.[81,82] With progress in identification of molecular pathways guiding embryonic stem cells toward the cardiac fate,[83,84] the possibility of engineering lineage-specified adult stem cells has recently come into view. Indeed, adult cardiogenic priming could be achieved if natural cues deciphered within the developing embryonic heart could be translated into a signaling paradigm capable of stimulating naïve stem cells to exogenously guide them toward a cardiac fate.[85,86]

Lineage Commitment of Embryonic Stem Cells

Stem cell commitment to the cardiac program is here termed *guided cardiopoiesis*, in which mimicry of natural cardiogenic signaling results in the generation of a cardiac progenitor population.[87] The molecular underpinnings of this process have been identified by genomic and proteomic characterization of natural cardioinductive signals, leading to the establishment of a recombinant approach to achieve "cardiopoietic guidance."[85] In addition to signaling molecules, this approach exploits synergism between growth and trophic factors to replicate the impact of the endodermal secretome to hone the unguided plasticity of pluripotent stem cells toward a specific myocardial pathway, nullifying the propensity for uncontrolled growth.[84,88,89]

Guided Cardiopoiesis in Adult Stem Cells

In contrast to embryonic stem cells, adult stem cells, particularly those harvested from patients, are sequestered in a state of plasticity, limiting their capacity for lineage specification.[90,91] Because of significant experience with its clinical use and characterization, the bone marrow is considered the archetypal adult stem cell source, containing different cell populations that have the potential to migrate and transdifferentiate into cells of diverse phenotypes.[82,92,93] However, until recently, the capacity of such stem cells to fully engage into the cardiac program remained uncertain.[73] The mononuclear phase of bone marrow consists of three major stem cell subsets: hematopoietic stem cells (HSCs), endothelial progenitors, and MSCs, which function in maintenance of tissue homeostasis and home during tissue injury aiding endogenous mechanisms of repair.[94] Such subpopulations are typically stratified through surface marker expression allowing isolation directly after marrow aspiration or recruitment from the peripheral circulation.[53,87,95]

The process of "guided lineage specification" was initially demonstrated on healthy donor adult stem cells, providing evidence for an in vitro capacity for cardiac commitment. Induction of lineage specification was demonstrated in bone marrow–derived MSCs exogenously subjected to endodermal signals deciphered during cardiogenesis.[90] In addition, a boost in cardiogenic potential was documented after co-culture of MSCs with neonatal cardiomyocytes.[96] These initial approaches, however, were found insufficient to guide patient-derived stem cells toward the cardiac fate because these cells were found latent, sequestered in a state of plasticity. To drive stem cells, derived from a morbid source, to the cardiogenic fate full humanization of the endodermal signaling paradigm that successfully guided embryonic lineage specification was needed.[97] Subjecting patient-derived stem cells to such a "boot camp" achieved full engagement toward a cardiac program, engineering a phenotype with regained repair aptitude.[68,96] With such stimulation before transplantation, the significant benefit variability noted with autologous transplantation of adult stem cells[30] is diminished with delivery of a uniformly primed population.[85,90,98,99]

Clinical Translation

Preclinical testing of growth factor–guided cardiopoietic specification of human bone marrow MSCs has documented reparative uniformity. Based on these findings, the C-CURE clinical trial was designed to assess the feasibility and safety of autologous cardiopoietic (CP) MSC therapy in ischemic heart failure. This is a first-in-human study assessing lineage-specified stem cells for cardiac repair in ischemic cardiomyopathy. Inclusion criteria included moderate to severe heart failure (New York Heart Association class II to III) with a left ventricular ejection fraction between 15 and 40 percent. Interim analysis has shown a favorable safety profile with no increase in the number of adverse clinical events, including ventricular dysrhythmia, compared with the control cohort. Ongoing analysis will determine efficacy signals and suitability for larger pivotal clinical trials.

Summary

Treatment of patients with stem cells has revealed fundamental challenges in the ex vivo procurement and release of derived products along with their packaging and delivery. In addition, variable outcome seen within treated patient populations has resulted in a need to uniformly augment therapeutic efficacy before transplantation. Subpopulations of stem cells are likely to be innately primed for cardiogenesis but insufficient in quantity to fully drive repair.[22,29] It is thus necessary to either derive endogenously prespecified or to exogenously guide patient-derived stem cells toward a cardiac fate.[98,100] In addition, optimization and standardized release of cellular harvest, procurement, and release are necessary to guarantee the highest level of quality in the translation from bench to bedside.[32]

Current State of the Art in Stem Cell–Based Myocardial Repair

Stem cell–based therapeutics for the injured heart have significantly advanced since the inaugural transplantation efforts with myoblasts and unfractionated blood or bone marrow mononuclear cells. With development of tools to aid successful delivery along with advance in dissection of mechanisms driving stem cell–based repair, regenerative medicine is poised to transit from proof of principle toward clinical validation. However, challenges, including a lack of consensus on cellular production, storage, and identity (which cell to use and what cell is really being transplanted); the site and method of delivery; the efficacy of autologous "sick patient"–derived stem cells versus allogeneic "healthy donor" cells; the mechanism and duration of benefit; the need for adjuvant growth factors; and the timing of delivery provide a formidable challenge that needs to be systematically addressed.[18]

Preclinical trials have established that adult stem cells, when recruited from young and healthy donors, have a strong capacity for repair. However, it is the patient population that is of interest clinically. Clinical trial evaluation of autologously derived and transplanted stem cells in this patient population has resulted in marginal benefit, significantly lower than predicted in preclinical trials.[29–31] High-throughput evaluation of adult stem cells demonstrating in vivo efficacy versus those that do not has been shown to allow identification of pathways to preemptively maximize cell capacity for repair during the time of harvest and expansion ex vivo before transplantation.[52,87,90,97,101] Such approaches are shown to guide naïve "first generation" stem cells to achieve a specific therapeutic objective within the organ of interest.[90,97]

Next Generation of Regenerative Therapy

To date, two methods have emerged in the derivation of lineage-specified adult stem cells to enhance repair of the injured heart. With identification resident C-kit$^+$ cardiac stem cells, the myocardium used as a reliable source for cell harvest. Furthermore, multipotent MSCs recruited from adipose or bone marrow tissue can be exogenously guided toward the cardiac fate to maximize repair efficacy. First-in-human safety and feasibility evaluation for these next generation stem cell therapeutics has been completed for lineage-specified stem cells (C-CURE clinical trial) or are under way for cardiac stem cells (SCIPIO and CADUCEUS). Such efforts to translate lineage-specified stem cells along with studies to clarify duration and mechanism of benefit and implications of repeat therapy mark the beginning of the second generation of stem cell therapeutics reduced to practice.

Induced pluripotency goes one step beyond multipotent stem cells by allowing reprogramming of somatic cells derived from an individual patient.[102–104] Novel iterations of the reprogramming paradigm have now been exercised to achieve successful lineage specification without the initial requirement of induced pluripotency.[105] As this principle has currently been demonstrated in nonhuman cell sources, further dissection and understanding of the molecular and signaling complexity that lay at the foundation of lineage commitment will pave the path toward translation to human samples.[106]

Thus, the challenge of translating cell-based therapeutics to practice has been increasingly answered with demonstrated clinical feasibility and safety for stem cell therapeutics now established in cardiovascular medicine.[107–111] Whether it is the cellular secretome that exerts a benefit or direct incorporation and function within the damaged heart, stem cell–based repair for the heart has now been independently documented across clinical trials.[29] Perhaps the best predictor of the road ahead is the one seen with heart transplantation. This effort began with Norman Shumway in 1958[112] with the first successful attempt a decade later in 1967 by Christiaan Barnard. However, broad clinical use was only seen in the 1980s after a multidisciplinary effort between clinicians and scientists yielded regimens to effectively suppress immunity. Early adoption of stem cell clinical translation has been criticized as premature.

However, the brisk pace of medical and scientific advance along with intimate inter-disciplinary collaborations will provide the foundation for success to bring the next generation of biologics, addressing the root cause of heart failure.

References

1. Gersh BJ, Sliwa K, Mayosi BM, Yusuf S. Novel therapeutic concepts: the epidemic of cardiovascular disease in the developing world: global implications. *Eur Heart J* 2010;31(6):642–8.
2. Lloyd-Jones D, Adams RJ, Brown TM, Carnethon M, Dai S, De Simone G, et al. Heart disease and stroke statistics–2010 update: a report from the American Heart Association. *Circulation* 2010;121(7):e46–e215.
3. Lloyd-Jones DM, Hong Y, Labarthe D, Mozaffarian D, Appel LJ, Van Horn L, et al. Defining and setting national goals for cardiovascular health promotion and disease reduction: the American Heart Association's strategic Impact Goal through 2020 and beyond. *Circulation* 2010;121(4):586–613.
4. Setoguchi S, Glynn RJ, Avorn J, Mittleman MA, Levin R, Winkelmayer WC. Improvements in long-term mortality after myocardial infarction and increased use of cardiovascular drugs after discharge: a 10-year trend analysis. *J Am Coll Cardiol* 2008;51(13):1247–54.
5. McMurray JJ. Clinical practice. Systolic heart failure. *N Engl J Med* 2010;362(3):228–38.
6. Beltrami AP, Barlucchi L, Torella D, Baker M, Limana F, Chimenti S, et al. Adult cardiac stem cells are multipotent and support myocardial regeneration. *Cell* 2003;114(6):763–76.
7. Hsieh PC, Segers VF, Davis ME, MacGillivray C, Gannon J, Molkentin JD, et al. Evidence from a genetic fate-mapping study that stem cells refresh adult mammalian cardiomyocytes after injury. *Nat Med* 2007;13(8):970–4.
8. Quaini F, Urbanek K, Beltrami AP, Finato N, Beltrami CA, Nadal-Ginard B, et al. Chimerism of the transplanted heart. *N Engl J Med* 2002;346(1):5–15.
9. Bergmann O, Bhardwaj RD, Bernard S, Zdunek S, Barnabe-Heider F, Walsh S, et al. Evidence for cardiomyocyte renewal in humans. *Science* 2009;324(5923):98–102.
10. Kajstura J, Urbanek K, Perl S, Hosoda T, Zheng H, Ogorek B, et al. Cardiomyogenesis in the adult human heart. *Circ Res* 2010;107(2):305–15.
11. Nelson TJ, Behfar A, Terzic A. Strategies for therapeutic repair: the "R(3)" regenerative medicine paradigm. *Clin Transl Sci* 2008;1(2):168–71.
12. Dimmeler S, Zeiher AM, Schneider MD. Unchain my heart: the scientific foundations of cardiac repair. *J Clin Invest* 2005;115(3):572–83.
13. Srivastava D, Ivey KN. Potential of stem-cell-based therapies for heart disease. *Nature* 2006;441(7097):1097–9.
14. Hansson EM, Lindsay ME, Chien KR. Regeneration next: toward heart stem cell therapeutics. *Cell Stem Cell* 2009;5(4):364–77.
15. Bartunek J, Vanderheyden M, Hill J, Terzic A. Cells as biologics for cardiac repair in ischaemic heart failure. *Heart* 2010;96(10):792–800.
16. Chien KR, Domian IJ, Parker KK. Cardiogenesis and the complex biology of regenerative cardiovascular medicine. *Science* 2008;322(5907):1494–7.
17. Tendera M, Wojakowski W. Cell therapy – success does not come easy. *Eur Heart J* 2009;30(6):640–1.
18. Forrester JS, White AJ, Matsushita S, Chakravarty T, Makkar RR. New paradigms of myocardial regeneration post-infarction: tissue preservation, cell environment, and pluripotent cell sources. *JACC Cardiovasc Interv* 2009;2(1):1–8.

19. Gnecchi M, He H, Liang OD, Melo LG, Morello F, Mu H, et al. Paracrine action accounts for marked protection of ischemic heart by Akt-modified mesenchymal stem cells. *Nat Med* 2005;11(4):367–8.

20. Passier R, van Laake LW, Mummery CL. Stem-cell-based therapy and lessons from the heart. *Nature* 2008;453(7193):322–9.

21. Johnston PV, Sasano T, Mills K, Evers R, Lee ST, Smith RR, et al. Engraftment, differentiation, and functional benefits of autologous cardiosphere-derived cells in porcine ischemic cardiomyopathy. *Circulation* 2009;120(12):1075–83, 7 p following 83.

22. Behfar A, Crespo-Diaz R, Nelson TJ, Terzic A, Gersh BJ. Stem cells: clinical trials results the end of the beginning or the beginning of the end? *Cardiovasc Hematol Disord Drug Targets.* 2010;10(3):186–201.

23. Wollert KC, Drexler H. Cell therapy for the treatment of coronary heart disease: a critical appraisal. *Nat Rev Cardiol* 2010;7(4):204–15.

24. Dib N, Dinsmore J, Lababidi Z, White B, Moravec S, Campbell A, et al. One-year follow-up of feasibility and safety of the first U.S., randomized, controlled study using 3-dimensional guided Catheter-based Delivery of Autologous Skeletal Myoblasts for Ischemic Cardiomyopathy (CAuSMIC study). *JACC Cardiovasc Interv* 2009;2(1): 9–16.

25. Dib N, McCarthy P, Campbell A, Yeager M, Pagani FD, Wright S, et al. Feasibility and safety of autologous myoblast transplantation in patients with ischemic cardiomyopathy. *Cell Transplant* 2005;14(1):11–9.

26. Menasche P, Alfieri O, Janssens S, McKenna W, Reichenspurner H, Trinquart L, et al. The Myoblast Autologous Grafting in Ischemic Cardiomyopathy (MAGIC) trial: first randomized placebo-controlled study of myoblast transplantation. *Circulation* 2008;117(9):1189–200.

27. Schuleri KH, Feigenbaum GS, Centola M, Weiss ES, Zimmet JM, Turney J, et al. Autologous mesenchymal stem cells produce reverse remodelling in chronic ischaemic cardiomyopathy. *Eur Heart J* 2009;30(22):2722–32.

28. Jiang M, He B, Zhang Q, Ge H, Zang MH, Han ZH, et al. Randomized controlled trials on the therapeutic effects of adult progenitor cells for myocardial infarction: meta-analysis. *Expert Opin Biol Ther* 2010;10(5):667–80.

29. Gersh BJ, Simari RD, Behfar A, Terzic CM, Terzic A. Cardiac cell repair therapy: a clinical perspective. *Mayo Clin Proc* 2009;84(10):876–92.

30. Rosenzweig A. Cardiac cell therapy – mixed results from mixed cells. *N Engl J Med* 2006;355(12):1274–7.

31. Abdel-Latif A, Bolli R, Tleyjeh IM, Montori VM, Perin EC, Hornung CA, et al. Adult bone marrow-derived cells for cardiac repair: a systematic review and meta-analysis. *Arch Intern Med* 2007;167(10):989–97.

32. Seeger FH, Tonn T, Krzossok N, Zeiher AM, Dimmeler S. Cell isolation procedures matter: a comparison of different isolation protocols of bone marrow mononuclear cells used for cell therapy in patients with acute myocardial infarction. *Eur Heart J* 2007;28(6):766–72.

33. Dietz AB, Padley DJ, Gastineau DA. Infrastructure development for human cell therapy translation. *Clin Pharmacol Ther* 2007;82(3):320–4.

34. Bieback K, Hecker A, Kocaomer A, Lannert H, Schallmoser K, Strunk D, et al. Human alternatives to fetal bovine serum for the expansion of mesenchymal stromal cells from bone marrow. *Stem Cells (Dayton, Ohio)* 2009;27(9):2331–41.

35. Doerr HW, Cinatl J, Sturmer M, Rabenau HF. Prions and orthopedic surgery. *Infection* 2003;31(3):163–71.

36. Cobo F, Talavera P, Concha A. Diagnostic approaches for viruses and prions in stem cell banks. *Virology* 2006;347(1):1–10.

37. Spees JL, Gregory CA, Singh H, Tucker HA, Peister A, Lynch PJ, et al. Internalized antigens must be removed to prepare hypoimmunogenic mesenchymal stem cells for cell and gene therapy. *Mol Ther* 2004;9(5):747–56.

38. Horwitz EM, Gordon PL, Koo WK, Marx JC, Neel MD, McNall RY, et al. Isolated allogeneic bone marrow-derived mesenchymal cells engraft and stimulate growth in children with osteogenesis imperfecta: implications for cell therapy of bone. *Proc Nat Acad Sci U S A* 2002;99(13):8932–7.

39. Selvaggi TA, Walker RE, Fleisher TA. Development of antibodies to fetal calf serum with arthus-like reactions in human immunodeficiency virus-infected patients given syngeneic lymphocyte infusions. *Blood* 1997;89(3):776–9.

40. Gregory CA, Reyes E, Whitney MJ, Spees JL. Enhanced engraftment of mesenchymal stem cells in a cutaneous wound model by culture in allogenic species-specific serum and administration in fibrin constructs. *Stem Cells (Dayton, Ohio)* 2006;24(10): 2232–43.

41. Mannello F, Tonti GA. Concise review: no breakthroughs for human mesenchymal and embryonic stem cell culture: conditioned medium, feeder layer, or feeder-free; medium with fetal calf serum, human serum, or enriched plasma; serum-free, serum replacement nonconditioned medium, or ad hoc formula? All that glitters is not gold! *Stem Cells (Dayton, Ohio)* 2007;25(7):1603–9.

42. Cobo F, Cabrera C, Catalina P, Concha A. General safety guidances in stem cell bank installations. *Cytotherapy* 2006;8(1):47–56.

43. Cobo F, Concha A. Application of microarray technology for microbial diagnosis in stem cell cultures: a review. *Cytotherapy* 2007;9(1):53–9.

44. Mackensen A, Drager R, Schlesier M, Mertelsmann R, Lindemann A. Presence of IgE antibodies to bovine serum albumin in a patient developing anaphylaxis after vaccination with human peptide-pulsed dendritic cells. *Cancer Immunol Immunother* 2000;49(3):152–6.

45. Muul LM, Tuschong LM, Soenen SL, Jagadeesh GJ, Ramsey WJ, Long Z, et al. Persistence and expression of the adenosine deaminase gene for 12 years and immune reaction to gene transfer components: long-term results of the first clinical gene therapy trial. *Blood* 2003;101(7):2563–9.

46. Tuschong L, Soenen SL, Blaese RM, Candotti F, Muul LM. Immune response to fetal calf serum by two adenosine deaminase-deficient patients after T cell gene therapy. *Hum Gene Ther* 2002;13(13):1605–10.

47. Reinisch A, Hofmann NA, Obenauf AC, Kashofer K, Rohde E, Schallmoser K, et al. Humanized large-scale expanded endothelial colony-forming cells function in vitro and in vivo. *Blood* 2009;113(26):6716–25.

48. Shahdadfar A, Fronsdal K, Haug T, Reinholt FP, Brinchmann JE. In vitro expansion of human mesenchymal stem cells: choice of serum is a determinant of cell proliferation, differentiation, gene expression, and transcriptome stability. *Stem Cells* 2005;23(9):1357–66.

49. Martin P. Wound healing–aiming for perfect skin regeneration. *Science* 1997;276(5309):75–81.

50. Wu Y, Chen L, Scott PG, Tredget EE. Mesenchymal stem cells enhance wound healing through differentiation and angiogenesis. *Stem Cells* 2007;25(10):2648–59.

51. Welt FG, Losordo DW. Cell therapy for acute myocardial infarction: curb your enthusiasm? *Circulation* 2006;113(10):1272–4.

52. Dimmeler S, Zeiher AM. Cell therapy of acute myocardial infarction: open questions. *Cardiology* 2008;113(3):155–60.

53. Sotiropoulou PA, Perez SA, Salagianni M, Baxevanis CN, Papamichail M. Characterization of the optimal culture conditions for clinical scale production of human mesenchymal stem cells. *Stem Cells* 2006;24(2):462–71.

54. Perin EC, Lopez J. Methods of stem cell delivery in cardiac diseases. *Nat Clin Pract Cardiovasc Med* 2006;3 Suppl 1:S110–3.

55. Bartunek J, Sherman W, Vanderheyden M, Fernandez-Aviles F, Wijns W, Terzic A. Delivery of biologics in cardiovascular regenerative medicine. *Clin Pharmacol Ther* 2009;85(5):548–52.

56. Lee RH, Pulin AA, Seo MJ, Kota DJ, Ylostalo J, Larson BL, et al. Intravenous hMSCs improve myocardial infarction in mice because cells embolized in lung are activated to secrete the anti-inflammatory protein TSG-6. *Cell Stem Cell* 2009;5(1):54–63.

57. Janssens S, Dubois C, Bogaert J, Theunissen K, Deroose C, Desmet W, et al. Autologous bone marrow-derived stem-cell transfer in patients with ST-segment elevation myocardial infarction: double-blind, randomised controlled trial. *Lancet* 2006;367(9505):113–21.

58. Schachinger V, Assmus B, Britten MB, Honold J, Lehmann R, Teupe C, et al. Transplantation of progenitor cells and regeneration enhancement in acute myocardial infarction: final one-year results of the TOPCARE-AMI Trial. *J Am Coll Cardiol* 2004;44(8):1690–9.

59. Britten MB, Abolmaali ND, Assmus B, Lehmann R, Honold J, Schmitt J, et al. Infarct remodeling after intracoronary progenitor cell treatment in patients with acute myocardial infarction (TOPCARE-AMI): mechanistic insights from serial contrast-enhanced magnetic resonance imaging. *Circulation* 2003;108(18): 2212–8.

60. Dill T, Schachinger V, Rolf A, Mollmann S, Thiele H, Tillmanns H, et al. Intracoronary administration of bone marrow-derived progenitor cells improves left ventricular function in patients at risk for adverse remodeling after acute ST-segment elevation myocardial infarction: results of the Reinfusion of Enriched Progenitor cells and Infarct Remodeling in Acute Myocardial Infarction study (REPAIR-AMI) cardiac magnetic resonance imaging substudy. *Am Heart J* 2009;157(3):541–7.

61. Bartunek J, Vanderheyden M, Vandekerckhove B, Mansour S, De Bruyne B, De Bondt P, et al. Intracoronary injection of CD133-positive enriched bone marrow progenitor cells promotes cardiac recovery after recent myocardial infarction: feasibility and safety. *Circulation* 2005;112(9 Suppl):I178–83.

62. Askari AT, Unzek S, Popovic ZB, Goldman CK, Forudi F, Kiedrowski M, et al. Effect of stromal-cell-derived factor 1 on stem-cell homing and tissue regeneration in ischaemic cardiomyopathy. *Lancet* 2003;362(9385):697–703.

63. De Falco E, Porcelli D, Torella AR, Straino S, Iachininoto MG, Orlandi A, et al. SDF-1 involvement in endothelial phenotype and ischemia-induced recruitment of bone marrow progenitor cells. *Blood* 2004;104(12):3472–82.

64. Yamaguchi J, Kusano KF, Masuo O, Kawamoto A, Silver M, Murasawa S, et al. Stromal cell-derived factor-1 effects on ex vivo expanded endothelial progenitor cell recruitment for ischemic neovascularization. *Circulation* 2003;107(9):1322–8.

65. Opie SR, Dib N. Surgical and catheter delivery of autologous myoblasts in patients with congestive heart failure. *Nat Clin Pract Cardiovasc Med* 2006;3 Suppl 1:S42–5.

66. Sherman W, Martens TP, Viles-Gonzalez JF, Siminiak T. Catheter-based delivery of cells to the heart. *Nat Clin Pract Cardiovasc Med* 2006;3 Suppl 1:S57–64.

67. Bollini S, Smart N, Riley PR. Resident cardiac progenitor cells: at the heart of regeneration. *J Mol Cell Cardiol* 2011;50(2):296–303.

68. Marban E, Malliaras K. Boot camp for mesenchymal stem cells. *J Am Coll Cardiol* 2010;56(9):735–7.

69. Messina E, De Angelis L, Frati G, Morrone S, Chimenti S, Fiordaliso F, et al. Isolation and expansion of adult cardiac stem cells from human and murine heart. *Circ Res* 2004;95(9):911–21.

70. Kajstura J, Urbanek K, Rota M, Bearzi C, Hosoda T, Bolli R, et al. Cardiac stem cells and myocardial disease. *J Mol Cell Cardiol* 2008;45(4):505–13.

71. Oh H, Bradfute SB, Gallardo TD, Nakamura T, Gaussin V, Mishina Y, et al. Cardiac progenitor cells from adult myocardium: homing, differentiation, and fusion after infarction. *Proc Natl Acad Sci U S A* 2003;100(21):12313–8.

72. Pfister O, Mouquet F, Jain M, Summer R, Helmes M, Fine A, et al. CD31- but Not CD31+ cardiac side population cells exhibit functional cardiomyogenic differentiation. *Circ Res* 2005;97(1):52–61.

73. Reinecke H, Minami E, Zhu WZ, Laflamme MA. Cardiogenic differentiation and transdifferentiation of progenitor cells. *Circ Res* 2008;103(10):1058–71.

74. Li TS, Cheng K, Lee ST, Matsushita S, Davis D, Malliaras K, et al. Cardiospheres recapitulate a niche-like microenvironment rich in stemness and cell-matrix interactions, rationalizing their enhanced functional potency for myocardial repair. *Stem Cells* 2010;28(11):2088–98.

75. Davis DR, Kizana E, Terrovitis J, Barth AS, Zhang Y, Smith RR, et al. Isolation and expansion of functionally-competent cardiac progenitor cells directly from heart biopsies. *J Mol Cell Cardiol* 2010;49(2):312–21.

76. Dawn B, Stein AB, Urbanek K, Rota M, Whang B, Rastaldo R, et al. Cardiac stem cells delivered intravascularly traverse the vessel barrier, regenerate infarcted myocardium, and improve cardiac function. *Proc Natl Acad Sci U S A* 2005;102(10):3766–71.

77. Urbanek K, Torella D, Sheikh F, De Angelis A, Nurzynska D, Silvestri F, et al. Myocardial regeneration by activation of multipotent cardiac stem cells in ischemic heart failure. *Proc Natl Acad Sci U S A* 2005;102(24):8692–7.

78. Tang XL, Rokosh G, Sanganalmath SK, Yuan F, Sato H, Mu J, et al. Intracoronary administration of cardiac progenitor cells alleviates left ventricular dysfunction in rats with a 30-day-old infarction. *Circulation* 121(2):293–305.

79. Deb A, Wang S, Skelding KA, Miller D, Simper D, Caplice NM. Bone marrow-derived cardiomyocytes are present in adult human heart: A study of gender-mismatched bone marrow transplantation patients. *Circulation* 2003;107(9):1247–9.

80. Hatzistergos KE, Quevedo H, Oskouei BN, Hu Q, Feigenbaum GS, Margitich IS, et al. Bone marrow mesenchymal stem cells stimulate cardiac stem cell proliferation and differentiation. *Circ Res* 2010;107(7):913–22.

81. Liechty KW, MacKenzie TC, Shaaban AF, Radu A, Moseley AM, Deans R, et al. Human mesenchymal stem cells engraft and demonstrate site-specific differentiation after in utero transplantation in sheep. *Nat Med* 2000;6(11):1282–6.

82. Jiang Y, Jahagirdar BN, Reinhardt RL, Schwartz RE, Keene CD, Ortiz-Gonzalez XR, et al. Pluripotency of mesenchymal stem cells derived from adult marrow. *Nature* 2002;418(6893):41–9.

83. Mummery C, Ward-van Oostwaard D, Doevendans P, Spijker R, van den Brink S, Hassink R, et al. Differentiation of human embryonic stem cells to cardiomyocytes: role of coculture with visceral endoderm-like cells. *Circulation* 2003;107(21):2733–40.

84. Behfar A, Perez-Terzic C, Faustino RS, Arrell DK, Hodgson DM, Yamada S, et al. Cardiopoietic programming of embryonic stem cells for tumor-free heart repair. *J Exp Med* 2007;204(2):405–20.

85. Behfar A, Faustino RS, Arrell DK, Dzeja PP, Perez-Terzic C, Terzic A. Guided stem cell cardiopoiesis: discovery and translation. *J Mol Cell Cardiol* 2008;45(4):523–9.

86. Spagnoli FM, Hemmati-Brivanlou A. Guiding embryonic stem cells towards differentiation: lessons from molecular embryology. *Curr Opin Genet Dev* 2006;16(5):469–75.

87. Bartunek J, Behfar A, Vanderheyden M, Wijns W, Terzic A. Mesenchymal stem cells and cardiac repair: principles and practice. *J Cardiovasc Transl Res* 2008;1(2): 115–9.

88. Arrell DK, Niederlander NJ, Faustino RS, Behfar A, Terzic A. Cardioinductive network guiding stem cell differentiation revealed by proteomic cartography of tumor necrosis factor alpha-primed endodermal secretome. *Stem Cells* 2008;26(2):387–400.

89. Faustino RS, Behfar A, Perez-Terzic C, Terzic A. Genomic chart guiding embryonic stem cell cardiopoiesis. *Genome Biol* 2008;9(1):R6.

90. Behfar A, Terzic A. Derivation of a cardiopoietic population from human mesenchymal stem cells yields cardiac progeny. *Nat Clin Pract Cardiovasc Med* 2006;3 Suppl 1:S78–82.

91. Dimmeler S, Leri A. Aging and disease as modifiers of efficacy of cell therapy. *Circ Res* 2008;102(11):1319–30.

92. Krause DS, Theise ND, Collector MI, Henegariu O, Hwang S, Gardner R, et al. Multi-organ, multi-lineage engraftment by a single bone marrow-derived stem cell. *Cell* 2001;105(3):369–77.

93. Orlic D, Kajstura J, Chimenti S, Jakoniuk I, Anderson SM, Li B, et al. Bone marrow cells regenerate infarcted myocardium. *Nature* 2001;410(6829):701–5.

94. Laird DJ, von Andrian UH, Wagers AJ. Stem cell trafficking in tissue development, growth, and disease. *Cell* 2008;132(4):612–30.

95. Asahara T, Murohara T, Sullivan A, Silver M, van der Zee R, Li T, et al. Isolation of putative progenitor endothelial cells for angiogenesis. *Science* 1997;275(5302):964–7.

96. Arminan A, Gandia C, Garcia-Verdugo JM, Lledo E, Mullor JL, Montero JA, et al. Cardiac transcription factors driven lineage-specification of adult stem cells. *J Cardiovasc Transl Res* 2010;3(1):61–5.

97. Behfar A, Yamada S, Crespo-Diaz R, Nesbitt JJ, Rowe LA, Perez-Terzic C, et al. Guided cardiopoiesis enhances therapeutic benefit of bone marrow human mesenchymal stem cells in chronic myocardial infarction. *J Am Coll Cardiol* 2010;56(9):721–34.

98. Seeger FH, Zeiher AM, Dimmeler S. Cell-enhancement strategies for the treatment of ischemic heart disease. *Nat Clin Pract Cardiovasc Med* 2007;4 Suppl 1:S110–3.

99. Mangi AA, Noiseux N, Kong D, He H, Rezvani M, Ingwall JS, et al. Mesenchymal stem cells modified with Akt prevent remodeling and restore performance of infarcted hearts. *Nat Med* 2003;9(9):1195–201.

100. Srivastava D. Making or breaking the heart: from lineage determination to morphogenesis. *Cell* 2006;126(6):1037–48.

101. Dimmeler S, Burchfield J, Zeiher AM. Cell-based therapy of myocardial infarction. *Arterioscler Thromb Vasc Biol* 2008;28(2):208–16.

102. Takahashi K, Narita M, Yokura M, Ichisaka T, Yamanaka S. Human induced pluripotent stem cells on autologous feeders. *PLoS One* 2009;4(12):e8067.

103. Takahashi K, Tanabe K, Ohnuki M, Narita M, Ichisaka T, Tomoda K, et al. Induction of pluripotent stem cells from adult human fibroblasts by defined factors. *Cell* 2007;131(5):861–72.

104. Takahashi K, Yamanaka S. Induction of pluripotent stem cells from mouse embryonic and adult fibroblast cultures by defined factors. *Cell* 2006;126(4):663–76.

105. Ieda M, Fu JD, Delgado-Olguin P, Vedantham V, Hayashi Y, Bruneau BG, et al. Direct reprogramming of fibroblasts into functional cardiomyocytes by defined factors. *Cell* 2010;142(3):375–86.

106. Ivey KN, Srivastava D. MicroRNAs as regulators of differentiation and cell fate decisions. *Cell Stem Cell* 2010;7(1):36–41.

107. Segers VF, Lee RT. Stem-cell therapy for cardiac disease. *Nature* 2008;451(7181):937–42.

108. Nelson T, Behfar A, Terzic A. Stem cells: biologics for regeneration. *Clin Pharmacol Ther* 2008;84(5):620–3.

109. van Ramshorst J, Bax JJ, Beeres SL, Dibbets-Schneider P, Roes SD, Stokkel MP, et al. Intramyocardial bone marrow cell injection for chronic myocardial ischemia: a randomized controlled trial. *JAMA* 2009;301(19):1997–2004.
110. Yoon CH, Koyanagi M, Iekushi K, Seeger F, Urbich C, Zeiher AM, et al. Mechanism of improved cardiac function after bone marrow mononuclear cell therapy: role of cardiovascular lineage commitment. *Circulation* 2010;121(18):2001–11.
111. Terzic A, Nelson TJ. Regenerative medicine advancing health care 2020. *J Am Coll Cardiol* 2010;55(20):2254–7.
112. Griepp RB, Stinson EB, Dong E, Jr., Clark DA, Shumway NE. Determinants of operative risk in human heart transplantation. *Am J Surg* 1971;122(2):192–7.

13

Wound Healing and Cell Therapy for Muscle Repair

J.B. VELLA AND JOHNNY HUARD

Muscle injury can result from insults that range from mechanical overloading, traumatic injury, metabolic disorders, ischemic events, and congenital dysfunction. Often these insults exceed the body's capacity to regenerate functional muscle. Cell therapies in which myogenic progenitors are transplanted to the muscle to promote regeneration remain a promising field of regenerative medicine. The field witnessed dramatic advances during the past decade in the form of myoblast transfer therapy (MTT) primarily for the treatment of Duchenne muscular dystrophy (DMD). DMD is the most common (one in 3,500 live male births) and severe of the congenital muscular dystrophies.[1] It is an X-linked muscle disease characterized by progressive muscle weakness caused by a lack of dystrophin expression at the sarcolemma of muscle fibers.[2–6] The lack of dystrophin in skeletal muscle disrupts the linkage between the subsarcolemmal cytoskeleton and the basal lamina, resulting in muscle fiber necrosis and progressive muscle weakness.[7,8] Although researchers have extensively investigated various approaches to deliver dystrophin in dystrophic muscle (e.g., cell and gene therapy), there is still no efficient treatment that alleviates the muscle weakness caused by DMD. Transplantation of normal myoblasts into dystrophin-deficient muscle can create a reservoir of normal myoblasts capable of fusing with dystrophic muscle fibers and restoring dystrophin.[9–33] Although myoblast transplantation can transiently deliver dystrophin and improve the strength of dystrophic muscle, clinical trials of this approach yielded various limitations, including immune rejection, poor cell survival rates, and the limited spread of the injected cells.[9–32] Isolation of muscle cells that can overcome these limitations would enhance the success of myoblast transplantation significantly. In this chapter, we briefly review the immunologic issues and transplanted cell phenotypes that affect the efficacy of cell-mediated transplantation. However, special attention will be given to the transplanted cell's ability to withstand inflammation and the deleterious effects of oxidative and inflammatory stress. Furthermore, we describe recent progress in our use of muscle-derived stem cells (MDSCs) for muscle regenerative therapy and the putative role of antioxidants in cell-mediated muscle regeneration.

In addition to its contractile function, skeletal muscle is designed to withstand and adapt to repeated cycles of mechanical loading throughout a person's lifetime. This loading exposes the tissue to injury that induces regeneration without any functional loss. In fact, muscle regeneration in this context often induces functional gain. This normal process of injury and regeneration follows a common pattern of interplay among the injured muscle cells, immune cells, and the satellite cells that are primarily responsible for skeletal muscle regeneration. However, pathologic muscle injury from insults such as traumatic injury, metabolic disorders, ischemic events, and genetic dysfunction may not always result in functional regeneration because of the severity of the insult or the compromised ability of the host to regenerate the damaged tissue.

One prominent model of chronic muscle degeneration is DMD, a devastating dystrophinopathy characterized by progressive muscle weakness and wasting caused by familial or spontaneous dystrophin gene mutations.[2–6,34] Dystrophin is a structural protein that concentrates at the myocyte z-line and forms a mechanical link between cytoplasmic actin to the basal lamina via a membrane-bound dystrophin associated complex. In this way, dystrophin transfers the force of contraction to the basal lamina.[7,8,35] In its absence, each contraction exposes the myocyte to membrane tearing, loss of cellular potential, and calcium ion leakage, initiating a cascade of cell necrosis, inflammation, and satellite cell activation.[36] Similar acute events of membrane tearing that occur during normal muscle loading should trigger regeneration with no loss of strength or satellite cell reserve. However, in DMD, this process is widespread, ongoing, and ultimately overwhelms the muscle's native capacity for repair. This disorder ultimately leads to cardiomyopathy, prominent kyphosis, and diaphragmatic and respiratory dysfunction. Current medical intervention is primarily supportive and targets delay of symptomatic progression.[37–39] Death results from respiratory insufficiency, pulmonary infection, and cardiac decompensation in the third decade of life.[35,39]

Considerable research effort has been devoted to efficient delivery of dystrophin to dystrophic muscle through various means such as cell and gene therapy; however, challenges remain before clinical translation can be realized. Although transplantation of normal myoblasts or other myogenic cells into dystrophin-deficient muscle can create a reservoir of normal myoblasts capable of fusing with dystrophic muscle fibers and restoring dystrophin, this approach has important limitations.[9–33] These include immune rejection, poor cell survival rates, and restricted spreading of the injected cells.[9–32]

The concept of loss of muscle progenitor reserve in the context of chronic muscle degeneration continues to motivate research into the efficacy of myogenic cell transplantation to augment or replenish this reserve. That is, the satellite cell reserve is unable regenerate at the same rate as the ongoing process of degeneration. However, by replenishing the progenitor cell reserve by allo- or autogenous transfer of myoblasts expanded in vitro, perhaps the pathology of degenerative muscle disorders could be alleviated. Furthermore, myoblasts could be genetically modified before transplantation to correct genetic disorders such as DMD, perhaps halting the ongoing pathology. Despite the isolation of numerous myogenic candidates, this cell therapy has so far proved elusive in DMD. One the most severe limitations is the high rate of cell death (up to 99 percent) within the first 48 hours of injection.[9-32] Researchers continue to explore explanations for this acute loss and to study methods to increase survival during this critical period.[40] It is encouraging to note, however, that the subpopulation of cells that do survive this initial period go on to fuse to existing myofibers and appear to trigger regeneration and angiogenesis in a paracrine fashion.[41-43]

Acute cell loss on transplantation appears to stem from a complex immune response to several simultaneous events, including the tissue damage of the injection, rejection of the foreign cells, and proinflammatory activity of host and even donor myoblasts. It may even involve local ischemia caused by disruption of capillary hemodynamics commonly seen in ischemia and reperfusion injury, which generates numerous reactive oxygen species (ROS).[44] The cause of this precipitous loss of transplanted cells is not entirely resolved. The temporal profile of the response suggests activity from the innate immune system, including inflammation and the influx of activated neutrophils,[45] macrophages,[46,47] and natural killer (NK) cells.[48,49] The injected cells are likely exposed to a storm of ROS and inflammatory cytokines. Recent studies have shown that the cells that survive and engraft also have increased oxidative and inflammatory stress tolerance.[50]

Physiologic Mechanism of Muscle Repair: Role of Satellite Cells and Other Myogenic Progenitors

The fundamental cellular unit of skeletal muscle is the myofiber, a linear, multinucleated cell whose contractile actin–myosin machinery is distributed serially along the length of the fiber. During contraction, these actin–myosin networks induce radical dimensional changes of the cell and therefore considerable shear strains in the sarcolemma. In cases of excessive loading or trauma, sarcolemmal tearing allows calcium ion leakage into the cytoplasm, which can lead to myofiber necrosis facilitated by calcium-dependent proteolysis (e.g., via calpains) and increased mitochondrial ROS production. Both events may trigger a cascade of acute immune cell activation, primarily of macrophages and neutrophils.[51-55] Although immune cell activation will initially promote further damage, it is critical for muscle regeneration with a particularly vital role for the macrophage.[36,56]

The cell primarily responsible for postnatal skeletal muscle regeneration is the satellite cell. The satellite cell is a quiescent, mononucleated cell that occupies a niche between the sarcolemma and basal lamina of the myofiber and comprises 2 to 7 percent of the nuclei associated with a myofiber.[57] On muscle injury or exercise, satellite cells are activated to asymmetrically divide to replicate themselves and form daughter cells that commit to a myoblast cell fate, expressing myogenic regulatory factors (MRFs) such as Myf-5, MyoD, α7 integrin, and desmin.[58] The precise molecular mechanism of satellite cell activation and cell fate commitment is not fully known, although it involves many of the same signals involved in prenatal somitic development, including early (myoD and Myf-5) and late (myogenin and MRF4) myogenic regulator factor (MRF) expression as well as Notch–Numb antagonism.[59–62] The MyoD- or Myf-5–expressing myoblast daughter cells proliferate and migrate to the site of muscle injury and either fuse with the damaged myofiber or fuse with one another to form new myofibers. Proliferation and differentiation of satellite cells is a tightly regulated process given the importance of maintaining a reservoir of myogenic cells in the event of future injury, with expression of the transcription factors Pax3 and Pax7 playing crucial roles.[63] The transforming growth factor-β (TGF-β) family members, including GDF8 and myostatin, have been shown to inhibit myogenic differentiation and thus muscle regeneration,[64,65] but growth factors such as insulin growth factor (IGF) and fibroblast growth factor (FGF6) stimulate differentiation into MyoD- and myogenin-positive cells.[66–68]

Studies have shown that the satellite cell is not the only myogenic cell that can be activated to induce skeletal muscle regeneration. Bone marrow–derived cells (mesenchymal stem cell or marrow stromal cell) can differentiate into myoblasts or even enter the satellite cell position and undergo myogenesis.[69–71] A number of multipotent progenitor cells have been isolated from muscle such as MDSCs,[42] side population cells,[72] Sk-DN/Sk-34 cells,[73] and CD133[+] progenitors.[74,75] There is growing evidence that these cells are intimately associated with or even share a common lineage with blood vessels.[76–78] Indeed, prospective isolation of pericytes,[79] mesangioblasts,[80] endothelial cells, and myoendothelial[81] cells have yielded myogenic differentiation in vitro and in vivo.[81–83] Given their multipotency, their ability to regenerate muscle may stem not only from their myogenic differentiation but their ability to promote nerve regeneration and angiogenesis, thus recapitulating a full complement of functioning muscle.[84,85] However, their contribution to normal muscle maintenance and regeneration appears to be quite small.[86] Perhaps these cells are held in reserve for when satellite cells are overwhelmed or depleted. It is also possible that not all of these cells participate in myogenesis during the repair process despite their capacity to do so.

Myogenic Progenitors as Candidates for Cell Therapy

Irrespective of their physiologic function, these myogenic cells have shown themselves to recapitulate myogenesis in vitro by undergoing myogenic differentiation and fusing into syncytial and contractile myotubes. More importantly, these cells, when transplanted, have demonstrated their ability to participate in skeletal and in many cases cardiac muscle regeneration. They do so by fusion with existing myofibers, generation of new myofibers by fusing with each other, or stimulating regeneration in a paracrine fashion. Therefore, we have accumulated a virtual library of cells to study possible cell therapies for muscle degeneration. Which of these cells offers the greatest ease of isolation and the greatest capacity for regeneration and how they are related to one another are all active areas of research.[57]

Work performed by our research group has shown that a population of murine MDSCs, isolated by a modified preplate technique, displays a high transplantation capacity in both skeletal and cardiac muscle.[42,43] The MDSCs' capacity for long-term proliferation, strong capacity for self-renewal, resistance to stress, ability to undergo multilineage differentiation, ability to induce neovascularization, and immune-privileged behavior at least partially explain the high regenerative capacity of these cells in skeletal and cardiac muscles. Although it appears that these cells may share lineage with vascular cells, it also is possible that these cells are derived from a subpopulation of satellite cells, the main muscle precursors involved in the regeneration of myofibers.[87,88] Evidence includes findings that satellite cells can self-renew and differentiate into other lineages, thus potentially representing a population of multipotent stem cells.[89–93]

Although the MDSCs isolated by our laboratory were derived from skeletal muscle, many sources must be considered, given previous studies in which pluripotent bone marrow stem cells[70,72,94–98]; blood vessel progenitors[99–103]; neural stem cells[104–106]; and cells from other connective tissues, including adipose tissue[107,108] and dermis,[109] have all shown the capacity to differentiate into myogenic cells. Many of these cell types appear to be able to undergo myogenic lineage in vitro, but their participation in the regeneration of skeletal muscle in vivo after injury or disease has been found to be extremely limited (especially the hematopoietic, bone marrow, and other circulating precursors).[110] Among all of these different cell types, it appears that blood vessel progenitors (including mesoangioblasts) share a number of features with the MDSCs identified by our group. In particular, they share cell-type marker profiles and have high myogenic potentials in vitro and in vivo, similarities that suggest a possible relationship among these types of cells.[57]

Challenges in Translating Myogenic Cell Transplantation to the Clinic

Early clinical trials of myogenic cell transplantation therapies were faced difficult challenges, including immune rejection, poor cell spreading (less than 200 μm from injection site), and rapid death on injection.[57] Many studies have generated novel ideas for ameliorating these obstacles and increasing efficiency of engraftment, but they have yet to translate into a clinically viable solution for DMD treatment.

The first major breakthrough in developing this therapy came with the validation of the *mdx* mouse model of DMD in addition to early evidence of engraftment of dystrophin-positive fibers in this model.[22,111] What followed were human clinical trials that demonstrated limited engraftment of dystrophin-positive myofibers.[10–12,23,28,30,112,113] Follow-up examination confirmed the limited therapeutic value of the procedure in terms of low efficiency of engraftment, delivery of dystrophin to the deficient muscle, and poor rates of improvement of muscle function. Mendell et al. attained a biceps muscle engraftment rate of about 10 percent using cyclosporine immunosuppression, yet muscle function test results were, again, disappointing.[28] Ironically, it was found that cyclosporine can induce apoptosis in differentiating myoblasts despite the survival benefit of immunosuppression.[112,113] Further studies confirmed that the poor engraftment efficiency arose because of immune rejection,[18,31,114] limited cell spreading,[115] and a phenomenon of rapid cell death within 48 hours of injection.[9,17,18,45,116,117]

Acute Immunogenicity of Myogenic Cell Transplantation

Upon injection into the host skeletal muscle, a number of simultaneous immune-related responses endanger the survival of the donor cells. Even independent of the presence of the donor cells, insertion of the needle and injection of fluid in the muscle induces tearing of multiple groups of myofibers and vascular structures, which initiates an immune reaction associated with myofiber damage and necrosis as well as a clotting cascade, both of which stimulate a state of inflammation. Inflammation rapidly alters the environment of the injection site in terms of the redox state, the nature and concentration of proinflammatory cytokines, the presence and activity of inflammatory cells, and consequently the phenotypic expression of host and donor cells. This complex interplay of host and donor cells, and our present knowledge of it will be very briefly reviewed.

The hallmarks of inflammation are increased vascular permeability, migration and activation of inflammatory cells, and change in the intra- and extracellular redox state. Rupturing the sarcolemmal membrane of the myofiber allows Ca^{++} influx and lysosomal enzyme efflux and exposes neighboring cells, including macrophages, to other cellular products of necrosis, which induce inflammation within seconds or minutes.[118]

Neutrophil and macrophage infiltration propagates inflammation by releasing cytotoxic chemicals and pro-inflammatory cytokines (e.g., tissue necrosis factor-α [TNF-α], interleukin-1 [IL-1], IL-10, IL-6). Degranulation of these cells releases ROS, such as superoxide (O_2^-), a highly reactive ROS that can be converted to H_2O_2 by superoxide dismutase, which can in turn be converted to the hydroxyl radical (OH^-), a far stronger oxidant.[119] This not only causes cellular damage via protein oxidation and lipid peroxidation but oxidizes intracellular nonenzymatic antioxidant molecules such as reduced glutathione (GSH) and alters the intracellular redox balance toward a proapoptotic state.[55] There are many putative mechanisms by which muscle cells sense changes in their intra- and extracellular environment[120,121]; however, one common signaling pathway upregulated by inflammation is nuclear factor kappa-B (NFκB) nuclear translocation.[122,123] Upregulation of NFκB has a number of potential effects, including upregulation of antioxidant defenses, quiescence, and apoptosis.[124,125] Its activity in muscle cells remains poorly understood, but recent studies of p65 (a class I member of the NFκB family) knockout MDSCs suggest that these cells have increased oxidative stress tolerance in vitro and yield increased rates of engraftment when injected into the *mdx* mouse gastrocnemius muscle (unpublished observation).

Studies of various muscle injuries, including eccentric loading and ischemia and reperfusion injuries, have shown that neutrophil infiltration occurs within 1 hour of injury and can remain for up to 5 days. The rapid sequence of events that precedes neutrophil invasion is not fully elucidated; however, evidence indicates that the muscle itself can promote inflammatory cell invasion. Human satellite cells have been shown to release factors that promote macrophage/monocyte endothelial transmigration in vitro.[118,126] Neutrophil invasion is important to healing insofar as neutrophils release proteases that help clear muscle debris created by injury; however, the cytotoxic enzymes such as superoxide anion released on neutrophil degranulation also cause damage to bystander cells, promoting further inflammation.

It is clear that macrophages also rapidly invade the injured muscle, but they have a far more complex role. They participate in cell lysis using a nitric oxide (NO)–dependent mechanism and phagocytose cell debris. They then take a mediating role in the inflammatory process by promoting further immune cell infiltration (e.g., neutrophils, NK cells); however, after necrotic cell debris has been cleared, they undergo a phenotypic change that allows them to participate in the healing and regeneration phase of injury.[36,46,47] This change in role is associated with its conversion from an inflammatory phenotype (M1) to that of a healing phenotype (M2).[127] In fact, macrophage depletion has been shown to greatly inhibit muscle healing.[36]

Damage of vasculature that is induced on injection of myoblasts is likely to stimulate activity of the clotting system, whose activity is proinflammatory through the protease activity of thrombin (factor IIa).[127] Thrombin binds protease-activated receptors (PARs), which are G protein–coupled receptors expressed on platelets and endothelial and smooth muscle cells. Binding induces several proinflammatory events, including production of chemokines and expression of leukocyte adhesion molecules necessary for leukocyte binding and diapedesis. However, to our knowledge, experiments exploring the utility of interrupting the clotting cascade on myoblast survival have not been pursued.

The timing of cell death immediately after transplantation suggests loss by the innate and nonspecific humoral immune system. One basic component of the nonspecific humoral immune system is complement activity, in which 20 complement proteins coordinate to form a membrane perforating membrane attack complex (MAC)[128] as well as activate B cells.[129] However, several of the complement proteins (C3a, C5a, and C4a) also act to stimulate resident mast cells to release histamine, which causes vasodilatation and increases vascular permeability. C5a is a powerful chemotactic agent for neutrophils, monocytes, eosinophils, and basophils and can also stimulate phospholipase activity, which initiates arachidonic acid production. However, complement depletion has been shown to only marginally improve myoblast survival.[130]

Subsequent detection of foreign cells by macrophages generates numerous chemotactic signals that trigger infiltration of NK cells. NK cells are lymphocytes that recognize and kill cells that do not express a "self" major histocompatibility complex class I (MHC-I) surface protein.[131] They target exogenous cells by secreting membrane perforating enzymes such as perforin and granzyme, which may induce apoptosis or proinflammatory necrosis. NK cells often coordinate with CD8$^+$ or cytotoxic T cells to kill foreign cells, which has also been a focus of myogenic cell transplantation optimization,[114] although these studies are inconclusive and offer conflicting conclusions on the importance and temporal profile of their infiltration.[49,132,133]

Transplanted Myogenic Cell Migration

Poor myoblast migration after intramuscular injection is likely a consequence of the connective tissue barriers that exist between muscle fibers. Skeletal muscle is packaged in fibrous connective tissue. At the finest scale, myofibers reside within endomysial tissue, groups of which are organized into fascicles by perimysium. At the largest scale, epimysium and a thick muscle fascia encase the entire muscle body. Each scale of connective tissue generates an increasing barrier to myoblast migration. Several studies have suggested that myoblast migration may be mediated by the production of metalloproteinases (MMPs), particularly MMP-1 and MMP-2.[134] Production of these MMPs could be stimulated by viral transfection or in the case of MMP-9 by simple treatment with basic fibroblast growth factor (bFGF) or TNF-α. Furthermore, soluble fibronectin yielded increases in MMP-1 activity. Interestingly and somewhat paradoxically, N-acetylcysteine, which may increase the antioxidant capacity of the myoblast, was shown to decrease MMP activity (particularly MMP-2 and MMP-9) and connective tissue transmigration in vitro.[134] Poor spreading can also be overcome by increasing the number and density of injection sites. In one monkey trial, engraftment was enhanced by injecting 30 million cells per mm.[2,115] Recent clinical trials of this "high-density" injection technique (~100 injections per cm^2 of muscle surface) with tacrolimus immunosuppression demonstrated the feasibility of long-term dystrophin expression (up to 18 months).[135,136] Although the prospect of receiving "high-density" injections to all dystrophic muscles would not seem clinically feasible as a standard treatment, it was well tolerated by the 11 patients enrolled in these

Canadian trials, which should be considered in light of the severity and progressive nature of DMD.

Intravascular delivery of myogenic cells may offer a more favorable distribution of dystrophin-expressing fibers especially in muscles such as the diaphragm. Capillary networks reach all myofibers of a given muscle, and cells could be selected to home to areas of inflammation. Several studies have demonstrated the feasibility of this delivery route.[74,75] The promise of this technique relies on the interaction of very late antigen 4 (VLA-4) in CD133+ stem cells with endothelial vascular cell adhesion molecule (VCAM-1) in areas of muscle inflammation.[57]

Immune Rejection of Transplanted Cells

Immune suppression is typically required to induce successful engraftment of allogenic myoblasts. Tacrolimus (or FK506) has often been used to control inflammation and graft rejection because it, like cyclosporine, interacts with calcineurin to inhibit both T-lymphocyte signal transduction and IL-2 transcription.[137] Chronic administration appears to be necessary because when it is withdrawn, the transplanted myoblasts die in short order.[138,139] The nephrotoxic and carcinogenic side effects of chronic tacrolimus, however, should be considered in this type of treatment. Immune tolerance can be induced either by nonmyeloablative irradiation treatments with anti-CD45RB to anti-CD154[140] or cyclophosphamide and busulfan[141] or central tolerance using whole-body irradiation and allogenic bone marrow transplant.[140] However, it has been found that this central tolerance does not seem to include all muscle neoantigens after myoblast engraftment.[142] It should be noted that some myogenic cells under study have demonstrated immune privilege such as MDSCs; thus, long-term allogenic cell engraftment without immune suppression may be possible.[42]

Reactive Oxygen Species and Antioxidant Capacity of Muscle-Derived Stem Cells

Our laboratory has focused considerable effort on isolating and characterizing skeletal muscle–derived multipotent cells, called MDSCs. This population of cells has been shown to be heterogeneous in terms of cell marker profiles because their marker profiles have a tendency to change during in vitro expansion.[42] Rather, they are isolated by a modified preplate technique in which cells that are slow to adhere to a collagen-coated flask have been shown to display stem cell markers and behavior.[143] We ascertained that MDSCs were not only multipotent but that their regenerative capacity in both skeletal and cardiac muscle consistently exceeded that of more differentiated myoblasts. In a sense, the failures of MTT paved the way for the discovery of MDSCs as the putative subpopulation of cells that survive the transplantation.[15,144]

Reactive oxygen species, in addition to reactive nitrogen species (RNS), have received a great deal of attention recently given their pathologic implications in aging, cancer, and inflammatory diseases as well as their important signaling functions. Clearly, the redox environment of the intramuscular injection site is altered by the action of granulocytes such as neutrophils and macrophages as they generate numerous cytolytic ROS and RNS species. Neutrophils rely on NADPH (reduced form of nicotinamide adenine dinucleotide phosphate) oxidase 2 (NOX2) to transfer electrons to oxygen to create the superoxide radical that is itself quite toxic but can be converted to far more reactive hypochlorous and hypobromous acids by the sequential action of superoxide dismutase (SOD) and myeloperoxidase.[145,146] These oxidizing species are extremely efficient in oxidizing thiols and other biomolecules that can shift the redox balance intra- and extracellularly. Similarly, macrophages induce cell lysis though production of NO via NO synthase (NOS2 or iNOS) rather than superoxide production.[147]

One intriguing characteristic of MDSCs that appears to correlate quite well with its regeneration capacity is its resistance to oxidative and inflammatory stress. We have found that these cells produce constitutively higher levels of GSH and SOD than their more differentiated myoblast counterparts.[50] They maintain their myogenic differentiation and proliferation capacity as well as their ability to resist apoptosis in the presence of oxidative (H_2O_2) and inflammatory challenge (TNF-α).[43,50] Furthermore, when GSH levels were depleted by diethyl maleate, the increased regenerative capacity in both cardiac and skeletal muscle was lost.[50] Recent studies have shown that the cells that survive and engraft also have increased oxidative and inflammatory stress tolerance in vitro.[50]

In fact, stress tolerance may be an essential attribute of stemness. This has been found in multiple lineages, including neural stem cells,[148] hematopoietic stem cells,[149] endothelial progenitor cells,[150,151] cancer stem cells,[152–154] and other circulating progenitors.[155] One may speculate that this is a consequence of a logical evolutionary drive to protect these rare and multipotent cells from senescence and dysfunction through oxidative damage. It also appears to be a signaling mechanism to preserve the progenitor phenotype.[156,157] Recent work in our laboratory has shown that sorting muscle-derived cells on a marker of their antioxidant activity such as aldehyde dehydrogenase (ALDH) yields a subpopulation of cells with not only increased stress tolerance but also increased rates of engraftment when injected in the *mdx* mouse.[178] From the perspective of regenerative medicine, this antioxidant capacity offers another critical benefit of stem cells for cell therapy and may prove to be a primary determinant of the efficacy of stem cell therapy.[50] ALDH plays an essential role in regulating retinoic acid production, which has been shown to mediate differentiation in a number of tissue-specific stem cell populations.[166–168] In hematopoietic stem cell populations, inhibition of ALDH activity has been shown to prevent differentiation and promote proliferation.[169] However, why ALDH production appears to be upregulated in a number of tissue specific stem cells is not entirely clear; however, its role in stem cell maintenance is likely to stimulate further study given its increasingly important role in stem cell sorting.

The cell's normal antioxidant defenses include enzymatic and nonenzymatic scavengers such as SOD, GSH, catalase, glutathione peroxidase, thioredoxin, and a peroxiredoxin family of proteins.[158] These molecules are responsible not only for protecting the cell from oxidative damage but also for maintaining a precise intracellular balance of redox potential given the important signaling role of ROS. Augmenting these normal antioxidant defenses may improve transplanted cell survival posttransplantation. Exogenous and synthetic SOD has been used to preserve function in isolating islet cell grafts and may prove useful for myogenic cell engraftment as well.[159,160] Thiol-based antioxidants are also of interest in improving engraftment such as N-acetylcysteine.[161–165]

Calcium Dysregulation and the Mitochondria

As stated previously with membrane damage through oxidative stress and other mechanisms, excess cytosolic calcium concentrations can activate Ca^{++} dependent proteases such as the calpains. However, Ca^{++} dysregulation can trigger other proapoptotic pathways by interactions with muscle mitochondria.[170] Ca^{++} plays a physiologic role in regulating mitochondrial dehydrogenases by increasing NADH supplies to fuel the respiratory chain. However, if the mitochondrial matrix becomes overloaded with Ca^{++}, it can trigger the opening of the mitochondrial permeability transition pore (mPTP), which destroys the proton motive force (pmf), including pH and mitochondrial ionic potential. This pore opening is further potentiated by oxidative stress.[171–173]

With the loss of pmf, mitochondrial ATPases are driven to reverse their adenosine triphosphate (ATP)–forming reactions such that they consume ATP to pump protons out of the mitochondria. ATP depletion leads to loss of ion homeostasis throughout the cell and ultimately necrotic cell death.[170] A further deleterious consequence of mPTP opening is mitochondrion swelling driven by colloidal osmotic pressure from matrix proteins. This can perforate the outer mitochondrial membrane and release proapoptotic proteins such as cytochrome C.[170] However, there are drugs, such as cyclosporin-A[174] and sanglifehrin-A,[175] that have been shown to inhibit mPTP opening through interactions with the matrix protein cyclophilin-D ,which may have some value in improving engraftment efficiency.[176,177] Other modes of prevention of mitochondrial swelling have been shown as well, such as using dantrolene[177] or fructose to induce D-glutaraldehyde production to engage mADLH.[177]

Conclusions

This chapter reviews briefly myogenic cell transplantation therapies for the treatment of DMD and other degenerative muscle injuries in all of its promise and continued challenges. We emphasize that an important aspect of transplanted cell survival lies in the cell's ability to withstand inflammation and the deleterious effects of oxidative and inflammatory stress. Furthermore, we describe recent progress in our use of MDSCs for muscle regenerative therapy and the putative role of stress resistance in transplanted cell-mediated tissue regeneration, a phenotypic behavior that may pave the way for a better approach for stem cell isolation.

References

1. Darras, B., et al. in *Neuromuscular Disorders of Infancy, Childhood, and Adolescence. A Clinician's Approach.* (ed. H. Jones, et al.) 649 (Elsevier Science, Philadelphia; 2003).
2. Hoffman, E.P., Brown, R.H., Jr., & Kunkel, L.M. Dystrophin: the protein product of the Duchenne muscular dystrophy locus. *Cell* 51, 919–928 (1987).
3. Watkins, S.C., Hoffman, E.P., Slayter, H.S., & Kunkel, L.M. Immunoelectron microscopic localization of dystrophin in myofibres. *Nature* 333, 863–866 (1988).
4. Arahata, K. et al. Immunostaining of skeletal and cardiac muscle surface membrane with antibody against Duchenne muscular dystrophy peptide. *Nature* 333, 861–863 (1988).
5. Bonilla, E. et al. Duchenne muscular dystrophy: deficiency of dystrophin at the muscle cell surface. *Cell* 54, 447–452 (1988).
6. Zubrzycka-Gaarn, E.E. et al. The Duchenne muscular dystrophy gene product is localized in sarcolemma of human skeletal muscle. *Nature* 333, 466–469 (1988).
7. Ervasti, J.M. & Campbell, K.P. Membrane organization of the dystrophin-glycoprotein complex. *Cell* 66, 1121–1131 (1991).
8. Ibraghimov-Beskrovnaya, O. et al. Primary structure of dystrophin-associated glycoproteins linking dystrophin to the extracellular matrix. *Nature* 355, 696–702 (1992).
9. Huard, J., Acsadi, G., Jani, A., Massie, B., & Karpati, G. Gene transfer into skeletal muscles by isogenic myoblasts. *Hum Gene Ther* 5, 949–958 (1994).
10. Huard, J. et al. Myoblast transplantation produced dystrophin-positive muscle fibres in a 16-year-old patient with Duchenne muscular dystrophy. *Clin Sci (Lond)* 81, 287–288 (1991).
11. Huard, J. et al. Human myoblast transplantation: preliminary results of 4 cases. *Muscle Nerve* 15, 550–560 (1992).
12. Huard, J. et al. Human myoblast transplantation between immunohistocompatible donors and recipients produces immune reactions. *Transplant Proc* 24, 3049–3051 (1992).
13. Huard, J. et al. Human myoblast transplantation in immunodeficient and immunosuppressed mice: evidence of rejection. *Muscle Nerve* 17, 224–234 (1994).
14. Huard, J., Verreault, S., Roy, R., Tremblay, M., & Tremblay, J.P. High efficiency of muscle regeneration after human myoblast clone transplantation in SCID mice. *J Clin Invest* 93, 586–599 (1994).
15. Beauchamp, J.R., Morgan, J.E., Pagel, C.N., & Partridge, T.A. Dynamics of myoblast transplantation reveal a discrete minority of precursors with stem cell-like properties as the myogenic source. *J Cell Biol* 144, 1113–1122 (1999).
16. Beauchamp, J.R., Morgan, J.E., Pagel, C.N., & Partridge, T.A. Quantitative studies of efficacy of myoblast transplantation. *Muscle Nerve* 18 (Suppl), 261 (1994).
17. Fan, Y., Maley, M., Beilharz, M., & Grounds, M. Rapid death of injected myoblasts in myoblast transfer therapy. *Muscle Nerve* 19, 853–860 (1996).
18. Guerette, B., Asselin, I., Skuk, D., Entman, M., & Tremblay, J.P. Control of inflammatory damage by anti-LFA-1: increase success of myoblast transplantation. *Cell Transplant* 6, 101–107 (1997).

19. Qu, Z. et al. Development of approaches to improve cell survival in myoblast transfer therapy. *J Cell Biol* 142, 1257–1267 (1998).
20. Partridge, T.A. Invited review: myoblast transfer: a possible therapy for inherited myopathies? *Muscle Nerve* 14, 197–212 (1991).
21. Karpati, G., Holland, P., & Worton, R.G. Myoblast transfer in DMD: problems in the interpretation of efficiency. *Muscle Nerve* 15, 1209–1210 (1992).
22. Karpati, G. et al. Dystrophin is expressed in mdx skeletal muscle fibers after normal myoblast implantation. *Am J Pathol* 135, 27–32 (1989).
23. Tremblay, J.P. et al. Results of a triple blind clinical study of myoblast transplantations without immunosuppressive treatment in young boys with Duchenne muscular dystrophy. *Cell Transplant* 2, 99–112 (1993).
24. Morgan, J.E., Hoffman, E.P., & Partridge, T.A. Normal myogenic cells from newborn mice restore normal histology to degenerating muscles of the *mdx* mouse. *J Cell Biol* 111, 2437–2449 (1990).
25. Morgan, J.E., Pagel, C.N., Sherratt, T., & Partridge, T.A. Long-term persistence and migration of myogenic cells injected into pre-irradiated muscles of *mdx* mice. *J Neurol Sci* 115, 191–200 (1993).
26. Morgan, J.E., Watt, D.J., Sloper, J.C., & Partridge, T.A. Partial correction of an inherited biochemical defect of skeletal muscle by grafts of normal muscle precursor cells. *J Neurol Sci* 86, 137–147 (1988).
27. Qu, Z. & Huard, J. Matching host muscle and donor myoblasts for myosin heavy chain improves myoblast transfer therapy. *Gene Ther* 7, 428–437 (2000).
28. Mendell, J.R. et al. Myoblast transfer in the treatment of Duchenne's muscular dystrophy. *N Engl J Med* 333, 832–838 (1995).
29. Gussoni, E., Blau, H.M., & Kunkel, L.M. The fate of individual myoblasts after transplantation into muscles of DMD patients. *Nat Med* 3, 970–977 (1997).
30. Gussoni, E. et al. Normal dystrophin transcripts detected in Duchenne muscular dystrophy patients after myoblast transplantation. *Nature* 356, 435–438 (1992).
31. Kinoshita, I. et al. Very efficient myoblast allotransplantation in mice under FK506 immunosuppression. *Muscle Nerve* 17, 1407–1415 (1994).
32. Vilquin, J.T., Wagner, E., Kinoshita, I., Roy, R., & Tremblay, J.P. Successful histocompatible myoblast transplantation in dystrophin-deficient *mdx* mouse despite the production of antibodies against dystrophin. *J Cell Biol* 131, 975–988 (1995).
33. Petersen, Z.Q. & Huard, J. The influence of muscle fiber type in myoblast-mediated gene transfer to skeletal muscles. *Cell Transplant* 9, 503–517 (2000).
34. Dalkilic, I. & Kunkel, L.M. Muscular dystrophies: genes to pathogenesis. *Curr Opin Genet Dev* 13, 231–238 (2003).
35. Anthony, C., Frosch, M., & De Girolami, U. in Robbins and Cotran: *Pathologic Basis of Disease*, Edn. 7th. (eds. Kumar, V., Fausto, N., and Abbas, A. K.) 1336–1338 (Elsevier, Philadelphia; 2005).
36. Segawa, M. et al. Suppression of macrophage functions impairs skeletal muscle regeneration with severe fibrosis. *Exp Cell Res* 314, 3232–3244 (2008).
37. Siegel, I.M. The management of muscular dystrophy: a clinical review. *Muscle Nerve* 1, 453–460 (1978).
38. Manzur, A.Y., Kuntzer, T., Pike, M., & Swan, A. Glucocorticoid corticosteroids for Duchenne muscular dystrophy. *Cochrane Database Syst Rev*, CD003725 (2008).
39. Brooke, M.H. et al. Duchenne muscular dystrophy: patterns of clinical progression and effects of supportive therapy. *Neurology* 39, 475–481 (1989).
40. Grounds, M.D. & Davies, K.E. The allure of stem cell therapy for muscular dystrophy. *Neuromusc Disord* 17, 206–208 (2007).
41. Qu, Z.Q. et al. Development of approaches to improve cell survival in myoblast transfer therapy. *J Cell Biol* 142, 1257–1267 (1998).

42. Qu-Petersen, Z. et al. Identification of a novel population of muscle stem cells in mice: potential for muscle regeneration. *J Cell Biol* 157, 851–864 (2002).

43. Oshima, H. et al. Differential myocardial infarct repair with muscle stem cells compared to myoblasts. *Mol Ther* 12, 1130–1141 (2005).

44. Gute, D.C., Ishida, T., Yarimizu, K., & Korthuis, R.J. Inflammatory responses to ischemia and reperfusion in skeletal muscle. *Mol Cell Biochem* 179, 169–187 (1998).

45. Guerette, B. et al. Prevention by anti-LFA-1 of acute myoblast death following transplantation. *J Immunol* 159, 2522–2531 (1997).

46. Lescaudron, L. et al. Blood borne macrophages are essential for the triggering of muscle regeneration following muscle transplant. *Neuromuscul Disord* 9, 72–80 (1999).

47. Arnold, L. et al. Inflammatory monocytes recruited after skeletal muscle injury switch into antiinflammatory macrophages to support myogenesis. *J Exp Med* 204, 1057–1069 (2007).

48. Hodgetts, S.I., Beilharz, M.W., Scalzo, A.A., & Grounds, M.D. Why do cultured transplanted myoblasts die in vivo? DNA quantification shows enhanced survival of donor male myoblasts in host mice depleted of CD4+ and CD8+ cells or Nk1.1+ cells. *Cell Transplant* 9, 489–502 (2000).

49. Hodgetts, S.I., Spencer, M.J., & Grounds, M.D. A role for natural killer cells in the rapid death of cultured donor myoblasts after transplantation. *Transplantation* 75, 863–871 (2003).

50. Urish, K.L. et al. Antioxidant levels represent a major determinant in the regenerative capacity of muscle stem cells. *Mol Biol Cell* 20, 509–520 (2009).

51. Dargelos, E., Poussard, S., Brule, C., Daury, L., & Cottin, P. Calcium-dependent proteolytic system and muscle dysfunctions: a possible role of calpains in sarcopenia. *Biochimie* 90, 359–368 (2008).

52. Kwak, K.B. et al. Increase in the level of m-calpain correlates with the elevated cleavage of filamin during myogenic differentiation of embryonic muscle cells. *Biochim Biophys Acta* 1175, 243–249 (1993).

53. Whitehead, N.P., Yeung, E.W., & Allen, D.G. Muscle damage in mdx (dystrophic) mice: role of calcium and reactive oxygen species. *Clin Exp Pharmacol Physiol* 33, 657–662 (2006).

54. Spencer, M.J. & Tidball, J.G. Calpain translocation during muscle fiber necrosis and regeneration in dystrophin-deficient mice. *Exp Cell Res* 226, 264–272 (1996).

55. Clutton, S. The importance of oxidative stress in apoptosis. *Br Med Bull* 53, 662–668 (1997).

56. Brunelli, S. & Rovere-Querini, P. The immune system and the repair of skeletal muscle. *Pharmacol Res* 58, 117–121 (2008).

57. Peault, B. et al. Stem and progenitor cells in skeletal muscle development, maintenance, and therapy. *Mol Ther* 15, 867–877 (2007).

58. Creuzet, S., Lescaudron, L., Li, Z.L., & Fontaine-Perus, J. MyoD, myogenin, and desmin-nls-lacZ transgene emphasize the distinct patterns of satellite cell activation in growth and regeneration. *Exp Cell Res* 243, 241–253 (1998).

59. Conboy, I.M. & Rando, T.A. The regulation of notch signaling controls satellite cell activation and cell fate determination in postnatal myogenesis. *Dev Cell* 3, 397–409 (2002).

60. Snider, L. & Tapscott, S.J. Emerging parallels in the generation and regeneration of skeletal muscle. *Cell* 113, 811–812 (2003).

61. Seale, P., Polesskaya, A., & Rudnicki, M.A. Adult stem cell specification by Wnt signaling in muscle regeneration. *Cell Cycle* 2, 418–419 (2003).

62. Seale, P. & Rudnicki, M.A. A new look at the origin, function, and "stem-cell" status of muscle satellite cells. *Dev Biol* 218, 115–124 (2000).

63. Relaix, F. et al. Pax3 and Pax7 have distinct and overlapping functions in adult muscle progenitor cells. *J Cell Biol* 172, 91–102 (2006).
64. McPherron, A.C., Lawler, A.M., & Lee, S.J. Regulation of skeletal muscle mass in mice by a new TGF-beta superfamily member. *Nature* 387, 83–90 (1997).
65. Li, Y. et al. Transforming growth factor-beta1 induces the differentiation of myogenic cells into fibrotic cells in injured skeletal muscle: a key event in muscle fibrogenesis. *Am J Pathol* 164, 1007–1019 (2004).
66. deLapeyriere, O. et al. Expression of the Fgf6 gene is restricted to developing skeletal muscle in the mouse embryo. *Development* 118, 601–611 (1993).
67. Florini, J.R., Ewton, D.Z., & Roof, S.L. Insulin-like growth factor-I stimulates terminal myogenic differentiation by induction of myogenin gene expression. *Mol Endocrinol* 5, 718–724 (1991).
68. Armand, A.S., Laziz, I., & Chanoine, C. FGF6 in myogenesis. *Biochim Biophys Acta* 1763, 773–778 (2006).
69. Krause, D.S. et al. Multi-organ, multi-lineage engraftment by a single bone marrow-derived stem cell. *Cell* 105, 369–377 (2001).
70. Pittenger, M.F. et al. Multilineage potential of adult human mesenchymal stem cells. *Science* 284, 143–147 (1999).
71. Prockop, D.J. Marrow stromal cells as stem cells for nonhematopoietic tissues. *Science* 276, 71–74 (1997).
72. Gussoni, E. et al. Dystrophin expression in the *mdx* mouse restored by stem cell transplantation. *Nature* 401, 390–394 (1999).
73. Tamaki, T. et al. Skeletal muscle-derived CD34(+)/45(−) and CD34(−)/45(−) stem cells are situated hierarchically upstream of Pax7(+) cells. *Stem Cells Dev* 17, 653–667 (2008).
74. Torrente, Y. et al. Human circulating AC133(+) stem cells restore dystrophin expression and ameliorate function in dystrophic skeletal muscle. *J Clin Invest* 114, 182–195 (2004).
75. Gavina, M. et al. VCAM-1 expression on dystrophic muscle vessels has a critical role in the recruitment of human blood-derived CD133+ stem cells after intra-arterial transplantation. *Blood* 108, 2857–2866 (2006).
76. Tamaki, T. et al. Identification of myogenic-endothelial progenitor cells in the interstitial spaces of skeletal muscle. *J Cell Biol* 157, 571–577 (2002).
77. Tavian, M. et al. The vascular wall as a source of stem cells. *Ann N Y Acad Sci* 1044, 41–50 (2005).
78. Crisan, M. et al. A perivascular origin for mesenchymal stem cells in multiple human organs. *Cell Stem Cell* 3, 301–313 (2008).
79. Dellavalle, A. et al. Pericytes of human skeletal muscle are myogenic precursors distinct from satellite cells. *Nat Cell Biol* 9, 255–267 (2007).
80. Sampaolesi, M. et al. Mesoangioblast stem cells ameliorate muscle function in dystrophic dogs. *Nature* 444, 574–579 (2006).
81. Zheng, B. et al. Prospective identification of myogenic endothelial cells in human skeletal muscle. *Nat. Biotechnol.* 25, 1025–1034 (2007).
82. Crisan, M. et al. Purification and long-term culture of multipotent progenitor cells affiliated with the walls of human blood vessels: myoendothelial cells and pericytes. *Methods Cell Biol* 86, 295–309 (2008).
83. Crisan, M. et al. Purification and culture of human blood vessel-associated progenitor cells. *Curr Protoc Stem Cell Biol* Chapter 2, Unit 2B 2 1–2B 2 13 (2008).
84. Lavasani, M., Lu, A., Peng, H., Cummins, J., & Huard, J. Nerve growth factor improves the muscle regeneration capacity of muscle stem cells in dystrophic muscle. *Hum Gene Ther* 17, 180–192 (2006).

85. Payne, T.R. et al. A relationship between vascular endothelial growth factor, angiogenesis, and cardiac repair after muscle stem cell transplantation into ischemic hearts. *J Am Coll Cardiol* 50, 1677–1684 (2007).

86. Perry, R.L. & Rudnick, M.A. Molecular mechanisms regulating myogenic determination and differentiation. *Front Biosci* 5, D750–767 (2000).

87. Bischoff, R. Proliferation of muscle satellite cells on intact myofibers in culture. *Dev Biol* 115, 129–139 (1986).

88. Bischoff, R. in *Myology: Basic and Clinical*, Edn. 2. (eds. A.G. Engel & C. Franzini-Armstrong) 97–118 (McGraw-Hill, New York; 1994).

89. Asakura, A., Komaki, M. & Rudnicki, M. Muscle satellite cells are multipotential stem cells that exhibit myogenic, osteogenic, and adipogenic differentiation. *Differentiation* 68, 245–253 (2001).

90. Collins, C.A. et al. Stem cell function, self-renewal, and behavioral heterogeneity of cells from the adult muscle satellite cell niche. *Cell* 122, 289–301 (2005).

91. Rando, T.A. The adult muscle stem cell comes of age. *Nat Med* 11, 829–831 (2005).

92. Taylor-Jones, J.M. et al. Activation of an adipogenic program in adult myoblasts with age. *Mech Ageing Dev* 123, 649–661 (2002).

93. Zammit, P. & Beauchamp, J. The skeletal muscle satellite cell: stem cell or son of stem cell? *Differentiation* 68, 193–204 (2001).

94. Ferrari, G. et al. Muscle regeneration by bone marrow-derived myogenic progenitors. *Science* 279, 1528–1530 (1998).

95. Bittner, R.E. et al. Recruitment of bone-marrow-derived cells by skeletal and cardiac muscle in adult dystrophic mdx mice. *Anat Embryol (Berl)* 199, 391–396 (1999).

96. Caplan, A.I. Mesenchymal stem cells. *J Orthop Res* 9, 641–650 (1991).

97. Young, H.E. et al. Pluripotent mesenchymal stem cells reside within avian connective tissue matrices. *In Vitro Cell Dev Biol Anim* 29A, 723–736 (1993).

98. Young, H.E. et al. Clonogenic analysis reveals reserve stem cells in postnatal mammals: I. Pluripotent mesenchymal stem cells. *Anat Rec* 263, 350–360 (2001).

99. De Angelis, L. et al. Skeletal myogenic progenitors originating from embryonic dorsal aorta coexpress endothelial and myogenic markers and contribute to postnatal muscle growth and regeneration. *J Cell Biol* 147, 869–878 (1999).

100. Sampaolesi, M. et al. Cell therapy of alpha-sarcoglycan null dystrophic mice through intra-arterial delivery of mesoangioblasts. *Science* 301, 487–492 (2003).

101. Cossu, G. & Mavilio, F. Myogenic stem cells for the therapy of primary myopathies: wishful thinking or therapeutic perspective? *J Clin Invest* 105, 1669–1674 (2000).

102. Cusella De Angelis, M.G. et al. Skeletal myogenic progenitors in the endothelium of lung and yolk sac. *Exp Cell Res* 290, 207–216 (2003).

103. Galvez, B.G. et al. Complete repair of dystrophic skeletal muscle by mesoangioblasts with enhanced migration ability. *J Cell Biol* 174, 231–243 (2006).

104. Clarke, D.L. et al. Generalized potential of adult neural stem cells. *Science* 288, 1660–1663 (2000).

105. Galli, R. et al. Skeletal myogenic potential of human and mouse neural stem cells. *Nat Neurosci* 3, 986–991 (2000).

106. Rietze, R.L. et al. Purification of a pluripotent neural stem cell from the adult mouse brain. *Nature* 412, 736–739 (2001).

107. Zheng, B., Cao, B., Li, G.H., & Huard, J. Mouse adipose-derived stem cells undergo multilineage differentiation in vitro but primarily osteogenic and chondrogenic differentiation in vivo. *Tissue Eng* 12, 1891–1901 (2006).

108. Zuk, P.A. et al. Multilineage cells from human adipose tissue: implications for cell-based therapies. *Tissue Eng* 7, 211–228 (2001).

109. Young, H.E. et al. Human reserve pluripotent mesenchymal stem cells are present in the connective tissues of skeletal muscle and dermis derived from fetal, adult, and geriatric donors. *Anat Rec* 264, 51–62 (2001).
110. Sherwood, R.I. et al. Isolation of adult mouse myogenic progenitors: functional heterogeneity of cells within and engrafting skeletal muscle. *Cell* 119, 543–554 (2004).
111. Partridge, T.A., Morgan, J.E., Coulton, G.R., Hoffman, E.P., & Kunkel, L.M. Conversion of *mdx* myofibres from dystrophin-negative to -positive by injection of normal myoblasts. *Nature* 337, 176–179 (1989).
112. Hardiman, O., Sklar, R.M., & Brown, R.H., Jr. Direct effects of cyclosporin A and cyclophosphamide on differentiation of normal human myoblasts in culture. *Neurology* 43, 1432–1434 (1993).
113. Hong, F. et al. Cyclosporin A blocks muscle differentiation by inducing oxidative stress and inhibiting the peptidyl-prolyl-cis-trans isomerase activity of cyclophilin A: cyclophilin A protects myoblasts from cyclosporin A-induced cytotoxicity. *FASEB J* 16, 1633–1635 (2002).
114. Guerette, B., Wood, K., Roy, R., & Tremblay, J.P. Efficient myoblast transplantation in mice immunosuppressed with monoclonal antibodies and CTLA4 Ig. *Transplant Proc* 29, 1932–1934 (1997).
115. Skuk, D., Roy, B., Goulet, M., & Tremblay, J.P. Successful myoblast transplantation in primates depends on appropriate cell delivery and induction of regeneration in the host muscle. *Exp Neurol* 155, 22–30 (1999).
116. Skuk, D. & Tremblay, J.P. Complement deposition and cell death after myoblast transplantation. *Cell Transplant* 7, 427–434 (1998).
117. Guerette, B., Asselin, I., Vilquin, J.T., Roy, R., & Tremblay, J.P. Lymphocyte infiltration following allo- and xenomyoblast transplantation in *mdx* mice. *Muscle Nerve* 18, 39–51 (1995).
118. Tidball, J.G. Inflammatory processes in muscle injury and repair. *Am J Physiol Regul Integr Comp Physiol* 288, R345–353 (2005).
119. Kamata, H. & Hirata, H. Redox regulation of cellular signalling. *Cell Signal* 11, 1–14 (1999).
120. Passarelli, C. et al. Myosin as a potential redox-sensor: an in vitro study. *J Muscle Res Cell Motil* 29, 119–126 (2008).
121. Eu, J.P., Sun, J.H., Xu, L., Stamler, J.S., & Meissner, G. The skeletal muscle calcium release channel: Coupled O-2 sensor and NO signaling functions. *Cell* 102, 499–509 (2000).
122. Ji, L.L. Antioxidant signaling in skeletal muscle: a brief review. *Exp Gerontol* 42, 582–593 (2007).
123. Valdes, J.A. et al. NF-kappaB activation by depolarization of skeletal muscle cells depends on ryanodine and IP3 receptor-mediated calcium signals. *Am J Physiol Cell Physiol* 292, C1960–1970 (2007).
124. Trachootham, D., Lu, W., Ogasawara, M.A., Nilsa, R.D., & Huang, P. Redox regulation of cell survival. *Antioxid Redox Signal* 10, 1343–1374 (2008).
125. Janssen-Heininger, Y.M.W. et al. Redox-based regulation of signal transduction: Principles, pitfalls, and promises. *Free Radic Biol Med* 45, 1–17 (2008).
126. Tidball, J.G. Inflammatory cell response to acute muscle injury. *Med Sci Sports Exerc* 27, 1022–1032 (1995).
127. Kumar, V., Abbas, A.K., & Fausto, N. in *Robbins and Cotran: Pathologic Basis of Disease*, Edn. 7th. (eds. V. Kumar, A.K. Abbas & N. Fausto) 48–78 (Elsevier, Philadelphia; 2005).
128. Carroll, M.C. The role of complement and complement receptors in induction and regulation of immunity. *Annu Rev Immunol* 16, 545–568 (1998).

129. Prodeus, A.P. et al. A critical role of complement in regulation of self-reactive B cells. *Mol Immunol* 35, 29 (1998).

130. Smythe, G.M., Hodgetts, S.I., & Grounds, M.D. Immunobiology and the future of myoblast transfer therapy. *Mol Ther* 1, 304–313 (2000).

131. Moretta, L. & Moretta, A. Unravelling natural killer cell function: triggering and inhibitory human NK receptors. *EMBO J* 23, 255–259 (2004).

132. Skuk, D. et al. Dynamics of the early immune cellular reactions after myogenic cell transplantation. *Cell Transplant* 11, 671–681 (2002).

133. Sammels, L.M. et al. Innate inflammatory cells are not responsible for early death of donor myoblasts after myoblast transfer therapy. *Transplantation* 77, 1790–1797 (2004).

134. Allen, D.L., Teitelbaum, D.H., & Kurachi, K. Growth factor stimulation of matrix metalloproteinase expression and myoblast migration and invasion in vitro. *Am J Physiol Cell Physiol* 284, C805–815 (2003).

135. Skuk, D. et al. First test of a "high-density injection" protocol for myogenic cell transplantation throughout large volumes of muscles in a Duchenne muscular dystrophy patient: eighteen months follow-up. *Neuromuscul Disord* 17, 38–46 (2007).

136. Skuk, D. et al. Dystrophin expression in muscles of duchenne muscular dystrophy patients after high-density injections of normal myogenic cells. *J Neuropathol Exp Neurol* 65, 371–386 (2006).

137. Liu, J. et al. Calcineurin is a common target of cyclophilin-cyclosporin A and FKBP-FK506 complexes. *Cell* 66, 807–815 (1991).

138. Irintchev, A., Zweyer, M., & Wernig, A. Cellular and molecularu reactions in mouse muscles after myoblast implantations. *J Neurocytol* 24, 319–331 (1995).

139. Wernig, A., Irintchev, A., & Lange, G. Functional effects of myoblast implantation into histoincompatible mice with or without immunosuppression. *J Physiol* 484 (Pt 2), 493–504 (1995).

140. Camirand, G., Rousseau, J., Ducharme, M.E., Rothstein, D.M., & Tremblay, J.P. Novel Duchenne muscular dystrophy treatment through myoblast transplantation tolerance with anti-CD45RB, anti-CD154 and mixed chimerism. *Am J Transplant* 4, 1255–1265 (2004).

141. Stephan, L. et al. Induction of tolerance across fully mismatched barriers by a nonmyeloablative treatment excluding antibodies or irradiation use. *Cell Transplant* 15, 835–846 (2006).

142. Camirand, G. et al. Central tolerance to myogenic cell transplants does not include muscle neoantigens. *Transplantation* 85, 1791–1801 (2008).

143. Gharaibeh, B. et al. Isolation of a slowly adhering cell fraction containing stems cells from murine skeletal muscle by the preplate technique. *Nat Protoc* 3, 1501–1509 (2008).

144. Urish, K.L., Kanda, Y., & Huard, J. Initial failure in myoblast transplantation therapy has led the way toward the isolation of muscle stem cells: Potential for tissue regeneration. *Curr Top Dev Biol* 68, 263–280 (2005).

145. Nauseef, W.M. How human neutrophils kill and degrade microbes: an integrated view. *Immunol Rev* 219, 88–102 (2007).

146. Behe, P. & Segal, A.W. The function of the NADPH oxidase of phagocytes, and its relationship to other NOXs. *Biochem Soc Trans* 35, 1100–1103 (2007).

147. MacMicking, J., Xie, Q.W., & Nathan, C. Nitric oxide and macrophage function. *Annu Rev Immunol* 15, 323–350 (1997).

148. Madhavan, L., Ourednik, V., & Ourednik, J. Grafted neural stem cells shield the host environment from oxidative stress. *Ann N Y Acad Sci* 1049, 185–188 (2005).

149. Pearce, D.J., Taussig, D., Simpson, C., & Bonnet, D. 4467 (Amer Soc Hematology, 2004).

150. Nagano, M. et al. Identification of functional endothelial progenitor cells suitable for the treatment of ischemic tissue using human umbilical cord blood. *Blood* 110, 151–160 (2007).

151. He, T.R. et al. Human endothelial progenitor cells tolerate oxidative stress due to intrinsically high expression of manganese superoxide dismutase. *Arterioscler Thromb Vasc Biol* 24, 2021–2027 (2004).

152. Ginestier, C. et al. ALDH1 is a marker of normal and malignant human mammary stem cells and a predictor of poor clinical outcome. *Cell Stem Cell* 1, 555–567 (2007).

153. Visus, C. et al. Identification of human aldehyde dehydrogenase 1 family member a1 as a novel CD8(+) T-Cell-Defined tumor antigen in squamous cell carcinoma of the head and neck. *Cancer Res* 67, 10538–10545 (2007).

154. Patel, M. et al. ALDH1A1 and ALDH3A1 expression in lung cancers: Correlation with histologic type and potential precursors. *Lung Cancer* 59, 340–349 (2008).

155. Povsic, T.J. et al. Circulating progenitor cells can be reliably identified on the basis of aldehyde dehydrogenase. *J Am Coll Cardiol* 50, 2243–2248 (2007).

156. Dernbach, E. et al. Antioxidative stress-associated genes in circulating progenitor cells: evidence for enhanced resistance against oxidative stress. *Blood* 104, 3591–3597 (2004).

157. Matsuzawa, A. & Ichijo, H. Redox control of cell fate by MAP kinase: physiological roles of ASK1-MAP kinase pathway in stress signaling. *Biochim Biophys Acta-Gen Subj* 1780, 1325–1336 (2008).

158. Finkel, T. Oxidant signals and oxidative stress. *Curr Opin Cell Biol* 15, 247–254 (2003).

159. Mysore, T.B. et al. Overexpression of glutathione peroxidase with two isoforms of superoxide dismutase protects mouse islets from oxidative injury and improves islet graft function. *Diabetes* 54, 2109–2116 (2005).

160. Bottino, R. et al. Preservation of human islet cell functional mass by anti-oxidative action of a novel SOD mimic compound. *Diabetes* 51, 2561–2567 (2002).

161. Amer, J., Atlas, D., & Fibach, E. N-acetylcysteine amide (AD4) attenuates oxidative stress in beta-thalassemia blood cells. *Biochim Biophys Acta* (2007).

162. Cotgreave, I.A. N-acetylcysteine: pharmacological considerations and experimental and clinical applications. *Adv Pharmacol* 38, 205–227 (1997).

163. Langen, R.C. et al. Tumor necrosis factor-alpha inhibits myogenesis through redox-dependent and -independent pathways. *Am J Physiol Cell Physiol* 283, C714–721 (2002).

164. Sadowska, A.M., Manuel, Y.K.B., & De Backer, W.A. Antioxidant and anti-inflammatory efficacy of NAC in the treatment of COPD: discordant in vitro and in vivo dose-effects: a review. *Pulm Pharmacol Ther* 20, 9–22 (2007).

165. Santangelo, F. Intracellular thiol concentration modulating inflammatory response: influence on the regulation of cell functions through cysteine prodrug approach. *Curr Med Chem* 10, 2599–2610 (2003).

166. Luo, P.H. et al. Intrinsic retinoic acid receptor alpha-cyclin-dependent kinase-activating kinase signaling involves coordination of the restricted proliferation and granulocytic differentiation of human hematopoietic stem cells. *Stem Cells* 25, 2628–2637 (2007).

167. Vasiliou, V., Pappa, A., & Petersen, D.R. Role of aldehyde dehydrogenases in endogenous and xenobiotic metabolism. *Chem Biol Interact* 129, 1–19 (2000).

168. Wang, J. et al. Retinoid-induced G1 arrest and differentiation activation are associated with a switch to cyclin-dependent kinase-activating kinase hypophosphorylation of retinoic acid receptor alpha. *J Biol Chem* 277, 43369–43376 (2002).

169. Chute, J.P. et al. Inhibition of aldehyde dehydrogenase and retinoid signaling induces the expansion of human hematopoietic stem cells. *Proc Natl Acad Sci U S A* 103, 11707–11712 (2006).

170. Halestrap, A.P. & Pasdois, P. The role of the mitochondrial permeability transition pore in heart disease. *Biochim Biophys Acta* (2009).

171. Halestrap, A.P., Woodfield, K.Y., & Connern, C.P. Oxidative stress, thiol reagents, and membrane potential modulate the mitochondrial permeability transition by affecting nucleotide binding to the adenine nucleotide translocase. *J Biol Chem* 272, 3346–3354 (1997).

172. Hajnoczky, G. et al. Mitochondrial calcium signalling and cell death: approaches for assessing the role of mitochondrial Ca2+ uptake in apoptosis. *Cell Calcium* 40, 553–560 (2006).

173. McStay, G.P., Clarke, S.J., & Halestrap, A.P. Role of critical thiol groups on the matrix surface of the adenine nucleotide translocase in the mechanism of the mitochondrial permeability transition pore. *Biochem J* 367, 541–548 (2002).

174. Crompton, M., Ellinger, H., & Costi, A. Inhibition by cyclosporin A of a Ca2+-dependent pore in heart mitochondria activated by inorganic phosphate and oxidative stress. *Biochem J* 255, 357–360 (1988).

175. Clarke, S.J., McStay, G.P., & Halestrap, A.P. Sanglifehrin A acts as a potent inhibitor of the mitochondrial permeability transition and reperfusion injury of the heart by binding to cyclophilin-D at a different site from cyclosporin A. *J Biol Chem* 277, 34793–34799 (2002).

176. Waldmeier, P.C., Zimmermann, K., Qian, T., Tintelnot-Blomley, M., & Lemasters, J.J. Cyclophilin D as a drug target. *Curr Med Chem* 10, 1485–1506 (2003).

177. Irwin, W.A. et al. Mitochondrial dysfunction and apoptosis in myopathic mice with collagen VI deficiency. *Nat Genet* 35, 367–371 (2003).

178. Vella, J.B., Thompson, S.D., Bucsek, M.J., Song, M., & Huard, J. Murine and Human Myogenic Cells Identified by Elevated Aldehyde Dehydrogenase Activity: Implications for Muscle Regeneration and Repair. *Plos ONE* 6, e29226 (2011).

14

Regenerative Pharmacology of Implanted Materials and Tissue-Engineered Constructs

EMILY ONGSTAD, MICHAEL J. YOST, RICHARD L. GOODWIN, HAROLD I. FRIEDMAN, STEPHEN A. FANN, GAUTAM S. GHATNEKAR, AND ROBERT G. GOURDIE

Synthetic and natural implants have been used for a variety of physiological and aesthetic purposes. Implants made of synthetic materials include pacemakers, various sensors, vascular stents, drug delivery pumps, and silicone implants used to augment body structure (e.g., breast implants, implants for facial reconstruction). Human transplant surgeries, in which a donated organ is used to replace a failing organ, date back to the first recorded successful corneal transplantation in 1905. More recently, the fields of tissue engineering and regenerative medicine have provided some level of success in engineered living tissue replacements spanning many of the body's tissues.

Every implant placed within the body will induce the immune response whether the implant serves a physiological role, such as a heart transplant, or serves an aesthetic purpose, such as a breast implant. The immune response can lead to rejection of a transplanted organ – causing mortality – or to the foreign body response and subsequent fibrous encapsulation. The formation of a fibrous capsule may cause reduced function of implanted sensors and pacemaker leads, disfigurement of breast implants, or ejection of the implant from the body.

The reaction of the immune system differs based on the composition of the implant. Synthetic materials incite components of innate immunity, leading to persistent macrophages and fibrous scar tissue. Natural materials may be antigenic but typically do not result in rejection, but cellular constructs and transplants can initiate the much harsher cellular adaptive immune response. Transplantation therapy requires the use of immunosuppressive agents to prevent rejection. Tissue-engineered replacements are also cellular and can provoke a wound-like response together with significant scar tissue differentiation after implantation.

A variety of pharmacological approaches have been investigated to reduce the immune response and implant rejection. These agents target all stages of the immune response and foreign body reaction [1]. Lessons taken from scar formation in the skin may also be applied to fibrous encapsulation of implants. One of these lessons is that of the ability of the αCT1 peptide to reduce scarring in excisional wounds and to reduce contraction capsule formation when applied to silicone implants. This chapter addresses wound healing and the foreign body reaction, the differences in adult and fetal wound healing, complications that occur in implantation, and pharmacological approaches taken to reduce the foreign body reaction and scarring. Lessons taken from the skin that can be applied to tissue engineering of skeletal muscle, and models for testing pharmacological therapies are also discussed.

Wound Healing and the Foreign Body Reaction

Many useful reviews on various aspects of wound healing and scar formation exist [2–13], so this subject will only be addressed briefly here. The function of wound healing is to close the wound and to replace any tissue that was lost to injury. The three stages in wound healing are (1) inflammation, (2) proliferation, and (3) matrix remodeling and scar formation. Inflammation is initiated after injury by an intense inflammatory cascade in which the cytokines and growth factors that affect scar formation are produced. Although the mechanism is unknown, it is thought that the early profile of inflammatory cytokines has a significant influence on the subsequent degree of scar formation. Neutrophils, and later macrophages, infiltrate the wound site and degrade and remodel the matrix through production of enzymes that include matrix metalloproteases. Fibroblasts migrate and proliferate into the wound site. During matrix remodeling and scar formation, angiogenesis occurs in the newly formed granulation tissue. This tissue acquires its label from the granular appearance imparted by the many newly formed blood vessels. New collagen synthesis (mostly by fibroblasts) is induced by the many growth factors and cytokines produced by macrophages, which can include basic fibroblast growth factor, transforming growth factors (TGFs), and insulin-like growth factors. Fibroblasts in granulation tissue may develop a myofibroblast phenotype. In the skin, myofibroblasts contribute to wound contraction. Myofibroblasts in the contraction capsule are also thought to provide the motive force leading to disfigurement of silicone breast implants and extrusion of subcutaneously implanted devices from the body [14]. The remodeling, collagen synthesis, and differentiation of a mature scar can continue for as long as 2 years after the initial injury. This process involves growth factors and cytokines that stimulate the production of extracellular matrix (ECM) proteins and enzymes involved in tissue turnover [15].

Implantation of devices and tissue-engineered constructs into the body are invasive surgical procedures that cause injury sufficient to trigger the wound healing response. Although it is much more difficult to visually evaluate the response to materials and devices implanted in the body, histologic evaluations have shown that granulation tissue formation, as occurs in the skin, and foreign body reaction is the normal wound healing response to implants. The degree and extent of the foreign body reaction depends on the composition, roughness, surface chemistry, and other properties of the device [16]. If the implant is cellular, fibrous deposition may occur within and surrounding the implant [18,19]. The final stage of the foreign body reaction involves deposition of a fibrous capsule surrounding the implant as the body attempts to isolate the implant from the local tissue environment. The fibrous capsule and foreign body reaction may persist at the tissue–implant interface for the life of the implant.

Repair versus Regeneration

Although small, there is a distinction between "repair" and "regeneration." An injury interrupts the function and morphology of a tissue. Continuity of the organ or tissue is reestablished when the tissue undergoes repair, whether the lost or damaged tissue is functionally and morphologically restored. Growth factors and cytokines that are produced during the wound healing process help support the most efficient healing mechanism. However, efficient wound closure almost never means fully functional wound closure and typically results in a scar. Cutaneous scars are functional in that they serve as a barrier. However, scars rarely attain mechanical properties that match native skin, nor do they completely replicate function of the native tissue [17]. In tissue regeneration, replacement of lost or damaged tissue completely restores both morphology and functionality. Outside of the liver, gut, and vascular system, mammals have negligible ability to regenerate. In some instances, such as skin, "partial regeneration" may be induced by the use of scaffolds and exogenous pharmacological agents [20]. In other tissues, repair is usually accompanied by scar formation.

The regenerative capacity of a tissue greatly influences the body's response to injury or an implanted material. Injury to tissues composed of nonproliferating cell types (e.g., nerve or cardiac tissue) typically results in scarring or fibrous encapsulation of an implant. Tissues composed of continuously proliferating cells (e.g., cells of the gut) or cells that have the capacity to proliferate after injury or in response to certain stimuli (e.g., liver) can theoretically accomplish perfect repair or be regenerated, although these tissue types often exhibit fibrotic responses to injury or implantation [16].

It is widely known that wound healing in early gestational fetal skin occurs with minimal scar formation, but wound healing in an adult almost always leads to scarring [21–24]. Differences in fetal cells, ECM, growth factor profiles, and gene expression affect the extent of scarring. Many of the pharmacological approaches taken to reduce scar formation in adult skin attempt to recapitulate the fetal wound environment and are discussed later. Also of note, the ability to regenerate tissue without scar formation is seen in fetal skin and fetal bone but does not exist to these extremes in other fetal tissues. The opportunity exists to use pharmacological agents, some of which are based on lessons learned from embryos, to reduce scar formation and promote functional integration of implanted materials and cells.

Implant-Associated Complications

A variety of complications can occur when a foreign object is placed in the body. These can include immune rejection, persistent foreign body reaction, and fibrous capsule formation. Because the wound healing environment within most adult tissues does not support complete regeneration, implanted tissue-engineered constructs often undergo significant fibrosis, leading to impairment of normal tissue function. Complications associated with patient comorbidities may also compromise the implant and lead to implant failure. Implant failure is defined as the loss of function of an implant. Implant failure often requires additional surgeries to replace the device or remove excessive fibrosis. Here we focus on the isolation and rejection of an implanted material or device and how pharmacological agents can be used to prevent isolation and rejection.

The Immune Response and Inflammation

The immune system is responsible for defending the body against infectious organisms. The body has two types of immunity: innate immunity, which makes it difficult for pathogens to enter the body, and acquired immunity, which includes mechanisms developed by the body in response to specific foreign organisms or stimuli. Every material that comes in contact with the body is subject to the immune response. Implantation causes injury to local tissues, so the initial wound healing response is mounted. Depending on the implanted material, the site of implantation, and the severity of the defect created, the body may undergo only a short inflammatory period or chronic inflammation and a subsequent foreign body reaction. The more highly reactive an implanted material is, the greater the degree of reaction the body mounts against it.

Capsule Formation, Persistent Foreign Body Reaction, and Extrusion

A greater effort will be made to isolate a highly reactive material from the body. This is done by creating a thicker fibrous, avascular capsule around the implant, often 50 to 200 μm thick. The absence of vascularization limits the potential for continued immune response. The capsule has contractile properties imparted by its constituent myofibroblasts, an α–smooth muscle actin-positive cell type. In some cases of percutaneous and subcutaneous implants, the implanted device can be extruded from the body by the action of the myofibroblasts in the contraction capsule.

Patient Comorbidities

Patient comorbidities that affect wound healing and the body's ability to mount an immune response also need to be addressed when implants are discussed [6,7]. Poor circulation, as can happen in individuals with diabetes mellitus, leads to a reduced wound healing response. Reduced immunity leaves patients more subject to wound infection. Low levels of human growth hormone (which reduces with age) can cause slow wound healing. Low levels of essential fatty acids in the diet and nutrient deficiencies in zinc; copper; and vitamins C, B5, A, and B-complex can all lead to impairment of the wound healing response. Although some of these issues can be addressed pharmacologically, many patients may be contraindicated from implants because of them.

Examples

The foreign body reaction that occurs in response to an implant is often detrimental to implant function. A stent placed in a coronary artery serves to keep the vessel lumen open after it has been occluded by plaque. Implantation of the stent causes injury to the vessel and the smooth muscle cells in the vessel wall undergo a fibroproliferative response. Although the proliferative response serves to somewhat incorporate the stent into the vessel wall, helping to fix the implant location, the sustained proliferation of cells may lead to vessel restenosis and implant failure [25].

This same type of reaction is seen when sensors are placed in the body. Blood glucose monitoring is essential for patients with diabetes. The standard procedure involves pricking a finger and using a digital meter to measure glucose levels. Using an implantable sensor would eliminate a patient's need for multiple finger pricks in a day. However, the implants currently under development would need to be replaced within 1 to 5 years of implantation because of fibrosis around the implant and surface fouling of the electrode, which can lead to instability in measurements.

Implantable drug delivery pumps, such as osmotic pumps, are used to obtain steady plasma concentrations of a desired drug. All drug pumps are faced with the common issue of fibrous capsule formation. Although the fibrous capsule helps immobilize the drug pump in its site of implantation, it can hinder the diffusion of the drug. Fibrosis may also lead to occlusion of the delivery port.

Pharmacological Modulation of Wound Healing and the Foreign Body Reaction

The foreign body reaction often leads to tissue repair and scarring instead of regeneration, functional wound healing, and implant tissue integration. There has been some research into pharmacological agents that can help in this area, but the field of cutaneous wound healing provides an abundance of research efforts using pharmacological agents to reduce fibrosis and scarring. Pharmacological agents that alter all stages of the immune response and wound healing have been used to reduce scarring and fibrosis. A few of the most widely studied agents, as well as some recent discoveries by our laboratory, will be discussed here.

Cyclooxygenase-2 Inhibitors

The enzymatic activity of cyclooxygenase (COX) results in the formation of prostanoids, which are mediators of inflammatory reactions [26]. Although COX-1 is constitutively expressed in most tissues, COX-2 undergoes immediate upregulation in response to an inflammatory stimulus. This leads to high levels of COX-2 at sites of inflammation. The prostaglandins that are subsequently produced control the induction of vascular permeability and the activation and infiltration of inflammatory cells [28]. COX-2 and its product prostaglandin E2 (PGE2) are known to critically mediate the inflammatory response. Because inflammation level and the resulting scar formation are thought to be related, reducing the inflammatory response may reduce scar formation. As such, it has been shown that inhibiting the COX-2 pathway can reduce neutrophil infiltration, PGE2 levels, TGF-β1, collagen deposition, and scar formation in full-thickness skin wounds in mice [29].

A novel approach to study the microenvironment of implants is through the use of implanted piezoelectric wafer active sensors (PWAS). The impedance of PWAS sensors changes as the mechanical properties of the associated tissue change, providing information about the relative viscosity in the local tissue [27]. Intramuscular implantation of a PWAS in rats with a COX-2 inhibitor led to decreased dampening of the PWAS waveform and delayed maturation of the wound healing response, including maturation of the collagen capsule, compared with control. Capsule formation in COX-2 inhibited animals at 20 weeks was indistinguishable from control. The authors concluded that PWAS sensors could be used to study the viscosity of wound exudate around soft tissue implants, a parameter that is indistinguishable by histologic examination.

Collagen Synthesis Inhibitors

The fibrous capsule that forms around the implant is composed primarily of collagen and fibrogenic cells. One approach to reducing fibrous encapsulation of implants is to inhibit synthesis of the collagen that makes up the fibrous capsule. Studies in hypertrophic scarring of animal skin have shown that inhibiting the excessive collagen synthesis that results in large, unsightly scars (e.g., keloids) can decrease the protrusion of the scar. Procollagen C-proteinase and prolyl 4-hydroxylase have been targeted to inhibit collagen deposition. Procollagen C-proteinase is the enzyme that catalyzes cleavage of the C-terminal propeptide from the collagen precursor molecule to form stable collagen fibrils. In other words, this enzyme is involved in the formation of mature collagen by fibrogenic cell types [30]. In studies of skin wounds in rabbits, inhibition of procollagen C-proteinase was able to decrease the elevation of the scar above the surrounding normal tissue when treated during late wound stages [31]. Prolyl 4-hydroxylase is an enzyme required for the hydroxylation of proline residues necessary for formation of a mature collagen molecule. When excisional skin wounds were treated with a prolyl 4-hydroxylase inhibitor, elevation of the scar was significantly decreased compared to control [32]. Inhibition of collagen fibril formation with antibodies to the telopeptide region of collagen has also been shown to reduce the number of collagen fibrils that form in an in vitro scar model [33].

Angiotensin-Converting Enzyme Inhibitors and Angiotensin Receptor Blockers

In the heart, upregulation of angiotensin-converting enzyme (ACE) is involved in fibrous cardiac remodeling. Whereas fibrous remodeling in the heart after infarction serves to strengthen the heart wall and prevent rupture, abnormal or excessive remodeling can lead to accumulation of ECM proteins. This can disrupt cardiomyocyte coupling, leading to electrical irregularities [34]. In skin, a local renin–angiotensin system may be present [35]. Exogenous angiotensin II analogs have been shown to accelerate repair in skin wounds in animal models [36, 37], and the activity level of ACE has been found to be elevated in scar tissue compared with normal skin [38]. The roles of angiotensin II in the inflammatory response include increasing vascular permeability and regulating cell growth and fibrosis, implicating it in scar formation [39]. Many other tissues in the body in addition to the skin and heart have been shown to have local renin–angiotensin systems, including blood vessels [40], brain [40], adipose tissue [41], liver [42], and kidney [40]. Because of the widespread action of angiotensin II, ACE inhibitors and angiotensin II receptor blockers may have potential for reducing fibrosis in implants in various tissues of the body.

Steroidal Anti-inflammatory Drugs

Glucocorticoids are steroid hormones that have been used to minimize foreign body reaction at the site of implants. Glucocorticoids exert their action on the immune system, inhibiting the formation and secretion of early inflammatory mediators such as prostanoids. The reduction in prostanoids leads to fewer inflammatory cells at the implant site, decreased vascular permeability, and suppressed fibroblast proliferation [43]. Long-term systemic use of glucocorticoids leads to unwanted side effects, so localized delivery via hydrogels, drug coatings, and microspheres have been investigated for delivery at implant sites [24, 44, 45]. Microsphere delivery of the glucocorticoid dexamethasone was able to reduce the inflammatory response in vivo as indicated by reduced inflammatory cells and reduced proliferation of fibroblasts at the implant site [46]. Although not yet tested in vivo, hydrogel delivery with various molecular weights of PLGA (polylactic co-glycolic acid) and PVA (polyvinyl alcohol) enable tailored release kinetics of dexamethasone [47]. Because corticosteroids are antiangiogenic, co-delivery of dexamethasone and vascular endothelial growth factor, which can stimulate growth of new blood vessels, was also investigated. This combined therapy was able to suppress inflammation and fibrosis while promoting angiogenesis [48].

Hyaluronan

Synthetic and natural coatings have been used for implanted devices to mask their surfaces from the immune system. A hydrophilic layer between the device and the tissue can minimize tissue reactions and improve device functionality and lifespan. Some natural materials that have been used for this purpose are dextran [49] and hyaluronan [50, 51]. Hyaluronan is a major component of skin and other tissues and is known to be involved in wound healing in adults and fetuses. Hyaluronan has been used as a wound dressing [50] and in drug delivery [51, 52]. Hyaluronan has been shown to accelerate wound healing in clinical trials [53] and to inhibit glial scar formation [54].

Osteopontin

Osteopontin has been shown to be upregulated in wound healing and to play a role in inflammation. This glycoprotein is involved in cell-matrix interactions and binds several integrin receptors on leukocytes. Osteopontin has also been shown to be elevated in fibrosis of lung [55], liver [56], and heart [57]. In PU.1 null mice, which lack myeloid cells, wound healing is improved, and osteopontin is found to be down-regulated [58]. Mori et al. report accelerated wound repair, decreased granulation tissue, and decreased fibrosis in skin wounds of mice with knockdown of osteopontin by antisense oligodeoxynucleotide delivery from pluronic gel [59]. They show that platelet-derived growth factor (PDGF) released from macrophages is responsible for osteopontin expression in wound fibroblasts. Because osteopontin-associated fibrosis is found in multiple tissues in the body, osteopontin or PDGF inhibition at the time of wound healing may be viable targets for reducing fibrosis in implanted materials and cells.

Transforming Growth Factor Beta

The secreted growth factors of the TGF-β family have numerous functions in cellular processes and are well known for their roles in scar formation and the inflammatory response. TGF-β is released after initial injury by platelets and is chemotactic for neutrophils, monocytes, and fibroblasts [23]. Macrophages, fibroblasts, keratinocytes, and endothelial cells continue to produce TGF-β in the wound environment. In normal wound healing, TGF-β1 and TGF-β2 upregulate collagen and fibronectin synthesis by dermal fibroblasts [60]. Not surprisingly, skin fibrillar collagen genes were found to be direct downstream targets of TGF-β [61]. Increased expression of TGF-β1 and

TGF-β2 has been shown to cause scarring in animal models [62, 63]. Because TGF-β1 and TGF-β2 lead to increased collagen gene expression and tissue fibrosis, they are considered fibrotic types of TGF-β [64]. TGF-β also plays a role in fibrosis of other organs [65].

The expression profiles of TGF-β differ greatly between adult and fetal wound healing, and TGF-β1, -β2, and -β3 have all been shown to have roles in fetal scar formation [66, 67]. In fetal wounds, high levels of TGF-β3 and low levels of TGF-β1 and TGF-β2 are expressed. Adult wounds exhibit high levels of TGF-β1 and TGF-β2 [67]. This suggests that the relative ratios of TGF-β are important for promoting scarless wound healing, although the precise molecular mechanism remains unclear.

The rationale for TGF-β targeting as a scar-reducing strategy is to imitate the scarless regeneration found in the fetal wound healing environment. Antibodies against TGF-β1 and TGF-β2 applied topically have led to decreased collagen production in vitro and reduced scarring in vivo [68, 69]. Antisense oligodeoxynucleotides against TGF-β1 and TGF-β2 have shown reduced scarring in rabbit and mouse models [70, 71]. Many animal studies have shown reduced scarring by increasing relative levels of TGF-β3 to TGF-β1 and TGF-β2 with either topical application of TGF-β3 or neutralizing TGF-β1 and TGF-β2. However, clinical trials for Juvista (recombinant human TGF-β3) showed no reduction in scarring [72]. Clinical trials using TGF-β targeting strategies have yet to be undertaken for implants.

Connexin43 and Gap Junctions

The gap junction is an aggregate of intercellular channels connecting the cytoplasm of two cells for the passage of molecules and ions less than 1000 Da. A gap junction channel is composed of two hexameric hemichannels of connexin proteins, each from an adjacent cell. Gap junctions serve to pass electrical signals in excitable tissues such as the heart and brain [73], to pass nutrients and metabolites [74], and to pass second messengers such as Ca^{2+} [75].

Intercellular communication between cells is essential for tissue repair after injury. Many connexins have been found to have roles in inflammatory response, tissue repair, and scar formation after injury [76, 77]. Connexin43 (Cx43) is just one of many connexins found in humans [78] and is thought to have a role in wound healing and the spread of injury signals. Cultured neural glial cells had an increasing rate of cell death in response to calcium, oxidative stress, or metabolic inhibition as the number and density of gap junctions between cells increased [79]. An increase in Cx43 levels has been found in glial scars [80] and in the fibrotic response to radiation in the lung [81]. In a cornea endothelial injury model, connexin43 knockdown via antisense oligodeoxynucleotide, small interfering RNA (siRNA), or adenovirus applied into the anterior chamber simultaneously with injury led to complete wound closure by day 3, but no closure was seen in controls by this stage [82]. Downregulation of Cx43 by anti-sense oligodeoxynucleotide has been shown to accelerate wound healing and reduce granulation tissue area in the mouse skin [83]. The upregulation of Cx43 in response to wounds and its implication in scar formation and fibrosis in many tissue types suggests that targeting of Cx43 may help reduce the degree of fibrous encapsulation of implants or encourage more functional integration of tissue-engineered constructs.

Lessons from Skin for Regenerative Integration of Tissue-Engineered Skeletal Muscle Replacement

Scarless Wound Regeneration in the Skin by aCT1 Peptide

Another approach to modulate wound healing based on Cx43 has been used in the Gourdie laboratory [84–87]. The α-connexin carboxyl-terminal peptide, or αCT1 peptide, was developed to inhibit interaction of the actin-binding protein Zonula Occludens-1 (ZO-1) with Cx43 [86]. This inhibitory peptide contains an antennapedia cell permeablization sequence linked to the last nine amino acids of the carboxyl-terminus of Cx43. ZO-1 normally localizes to the edges of gap junction plaques, but the αCT1 peptide is able to inhibit this interaction, leading to an increase in gap junction plaque size.

αCT1 has since been shown to have benefits in healing of skin wounds [85]. In excisional skin wounds in mice, the αCT1 peptide was able to increase the rate of wound healing and promote skin structure more similar to normal skin after wound closure. Wound strength at 90 days was greater in αCT1 treatment than control. In neonatal skin wounds in CD-1 mice, αCT1 application resulted in faster healing and less scarring. A similar trend was seen in skin wounds in adult mice. A significant reduction in neutrophil content in skin wounds was seen in both adults and neonates. The histologic complexity (e.g., rete pegs) with αCT1 treatment was reproduced in skin wounding in swine.

aCT1 in the Silicone Disk Contraction Capsule

Implants are subject to the foreign body reaction, which typically results in the formation of a fibrous capsule surrounding the implant. Mechanically active cell types, such as myofibroblasts, are often found within this fibrous capsule. These cells types can lead to deformation of the implant and impairment of its function. Removal or revision may be required depending on the extent to which encapsulation and contraction affect the function of the implant.

Originally developed to examine the effects of inhibiting Cx43-ZO-1 interaction on gap junction organization, the αCT1 peptide showed shorter healing time and reduced scarring in studies of cutaneous wound healing. αCT1 has the potential for application in reduction of the contraction capsule that forms in response to implants [87].

When delivered in a pluronic gel vehicle surrounding a silicone implant in rats, αCT1 was shown to reduce neutrophil counts in the tissue surrounding the implants at early time points compared with vehicle controls, possibly by impeding neutrophil recruitment [88]. αCT1 also increased the number of α–smooth muscle actin positive blood vessels surrounding the implant, and fewer nonvascular α–smooth muscle actin positive cells. This indicated that the tissue was better vascularized and had less contractile activity owing to myofibroblasts. Less collagen and fibrous protein were found in the capsule around αCT1-treated implants than in vehicle controls at 4 weeks. The reduction in nonvascular α–smooth muscle actin positive cells in the αCT1-treated group persisted at 4 weeks [88]. In line with this cellular composition, intramuscular implantation of an αCT1-treated PWAS biosensor led to decreased dampening of the piezoelectric sensor waveform compared with controls, consistent with the differentiation of a less contractile capsule around the implanted device (Fig. 14-1).

Limitations to Skeletal Muscle Tissue Engineering

The implantation of tissue-engineered devices into the body is an area of intense current interest. Unfortunately, there is no pass on a wound healing response or foreign body reaction to engrafted cells or implanted cellularized devices. Promoting regenerative integration of tissue-engineered devices thus remains a significant challenge and is a problem that may benefit from novel pharmacological strategies. Numerous tissue-engineered devices are under different stages of development and testing [89–96]. One of most widely known is the tissue-engineered bladder from Atala's group [97]. Experience of our own group has focused on development of cellularized constructs for skeletal muscle repair. In the closing section, we summarize aspects of this work, including insights gained from animal models on the challenges that the foreign body response poses to translation of tissue-engineered implants into the clinic.

Skeletal muscle tissue is known to contain a population of progenitor cells, the satellite cells. These progenitor cells remain quiescent until the muscle tissue sustains injury, at which point they migrate and proliferate into the injury site and differentiate into myoblast cells. Myoblasts then form new muscle by generating multinucleated myofibers or repair muscle by fusing to damaged myofibers [98]. If skeletal muscle sustains massive injury, satellite cells are not able to compensate for the defect, and fibrosis occurs. Because of this inability to regenerate, the repair of skeletal muscle through tissue engineering approaches would represent a clinically significant advance [107,108]. Strategies subject to experimental study include the use of scaffolds composed of various kinds of polyesters, including polycaprolactone (PCL), poly(lactic acid) (PLA), poly(glycolic acid) (PGA), and poly(lactic-*co*-glycolic acid (PLGA), [99] seeded with either skeletal muscle cells [100] or satellite cells [101], as well as

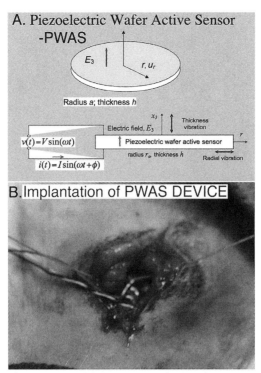

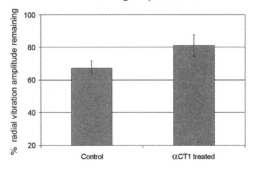

Figure 14-1. Mechanical testing of αCT1-treated contraction capsules around silicone implants. (**A**) Principal modes of vibration of a circular piezoelectric wafer under oscillatory voltage excitation. (**B**) Subdermal or intramuscular implantation of wired piezoelectric wafer active sensor (PWAS) device in vivo in a rat. (**C**) αCT1 reduces dampening of the PWAS amplitude indicative of a less contracted capsule. (PWAS data obtained in collaboration with Victor Giurgiutiu PhD USC – Mechanical Engineering.) (See color plate 30.)

an approach using aligned collagen matrices woven into a tubelike construct that was developed by the Yost laboratory (Fig. 14-2) [102]. Our work with the collagen tube has achieved significant progress in both new muscle differentiation and neovascularization in animal models. In particular, we have found that our tube, when cellularized

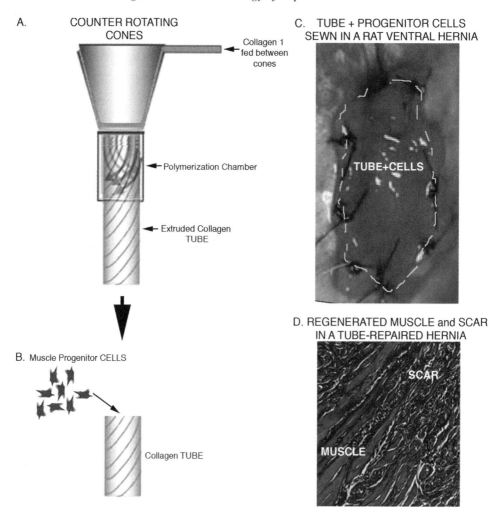

Figure 14-2. Tissue-engineered device for hernia repair. (**A**) Schema for device generating collagen tubes. (**B**) Skeletal muscle progenitor cells (satellite cells) are added to the collagen tube generating the tissue-engineered device. (**C**) The collagen tube with added muscle progenitor cells sewn into a ventral hernia in a rat. (**D**) Histologic section of a repaired ventral hernia 4 weeks after sewing in the tissue-engineered device. The device mediated a partial repair of the muscle defect. However, it did so imperfectly because the repair exhibited a mixture of regenerated muscle and scar tissue. Pharmacological approaches such as αCT1 may further decrease fibrosis, increasing the proportion of muscle to scar in the repaired hernia. (See color plate 31.)

with autologous satellite cells, provides improvement in regenerative repair of ventral hernia in a rat model over controls. Despite this progress, fibrotic scar tissue is seen between regenerated skeletal muscle fibers in the implanted construct. Observations similar to ours are not widely reported in the literature. However, anecdotally, it is widely acknowledged that "scarring up" of tissue-engineered constructs, including intermixing of scar and regenerated tissue in the implant, remains an ongoing concern.

A pharmacological approach that we are presently testing to reduce scar tissue in implanted muscle sheets in the model of ventral hernia repair is to use αCT1 peptide, the application of which has been previously shown to reduce fibrous contraction capsule formation around silicone implants. As already described in this review, numerous other drugs and biologics are available in addition to αCT1, including compounds thought to promote scarless healing via mechanisms analogous to those occurring in fetal tissues. Such compounds represent alternative prospects for testing in the regenerative integration of tissue-engineered devices in vivo.

Animal and Cellular Models for Regenerative Integration

Because of the patient comorbidities discussed earlier, many patients may have an impaired wound healing response. Various animal models, including mouse transgenics, are available for testing tissue-engineered constructs [109]. Severe combined immunodeficiency immunocompromised mice are commonly used to test cell or tissue transplantation. Although the absence of T and B cells in these mice prevents the transplanted cells or tissue from being rejected [110], there may be better models available for studying wound healing and the foreign body reaction. Because transplants and implants are not performed in perfect tissue, studying the reaction to an implant in a compromised environment may give a more accurate representation of the patient population. There are many murine models of diabetes in use today. Diabetic (Db/db) mice have been shown to have impairment in wound healing compared with other murine models of diabetes, making it one of the preferred models for studying wound healing in diabetes [111]. Doxorubicin, a commonly used cancer chemotherapeutic, has been shown to inhibit healing of skin wounds [112] and has been used to investigate therapies for wound healing [36]. Because regenerative repair and wound healing is known to slow with age [113], testing regenerative integration of tissue-engineered constructs in aged animal models is also of relevance.

A variety of stem cells are used for tissue engineering and include embryonic stem (ES) cells; bone marrow stem cells; and, more recently, induced pluripotent stem (iPS) cells [114–116]. Although ES cells provide the greatest regenerative capacity, there are ethical debates on their use. ES cells also have the limitation of potentially leading to teratoma formation [117, 118]. In a promising finding, nonautologous bone marrow stem cells appear to have a degree of immune privilege when implanted and may even convey such privilege on co-engrafted cells [119]. This being said, recent findings on tissue rejection in immunocompromised animal models of nonautologous bone marrow cell implantation indicate that further preclinical evaluation will be required before clinical implementation [120]. The use of autologous bone marrow cells eliminates the problem of immune rejection but is challenged by attaining sufficient numbers of cells to be used therapeutically. iPS cells can be produced in abundance, can be generated autologously, and may also mitigate ethical concerns.

Table 14-1. *Challenges to regenerative integration of implanted cells and materials*

Obstacles to regenerative integration	Need
Minimal regenerative capacity of most tissues in humans	Determination of healing process or foreign body response in various human tissues
Obtaining sufficient cell number to generate tissue for large defects	Optimization of various cell proliferating techniques
High cost to patient	Optimization of production process to decrease costs
Patient drug reactions	
Patient comorbidities that affect wound healing	Generating a number of viable tissue-engineered constructs for one tissue type with a variety of drugs
Inflammation-associated fibrosis after implantation	Testing of tissue-engineered constructs in animal models of patient comorbidities (e.g., impaired wound healing, diabetes)
Rejection of implanted tissue-engineered constructs	Application of strategies to reduce inflammation or fibrosis
Appropriate cell source to provide best regenerative integration with minimal fibrosis	Use of autologous cell sources (e.g., autologous bone marrow or iPS cells)
	Testing various cell sources for best regenerative capability and limited fibrosis

iPS = induced pluripotent stem.

However, the transforming potential of viral vectors presently required for efficient transduction of cells to an iPS state has raised safety concerns.

Summary

The fields of tissue engineering and regenerative medicine have had modest success in recent years with respect to replacing lost or damaged body tissues and organs. Controlling the complex foreign body reaction remains a challenge in the implantation of tissue-engineered scaffolds because most tissue-engineered replacements result in some degree of fibrosis after implantation. Induction of the wound healing response can be expected because a certain level of tissue injury must be created during the implantation of a tissue-engineered construct. Years of study in the skin have shown that attaining appropriate control of inflammation and the wound healing response can lead to faster healing and reduction of scarring after cutaneous wounding. Modulation of the foreign body reaction and wound healing by various pharmacological agents has led to reduction in the degree of fibrous capsule formation around synthetic implants in various tissues. Application of these approaches in the implantation of tissue-engineered constructs may lead to better integration and improved function of the targeted tissue. Although the prospect for advancement is good, a number of obstacles still need to be overcome. Table 14-1 provides a summary of some of these challenges to progress.

References

1. Anderson, J.M., A. Rodriguez, and D.T. Chang, *Foreign body reaction to biomaterials.* Semin Immunol, 2008. 20(2): p. 86–100.

2. Clark, R., *Wound Repair Overview and General Considerations.* The Molecular and Cellular Biology of Wound Repair, ed. R. Clark. 1996, New York: Plenum Press. 3–50.

3. Singer, A.J. and R.A. Clark, *Cutaneous wound healing.* N Engl J Med, 1999. 341(10): p. 738–46.

4. Werner, S. and R. Grose, *Regulation of wound healing by growth factors and cytokines.* Physiol Rev, 2003. 83(3): p. 835–70.

5. Wells, A., A. Huttenlocher, and D.A. Lauffenburger, *Calpain proteases in cell adhesion and motility.* Int Rev Cytol, 2005. 245: p. 1–16.

6. Nanney, L.B., et al., *Novel approaches for understanding the mechanisms of wound repair.* J Investig Dermatol Symp Proc, 2006. 11(1): p. 132–9.

7. Li, J., J. Chen, and R. Kirsner, *Pathophysiology of acute wound healing.* Clin Dermatol, 2007. 25(1): p. 9–18.

8. Doshi, B.M., G.A. Perdrizet, and L.E. Hightower, *Wound healing from a cellular stress response perspective.* Cell Stress Chaperones, 2008. 13(4): p. 393–9.

9. Shaw, T.J. and P. Martin, *Wound repair at a glance.* J Cell Sci, 2009. 122(Pt 18): p. 3209–13.

10. Kwan, P., et al., *Scar and contracture: biological principles.* Hand Clin, 2009. 25(4): p. 511–28.

11. Guo, S. and L.A. Dipietro, *Factors affecting wound healing.* J Dent Res. 89(3): p. 219–29.

12. Palatinus, J.A., J.M. Rhett, and R.G. Gourdie, *Translational lessons from scarless healing of cutaneous wounds and regenerative repair of the myocardium.* J Mol Cell Cardiol. 48(3): p. 550–7.

13. Hocking, A.M. and N.S. Gibran, *Mesenchymal stem cells: paracrine signaling and differentiation during cutaneous wound repair.* Exp Cell Res. 316(14): p. 2213–9.

14. Lossing, C. and H.A. Hansson, *Peptide growth factors and myofibroblasts in capsules around human breast implants.* Plast Reconstr Surg, 1993. 91(7): p. 1277–86.

15. Reish, R.G. and E. Eriksson, *Scar treatments: preclinical and clinical studies.* J Am Coll Surg, 2008. 206(4): p. 719–30.

16. Ratner, B.D., *Biomaterials science: an introduction to materials in medicine.* 2nd ed. 2004, Amsterdam; Boston: Elsevier Academic Press. xii, 851 p.

17. Corr, D.T., et al., *Biomechanical behavior of scar tissue and uninjured skin in a porcine model.* Wound Repair Regen, 2009. 17(2): p. 250–9.

18. Kalfa, D., et al., *A polydioxanone electrospun valved patch to replace the right ventricular outflow tract in a growing lamb model.* Biomaterials, 2010. 31(14): p. 4056–63.

19. Kim, S.M., S.K. Lee, and J.H. Lee, *Peripheral nerve regeneration using a three dimensionally cultured schwann cell conduit.* J Craniofac Surg, 2007. 18(3): p. 475–88.

20. Murphy, G.F., D.P. Orgill, and I.V. Yannas, *Partial dermal regeneration is induced by biodegradable collagen-glycosaminoglycan grafts.* Lab Invest, 1990. 62(3): p. 305–13.

21. Ferguson, M.W. and S. O'Kane, *Scar-free healing: from embryonic mechanisms to adult therapeutic intervention.* Philos Trans R Soc Lond B Biol Sci, 2004. 359(1445): p. 839–50.

22. Martin, P. and S.M. Parkhurst, *Parallels between tissue repair and embryo morphogenesis.* Development, 2004. 131(13): p. 3021–34.

23. Bullard, K.M., M.T. Longaker, and H.P. Lorenz, *Fetal wound healing: current biology.* World J Surg, 2003. 27(1): p. 54–61.

24. Buchanan, E.P., M.T. Longaker, and H.P. Lorenz, *Fetal skin wound healing*. Adv Clin Chem, 2009. 48: p. 137–61.

25. Strecker, E.P., et al., *Effect on intimal hyperplasia of dexamethasone released from coated metal stents compared with non-coated stents in canine femoral arteries.* Cardiovasc Intervent Radiol. 1998. 21(6) p. 487–96.

26. Wu, K.K., *Cyclooxygenase 2 induction: molecular mechanism and pathophysiologic roles*. J Lab Clin Med, 1996. 128(3): p. 242–5.

27. Friedman, H.I., et al., *A biomechanical and morphologic analysis of capsule formation around implanted piezoelectric wafer active sensors in rats treated with cyclooxygenase-2 inhibition*. Ann Plast Surg, 2008. 60(2): p. 198–203.

28. Wilgus, T.A., et al., *Topical application of a selective cyclooxygenase inhibitor suppresses UVB mediated cutaneous inflammation*. Prostaglandins Other Lipid Mediat, 2000. 62(4): p. 367–84.

29. Wilgus, T.A., et al., *Reduction of scar formation in full-thickness wounds with topical celecoxib treatment*. Wound Repair Regen, 2003. 11(1): p. 25–34.

30. Panchenko, M.V., et al., *Metalloproteinase activity secreted by fibrogenic cells in the processing of prolysyl oxidase. Potential role of procollagen C-proteinase*. J Biol Chem, 1996. 271(12): p. 7113–9.

31. Reid, R.R., et al., *Inhibition of procollagen C-proteinase reduces scar hypertrophy in a rabbit model of cutaneous scarring*. Wound Repair Regen, 2006. 14(2): p. 138–41.

32. Kim, I., et al., *Inhibition of prolyl 4-hydroxylase reduces scar hypertrophy in a rabbit model of cutaneous scarring*. Wound Repair Regen, 2003. 11(5): p. 368–72.

33. Chung, H.J., et al., *Collagen fibril formation. A new target to limit fibrosis*. J Biol Chem, 2008. 283(38): p. 25879–86.

34. Schnee, J.M. and W.A. Hsueh, *Angiotensin II, adhesion, and cardiac fibrosis*. Cardiovasc Res, 2000. 46(2): p. 264–8.

35. Steckelings, U.M., et al., *Human skin: source of and target organ for angiotensin II*. Exp Dermatol, 2004. 13(3): p. 148–54.

36. Abiko, M., et al., *Acceleration of dermal tissue repair by angiotensin II*. Wound Repair Regen, 1997. 5(2): p. 175–83.

37. Takeda, H., et al., *Effects of angiotensin II receptor signaling during skin wound healing*. Am J Pathol, 2004. 165(5): p. 1653–62.

38. Morihara, K., et al., *Cutaneous tissue angiotensin-converting enzyme may participate in pathologic scar formation in human skin*. J Am Acad Dermatol, 2006. 54(2): p. 251–7.

39. Suzuki, Y., et al., *Inflammation and angiotensin II*. Int J Biochem Cell Biol, 2003. 35(6): p. 881–900.

40. Bader, M., et al., *Tissue renin-angiotensin systems: new insights from experimental animal models in hypertension research*. J Mol Med, 2001. 79(2–3): p. 76–102.

41. Engeli, S., R. Negrel, and A.M. Sharma, *Physiology and pathophysiology of the adipose tissue renin-angiotensin system*. Hypertension, 2000. 35(6): p. 1270–7.

42. Bataller, R., et al., *Activated human hepatic stellate cells express the renin-angiotensin system and synthesize angiotensin II*. Gastroenterology, 2003. 125(1): p. 117–25.

43. Perretti, M. and A. Ahluwalia, *The microcirculation and inflammation: site of action for glucocorticoids*. Microcirculation, 2000. 7(3): p. 147–61.

44. Galeska, I., et al., *Controlled release of dexamethasone from PLGA microspheres embedded within polyacid-containing PVA hydrogels*. AAPS J, 2005. 7(1): p. E231–40.

45. Quinn, C.A., R.E. Connor, and A. Heller, *Biocompatible, glucose-permeable hydrogel for in situ coating of implantable biosensors*. Biomaterials, 1997. 18(24): p. 1665–70.

46. Hickey, T., et al., *In vivo evaluation of a dexamethasone/PLGA microsphere system designed to suppress the inflammatory tissue response to implantable medical devices*. J Biomed Mater Res, 2002. 61(2): p. 180–7.

47. Bhardwaj, U., et al., *PLGA/PVA hydrogel composites for long-term inflammation control following s.c. implantation.* Int J Pharm, 2010. 384(1–2): p. 78–86.

48. Patil, S.D., F. Papadmitrakopoulos, and D.J. Burgess, *Concurrent delivery of dexamethasone and VEGF for localized inflammation control and angiogenesis.* J Control Release, 2007. 117(1): p. 68–79.

49. Draye, J.P., et al., *In vitro and in vivo biocompatibility of dextran dialdehyde cross-linked gelatin hydrogel films.* Biomaterials, 1998. 19(18): p. 1677–87.

50. Vercruysse, K.P. and G.D. Prestwich, *Hyaluronate derivatives in drug delivery.* Crit Rev Ther Drug Carrier Syst, 1998. 15(5): p. 513–55.

51. Morra, M., *Engineering of biomaterials surfaces by hyaluronan.* Biomacromolecules, 2005. 6(3): p. 1205–23.

52. Yadav, A.K., P. Mishra, and G.P. Agrawal, *An insight on hyaluronic acid in drug targeting and drug delivery.* J Drug Target, 2008. 16(2): p. 91–107.

53. Price, R.D., et al., *A comparison of tissue-engineered hyaluronic acid dermal matrices in a human wound model.* Tissue Eng, 2006. 12(10): p. 2985–95.

54. Lin, C.M., et al., *Hyaluronic acid inhibits the glial scar formation after brain damage with tissue loss in rats.* Surg Neurol, 2009. 72 Suppl 2: p. S50–4.

55. Pardo, A., et al., *Up-regulation and profibrotic role of osteopontin in human idiopathic pulmonary fibrosis.* PLoS Med, 2005. 2(9): p. e251.

56. Lee, S.H., et al., *Effects and regulation of osteopontin in rat hepatic stellate cells.* Biochem Pharmacol, 2004. 68(12): p. 2367–78.

57. Singh, M., et al., *Osteopontin: role in extracellular matrix deposition and myocardial remodeling post-MI.* J Mol Cell Cardiol, 2010. 48(3): p. 538–43. 42.

58. Cooper, L., et al., *Wound healing and inflammation genes revealed by array analysis of 'macrophageless' PU.1 null mice.* Genome Biol, 2005. 6(1): p. R5.

59. Mori, R., T.J. Shaw, and P. Martin, *Molecular mechanisms linking wound inflammation and fibrosis: knockdown of osteopontin leads to rapid repair and reduced scarring.* J Exp Med, 2008. 205(1): p. 43–51.

60. Bettinger, D.A., et al., *The effect of TGF-beta on keloid fibroblast proliferation and collagen synthesis.* Plast Reconstr Surg, 1996. 98(5): p. 827–33.

61. Verrecchia, F., M.L. Chu, and A. Mauviel, *Identification of novel TGF-beta /Smad gene targets in dermal fibroblasts using a combined cDNA microarray/promoter transactivation approach.* J Biol Chem, 2001. 276(20): p. 17058–62.

62. Wang, X., et al., *Exogenous transforming growth factor beta(2) modulates collagen I and collagen III synthesis in proliferative scar xenografts in nude rats.* J Surg Res, 1999. 87(2): p. 194–200.

63. Lanning, D.A., et al., *TGF-beta1 alters the healing of cutaneous fetal excisional wounds.* J Pediatr Surg, 1999. 34(5): p. 695–700.

64. Peltonen, J., et al., *Evaluation of transforming growth factor beta and type I procollagen gene expression in fibrotic skin diseases by in situ hybridization.* J Invest Dermatol, 1990. 94(3): p. 365–71.

65. Blobe, G.C., W.P. Schiemann, and H.F. Lodish, *Role of transforming growth factor beta in human disease.* N Engl J Med, 2000. 342(18): p. 1350–8.

66. Chen, W., et al., *Ontogeny of expression of transforming growth factor-beta and its receptors and their possible relationship with scarless healing in human fetal skin.* Wound Repair Regen, 2005. 13(1): p. 68–75.

67. Cowin, A.J., et al., *Expression of TGF-beta and its receptors in murine fetal and adult dermal wounds.* Eur J Dermatol, 2001. 11(5): p. 424–31.

68. Lu, L., et al., *The temporal effects of anti-TGF-beta1, 2, and 3 monoclonal antibody on wound healing and hypertrophic scar formation.* J Am Coll Surg, 2005. 201(3): p. 391–7.

69. Shah, M., D.M. Foreman, and M.W. Ferguson, *Control of scarring in adult wounds by neutralising antibody to transforming growth factor beta.* Lancet, 1992. 339(8787): p. 213–4.

70. Choi, B.M., et al., *Control of scarring in adult wounds using antisense transforming growth factor-beta 1 oligodeoxynucleotides.* Immunol Cell Biol, 1996. 74(2): p. 144–50.

71. Cordeiro, M.F., et al., *Novel antisense oligonucleotides targeting TGF-beta inhibit in vivo scarring and improve surgical outcome.* Gene Ther, 2003. 10(1): p. 59–71.

72. Occleston, N.L., et al., *Prevention and reduction of scarring in the skin by transforming growth factor beta 3 (TGFbeta3): from laboratory discovery to clinical pharmaceutical.* J Biomater Sci Polym Ed, 2008. 19(8): p. 1047–63.

73. Kirchhoff, S., et al., *Reduced cardiac conduction velocity and predisposition to arrhythmias in connexin40-deficient mice.* Curr Biol, 1998. 8(5): p. 299–302.

74. Goldberg, G.S., P.D. Lampe, and B.J. Nicholson, *Selective transfer of endogenous metabolites through gap junctions composed of different connexins.* Nat Cell Biol, 1999. 1(7): p. 457–9.

75. Saez, J.C., et al., *Hepatocyte gap junctions are permeable to the second messenger, inositol 1,4,5-trisphosphate, and to calcium ions.* Proc Natl Acad Sci U S A, 1989. 86(8): p. 2708–12.

76. Chanson, M., et al., *Gap junctional communication in tissue inflammation and repair.* Biochim Biophys Acta, 2005. 1711(2): p. 197–207.

77. Cook, J.E. and D.L. Becker, *Gap-junction proteins in retinal development: new roles for the "nexus."* Physiology (Bethesda), 2009. 24: p. 219–30.

78. Giepmans, B.N., *Gap junctions and connexin-interacting proteins.* Cardiovasc Res, 2004. 62(2): p. 233–45.

79. Lin, J.H., et al., *Gap-junction-mediated propagation and amplification of cell injury.* Nat Neurosci, 1998. 1(6): p. 494–500.

80. Haupt, C., O.W. Witte, and C. Frahm, *Up-regulation of Connexin43 in the glial scar following photothrombotic ischemic injury.* Mol Cell Neurosci, 2007. 35(1): p. 89–99.

81. Kasper, M., et al., *Upregulation of gap junction protein connexin43 in alveolar epithelial cells of rats with radiation-induced pulmonary fibrosis.* Histochem Cell Biol, 1996. 106(4): p. 419–24.

82. Nakano, Y., et al., *Connexin43 knockdown accelerates wound healing but inhibits mesenchymal transition after corneal endothelial injury in vivo.* Invest Ophthalmol Vis Sci, 2008. 49(1): p. 93–104.

83. Qiu, C., et al., *Targeting connexin43 expression accelerates the rate of wound repair.* Curr Biol, 2003. 13(19): p. 1697–703.

84. Gourdie, R.G., et al., *The unstoppable connexin43 carboxyl-terminus: new roles in gap junction organization and wound healing.* Ann N Y Acad Sci, 2006. 1080: p. 49–62.

85. Ghatnekar, G.S., et al., *Connexin43 carboxyl-terminal peptides reduce scar progenitor and promote regenerative healing following skin wounding.* Regen Med, 2009. 4(2): p. 205–23.

86. Hunter, A.W., et al., *Zonula occludens-1 alters connexin43 gap junction size and organization by influencing channel accretion.* Mol Biol Cell, 2005. 16(12): p. 5686–98.

87. Rhett, J.M., et al., *Novel therapies for scar reduction and regenerative healing of skin wounds.* Trends Biotechnol, 2008. 26(4): p. 173–80.

88. Soder, B.L., et al., *The connexin43 carboxyl-terminal peptide ACT1 modulates the biological response to silicone implants.* Plast Reconstr Surg, 2009. 123(5): p. 1440–51.

89. Nomi, M., et al., *Principals of neovascularization for tissue engineering.* Mol Aspects Med, 2002. 23(6): p. 463–83.

90. Vunjak-Novakovic, G., et al., *Challenges in cardiac tissue engineering.* Tissue Eng Part B Rev. 16(2): p. 169–87.

91. Badylak, S.F., *The extracellular matrix as a biologic scaffold material.* Biomaterials, 2007. 28(25): p. 3587–93.

92. Pfister, B.J., et al., *Neural engineering to produce in vitro nerve constructs and neurointerface.* Neurosurgery, 2007. 60(1): p. 137–41; discussion 141–2.

93. Dallon, J.C. and H.P. Ehrlich, *A review of fibroblast-populated collagen lattices.* Wound Repair Regen, 2008. 16(4): p. 472–9.

94. Frohlich, M., et al., *Tissue engineered bone grafts: biological requirements, tissue culture and clinical relevance.* Curr Stem Cell Res Ther, 2008. 3(4): p. 254–64.

95. Jackson, W.M., L.J. Nesti, and R.S. Tuan, *Potential therapeutic applications of muscle-derived mesenchymal stem and progenitor cells.* Expert Opin Biol Ther. 10(4): p. 505–17.

96. Visconti, R.P., et al., *Towards organ printing: engineering an intra-organ branched vascular tree.* Expert Opin Biol Ther. 10(3): p. 409–20.

97. Atala, A., *Recent applications of regenerative medicine to urologic structures and related tissues.* Curr Opin Urol, 2006. 16(4): p. 305–9.

98. Ten Broek, R.W., S. Grefte, and J.W. Von den Hoff, *Regulatory factors and cell populations involved in skeletal muscle regeneration.* J Cell Physiol, 2010. 224(1): p. 7–16.

99. Aviss, K.J., J.E. Gough, and S. Downes, *Aligned electrospun polymer fibres for skeletal muscle regeneration.* Eur Cell Mater, 2010. 19: p. 193–204.

100. Choi, J.S., et al., *The influence of electrospun aligned poly(epsilon-caprolactone)/collagen nanofiber meshes on the formation of self-aligned skeletal muscle myotubes.* Biomaterials, 2008. 29(19): p. 2899–906.

101. Thorrez, L., et al., *Growth, differentiation, transplantation and survival of human skeletal myofibers on biodegradable scaffolds.* Biomaterials, 2008. 29(1): p. 75–84.

102. Fann, S.A., et al., *A model of tissue-engineered ventral hernia repair.* J Invest Surg, 2006. 19(3): p. 193–205.

103. Custer, R.P., G.C. Bosma, and M.J. Bosma, *Severe combined immunodeficiency (SCID) in the mouse.* Pathology, reconstitution, neoplasms. Am J Pathol, 1985. 120(3): p. 464–77.

104. Michaels, J.T., et al., *Db/db mice exhibit severe wound-healing impairments compared with other murine diabetic strains in a silicone-splinted excisional wound model.* Wound Repair Regen, 2007. 15(5): p. 665–70.

105. Devereux, D.F., et al., *The quantitative and qualitative impairment of wound healing by adriamycin.* Cancer, 1979. 43(3): p. 932–8.

106. Costa, R.A., et al., *Effects of strain and age on ear wound healing and regeneration in mice.* Braz J Med Biol Res, 2009. 42(12): p. 1143–9.

107. Li, Y., H. Pan, and J. Huard, *Isolating stem cells from soft musculoskeletal tissues.* J Vis Exp, 2010; 41: pii: 2011. (video).

108. Kwan, M.D., et al., *Cell-based therapies for skeletal regenerative medicine.* Hum Mol Genet, 2008. 17(R1): p. R93–8.

109. Fang, R.C. and T.A. Mustoe, *Animal models of wound healing: utility in transgenic mice.* J Biomater Sci Polym Ed, 2008. 19(8): p. 989–1005.

110. Custer, R.P., G.C. Bosma, and M.J. Bosma, *Severe combined immunodeficiency (SCID) in the mouse.* Pathology, reconstitution, neoplasms. Am J Pathol, 1985. 120(3): p. 464–77.

111. Michaels, J.t., et al., *db/db mice exhibit severe wound-healing impairments compared with other murine diabetic strains in a silicone-splinted excisional wound model.* Wound Repair Regen, 2007. 15(5): p. 665–70.

112. Devereux, D.F., et al., *The quantitative and qualitative impairment of wound healing by adriamycin.* Cancer, 1979. 43(3): p. 932–8.

113. Costa, R.A., et al., *Effects of strain and age on ear wound healing and regeneration in mice*. Braz J Med Biol Res, 2009. 42(12): p. 1143–9.
114. Lengner, C.J., *iPS cell technology in regenerative medicine*. Ann N Y Acad Sci. 1192(1): p. 38–44.
115. McDevitt, T.C. and S.P. Palecek, *Innovation in the culture and derivation of pluripotent human stem cells*. Curr Opin Biotechnol, 2008. 19(5): p. 527–33.
116. Brignier, A.C. and A.M. Gewirtz, *Embryonic and adult stem cell therapy*. J Allergy Clin Immunol. 125(2 Suppl 2): p. S336–44.
117. Teramoto, K., et al., *Teratoma formation and hepatocyte differentiation in mouse liver transplanted with mouse embryonic stem cell-derived embryoid bodies*. Transplant Proc, 2005. 37(1): p. 285–6.
118. Brederlau, A., et al., *Transplantation of human embryonic stem cell-derived cells to a rat model of Parkinson's disease: effect of in vitro differentiation on graft survival and teratoma formation*. Stem Cells, 2006. 24(6): p. 1433–40.
119. Vassalli, G., et al., *Modalities and future prospects of gene therapy in heart transplantation*. Eur J Cardiothorac Surg, 2009. 35(6): p. 1036–44.
120. Sbano, P., et al., *Use of donor bone marrow mesenchymal stem cells for treatment of skin allograft rejection in a preclinical rat model*. Arch Dermatol Res, 2008. 300(3): p. 115–24.

15

The Past, Present, and Future of Tissue Regeneration

M. NATALIA VERGARA AND PANAGIOTIS A. TSONIS

The study of regeneration is probably one of the most fascinating and ancient human quests, one that holds the potential of impacting human life not only by providing novel medical strategies but also by challenging our understanding of biology and evolution in general.

The idea of regenerating an amputated body part has been engrained in human imagination since the beginnings of civilization, and testimonies to that account can be found from the texts of ancient Egypt to Greek mythology to Middle Age writings (Sanchez Alvarado, 2000; Tsonis, 2000; Stocum, 2004). The eighteenth-century natural philosopher René-Antoine Ferchault de Reaumur was probably the first to scientifically describe the regeneration of crayfish limbs and claws (reviewed in Dinsmore, 1992; Okada, 1996). He was followed in the 1740s by the works of the Swiss scientists Abraham Trembley and Charles Bonet, who described the complete regeneration of hydra and earthworms upon resection (Galliot, 2012). And in the 1760s, Lazzaro Spallanzani published the first work on the ability of salamanders to regenerate their limbs, jaws, and tails (Dinsmore, 1991; Okada, 1996; Sanchez Alvarado, 2000; Tsonis and Fox, 2009). Since then, the field of regenerative biology has made remarkable progress, making significant contributions along its way to the study of embryology and genetics (Dinsmore, 1992; Okada, 1996). Still, it is interesting to ponder that the fundamental questions have remained the same: What determines the capacity of a tissue to regenerate? Why don't different tissues adopt similar regenerative strategies? Why can newts regenerate almost any body part but humans cannot? Can we harness such potential?

In addition, the advent of the evolutionary theory in the nineteenth century brought about further questions to the study of regeneration. This is because, as complex and diverse as a biologic phenomenon can be, regeneration is intriguingly widespread in the animal world. However, the fact that this ability is not universal and that closely related species can vary extensively in their response to injury has made the issue of the evolution of the regenerative capacity a controversial one (Sanchez

311

Alvarado, 2000; Brockes et al., 2001; Brockes and Kumar, 2008; Bely and Nyberg, 2010).

To facilitate this discussion, we will resort to a broad definition of regeneration as the morphologic and functional restoration of an injured tissue or body part. This restoration can be achieved to varying degrees depending on the type of tissue; the size of the lesion; the age of the animal; and, as mentioned before, the animal species (Tsonis, 2000; Vergara et al., 2005; Sanchez Alvarado and Tsonis, 2006; Cai et al., 2007; Brockes and Kumar, 2008; Bely and Nyberg, 2010). Correspondingly, different strategies are used in the different scenarios, from simple proliferation of mature cells such as that observed in liver regeneration in mammals, to the use of stem cells to reconstitute amputated body parts in planarias, to the more dramatic process of transdifferentiation observed in lens regeneration in salamanders (Tsonis, 2000; Vergara et al., 2005; Sanchez Alvarado and Tsonis, 2006; Cai et al., 2007; Brockes and Kumar, 2008; Bely and Nyberg, 2010; Eguchi et al., 2011). This diversity points to the complexity of the regenerative phenomenon as a multistep process and to the numerous mechanisms that have to be in place to modulate each of its stages. However, common ground has been found among these different mechanisms, and that understanding has driven us closer than we have ever been to translating the basic science of regeneration into clinical applications. This is in no small part because of the development over the past few decades of the new field of regenerative medicine, which combines aspects of biomedical engineering, materials science, and regenerative biology with the aim of repairing or replacing damaged body parts (Cai et al., 2007; Tsonis, 2007; Baddour et al., 2012).

In this chapter, we will attempt to give a general overview of the current knowledge in the field of regenerative biology, its implications about the past, and its applications to the future.

Lessons from the Past: The Evolution of Regeneration

Broadly defined, regeneration is a prevalent phenomenon throughout the animal kingdom, and examples can be found in almost every phylum (Sanchez Alvarado, 2000; Tsonis, 2000; Brockes et al., 2001; Brockes and Kumar, 2008; Bely and Nyberg, 2010). However, a closer look at the variety of mechanisms that operate under that name can obscure the drawing of definitive conclusions.

Several events need to take place if the functional restoration of an injured body part is to be achieved. First, there needs to be a response to the injury, that is, a mechanism that senses the extent of the loss and initiates a wound healing process. Second, cellular precursors have to be generated or recruited in response to that stimulus. And third, a morphogenetic process has to occur to restore the morphology and physiological properties of the lost tissue (Brockes and Kumar, 2008). At each step, finely regulated control mechanisms must be in place to ensure the regeneration of the correct number and size of structures, in the right position and orientation, and without the concomitant generation of unwanted side effects such as excessive growth or tumor formation.

The animal world has made use of an array of strategies to achieve this goal. Is that an indication that the regenerative capacity evolved independently in the different phyla (also known as convergent evolution)? Not necessarily because some common ground has been found among such strategies that could point to the alternative hypothesis: that regeneration is a primordial characteristic of metazoans (Goss, 1992; Sanchez Alvarado, 2000; Brockes et al., 2001; Brockes and Kumar, 2002, 2008; Bely and Nyberg, 2010). We will discuss the evidence supporting these hypotheses in the context of the different steps involved in the regenerative process.

Response to Injury

The mechanisms of response to injury are probably the least clearly understood because they could involve many potential signals (Brockes and Kumar, 2008; Yokoyama, 2008). To illustrate this point, one intriguing example of a seemingly conserved mechanism is the use of bioelectrical signals (Levin, 2007). In this regard, reducing the transepithelial potential after limb amputation in newts resulted in a certain level of inhibition of regeneration, as did the inhibition of a V-ATPase proton pump during tail regeneration in larval *Xenopus*, which also altered the membrane voltage at the injury site (Jenkins et al., 1996; Adams et al., 2007; Levin, 2007). Moreover, in planaria, the polarity of regeneration could be altered by the application of an electric field (Carlson, 2007). Are these phenomena mechanistically related, and if so, do they remain true in other animal species? If the answer to these questions is yes, then this would provide some indirect support to the hypothesis of a single evolutionary origin of regeneration. However, until further studies are done to elucidate the underlying mechanisms of action of bioelectrical signals, this issue will remain in the realm of speculation.

Generation of Precursors

In contrast to the injury response, the origin of the cellular precursors that regenerate lost tissues has been better characterized in most cases. Already in 1901, T.H. Morgan identified two modes of regeneration according to their cellular source: morphallaxis, in which existing cells are redeployed without proliferation, and epimorphosis or regeneration, which requires cell proliferation (Morgan, 1901; Sanchez Alvarado, 2000; Brockes et al., 2001). The latter could be subsequently divided into three different subtypes: proliferation of differentiated cells; recruitment, proliferation, and differentiation of resident stem cells; and transdifferentiation or dedifferentiation of mature cell types involving reprogramming (Sanchez Alvarado, 2000; Tsonis, 2000; Brockes et al., 2001; Stocum, 2004; Sanchez Alvarado and Tsonis, 2006).

Hydra regeneration is the prototypical example of morphallaxis. When these microscopic fresh-water Cnidarians are cut into pieces, each segment is able to generate an entire, albeit smaller, body without creating new material (Galliot, 1997, 2012; Sanchez Alvarado and Tsonis, 2006; Bosch, 2007). This capacity, which generated controversies about the concept of identity when it was first described in 1744, has been one of the main arguments attempting to link the evolutionary origins of regeneration to asexual reproduction (Sanchez Alvarado, 2000; Tsonis, 2000; Brockes and Kumar, 2008). On the other hand, examples of regeneration through proliferation of differentiated cells are given by liver and gastrointestinal mucosa regeneration in mammals (Michalopoulos and DeFrances, 1997; Jones et al., 1999; Tsonis, 2000; Sanchez Alvarado and Tsonis, 2006).

Epimorphic regeneration using undifferentiated stem or progenitor cells is observed in organisms such as planarias, in which bisection of the body leads to the recruitment of undifferentiated cells called neoblasts to the injury site, where they form a specialized structure known as the regeneration blastema (Baguna, 1998; Agata and Watanabe, 1999; Newmark and Alvarado, 2000). The blastema consists of an outer epithelial layer or wound epithelium covering the mass of undifferentiated cells. Those cells then proliferate and differentiate to form the missing body structures. In planarias, the end result is the formation of a complete animal from each body fragment (Baguna, 1998; Agata and Watanabe, 1999; Newmark and Alvarado, 2000). Another example of this mechanism seems to be heart regeneration in zebrafish, in which resident stem cells have been proposed to regenerate the missing tissue through blastema formation (Lepilina et al., 2006).

The third type of epimorphic regeneration is probably the most striking, and it involves reprogramming of already differentiated cells that revert to a progenitor stem cell-like state. We can see this type during newt limb regeneration in which, for example, muscle de-differentiates to form muscle or bone de-differentiates to form bone. Newts can also regenerate body parts through a process of transdifferentiation – after de-differentiation, the original cell changes to another cell type. This is clear during lens regeneration when the pigmented epithelial cells from the iris de-differentiate and then transdifferentiate to lens, a process that is faithfully reproduced independently of the age of the animal or the number of times that the lens is removed (Eguchi et al., 2011).

In any case, when discussing cellular sources of regeneration, it should be noted that even though the prevalent contribution of one cellular source has been established in most situations, the possible involvement of other mechanisms cannot usually be discarded. Moreover, different regenerative strategies can be used by the same animal to restore different tissues (Tsonis, 2000; Del Rio-Tsonis and Tsonis, 2003).

As for the evolutionary relationship of these mechanisms, questions abound, but there is no definitive answer to be found at this time. However, the pursuit of those answers is bound to bring interesting insights to our understanding of evolutionary relationships and therefore to the fundamental question of why some animal species can regenerate but others are more limited in that capacity. Still, some light can be shed on this issue by comparative analysis. In this regard, one noteworthy example of conservation of regenerative strategy is the case of blastema formation. This structure has a striking morphologic, molecular, and functional resemblance to the vertebrate embryonic limb bud (Imokawa and Yoshizato, 1997). The formation of a blastema during regeneration in a variety of organisms, such as the aforementioned planarias and mollusks; tail regeneration in newts and *Xenopus*; fin regeneration in zebrafish; wing regeneration in chicks; and limb regeneration in *Xenopus*, newts, axolotls, and embryonic mice, speaks to the importance of this structure as a common feature of regeneration (Geraudie and Singer, 1992; Reginelli et al., 1995; Tsonis, 1996, 2000; Christen and Slack, 1997; Sanchez Alvarado, 2000; Sanchez Alvarado and Tsonis, 2006; Mochii et al., 2007). Even though the same strategy could have been reinvented several times throughout evolution, the widespread distribution across such different phyla is more supportive of the idea that regeneration is a primordial trait of metazoans.

Morphogenesis

Finally, after the issue of generating appropriate progenitors is overcome, there is the problem of morphogenesis. Successful regeneration needs to reestablish the functional properties of the lost structure, which in most cases requires concomitant morphologic restoration. In this phase, the similarities with developmental processes cannot be overlooked. Even though the existence of a unique regenerative process of morphogenesis could be proposed, this possibility seems highly unlikely. It is more reasonable to assume that this phase of regeneration might co-opt mechanisms that existed during the ontogeny of the missing structure.

Morphogenesis involves the specification of positional information in every cell, the establishment of gradients of signaling molecules to define body axes, and the precise expression of transcription factors that lead to appropriate cellular differentiation, a process that by nature requires multiple steps. In this context, there is a high level of conservation of developmental pathways across many animal species, and numerous examples exist of reactivation of such pathways during tissue regeneration. One such example is the case of the products of *Hox* genes, which have been demonstrated to determine positional identity during the development of a wide range of animals and are reexpressed during regeneration in hydra, planarias, newt limbs, and zebrafish fins (Schummer et al., 1992; Bayascas et al., 1997; Gauchat et al., 2000; Tsonis, 2000; Sanchez Alvarado and Tsonis, 2006). A particularly interesting case is that of the homeobox-containing gene *Pax-6*, which encodes a transcription factor responsible for controlling eye development in organisms ranging from flat worms to *Drosophila* to humans. This transcription factor is reexpressed during eye regeneration in planaria, retina regeneration in newts and chicks, and lens regeneration in newts and *Xenopus*, just to name a few (Del Rio-Tsonis et al., 1995; Callaerts et al., 1999; Kaneko et al., 1999; Mizuno et al., 1999; Makar'ev et al., 2002; Spence et al., 2007).

In addition to transcription factors, secreted morphogenetic signaling molecules such as Hedgehog, bone morphogenetic proteins (BMPs), retinoic acid (RA), fibroblast growth factors (FGFs) and Wnt, all of which play numerous roles in the establishment of axes and cell type specification during development, are recruited again to regulate regeneration in a variety of cases (Lawrence, 2001; Vergara et al., 2005). Just to give some examples, Hedgehog signaling has been shown to play crucial roles in lens regeneration in newts; limb regeneration in newts, axolotls, and *Xenopus* tadpoles; fin regeneration in zebrafish; tail regeneration in axolotls and *Xenopus*; and retina regeneration in chicks and mice (Imokawa and Yoshizato, 1997; Endo et al., 1999; Torok et al., 1999; Spence et al., 2004, 2007; Tsonis et al., 2004; Schnapp et al., 2005; Avaron et al., 2007; Mochii et al., 2007). BMP signaling, another highly conserved morphogenetic pathway with important roles in development, has also been found to play fundamental roles in lens regeneration in newts, digit tip regeneration in mice, and tail regeneration in *Xenopus* (Beck et al., 2003; Han et al., 2003; Grogg et al., 2005). Similar examples exist for the other aforementioned signaling molecules, making a strong the case for the argument that this phase of the regenerative process is as phylogenetically conserved as its developmental counterparts. Therefore, the likelihood that such mechanisms could have arisen independently during evolution is improbable.

Our understanding of the molecular mechanisms of regeneration has benefited tremendously from the rapid progress in the fields of development and genetics. However, the search for animal models that could be easily maintained in laboratory conditions, amenable to genetic manipulation, with large numbers and rapid generation of progeny to be used in scientific research, has generated a significant imbalance in the amount of knowledge accumulated on the now called "traditional" animal models in detriment of others. Unfortunately, the species that exhibit the best regenerative capacities are generally not included among the most favored models (Sanchez Alvarado, 2000). The discussions on the evolution of regeneration have been largely powered by comparative analysis across phylogeny, and the field would benefit greatly if the molecular tools now available for traditional models were applied to a broader range of organisms (Sanchez Alvarado, 2000; Sanchez Alvarado and Tsonis, 2006).

The Present and Future of Regeneration: Contributions to Regenerative Medicine

We are now at an unprecedented point in the history of regenerative biology. Despite the limitations already described, the scientific advances over the past few decades have exponentially increased our understanding of the mechanisms of regeneration

(Stoick-Cooper et al., 2007; Barbosa-Sabanero et al., 2012), and the advent of regenerative medicine is providing for the first time the opportunity to apply this knowledge to the improvement of human health.

Learning from the Similarities

As was the case with evolution, the molecular biology of regeneration is also gaining crucial insights from the comparison of similarities among animal species that possess regenerative abilities. For example, the development of RNAi screening technology applied to planarian regeneration has uncovered 240 genes that have roles in this process, 85 percent of which are conserved in other animals (Reddien et al., 2005a). One case is that of smedwi2, which belongs to the argonaute/PIWI family of proteins known to regulate stem cells in various organisms. Downregulation of this gene in planaria led to an inhibition of the ability of neoblasts to form a regeneration-competent blastema (Reddien et al., 2005b). Members of this family of proteins in mouse have been shown to be essential for the differentiation of germ cells into spermatocytes (Deng and Lin, 2002; Kuramochi-Miyagawa et al., 2004). These proteins represent interesting candidates to be tested for their involvement in other regenerating systems.

Another instance in which molecular similarities in regenerative mechanisms have been found in different species is that of retina regeneration through transdifferentiation. In embryonic chicks, upon retina removal, FGF signaling is able to induce the regeneration of a neural retina by stimulation of stem cells present in the ciliary body/ciliary marginal zone of the eye and by transdifferentiation of the retinal pigmented epithelial (RPE) cells in the posterior part of the eye. FGF administration leads to the activation of the mitogen-activated protein kinase (MAPK) pathway in the RPE cells, which lose their pigment, proliferate, and eventually give rise to a multilayered retina composed of all the different types of neurons and glia present in the normal one (Spence et al., 2007). The MAPK signaling pathway is also involved in the activation of RPE cells necessary for retina regeneration in adult newts, which takes place through a similar transdifferentiation process (Mizuno et al., 2012). Taking advantage of this knowledge, a new model of retina regeneration has recently been developed in which *Xenopus* tadpoles were successfully induced to regenerate a neural retina after complete removal by exogenous administration of FGF-2 (Vergara and Del Rio-Tsonis, 2009). Such regeneration seemed to take place through transdifferentiation of the pigmented epithelia of the eye and was shown to be mediated by the activation of the MAPK pathway by FGF receptors as well, demonstrating that the knowledge acquired in some systems can be applied to others (Vergara and Del Rio-Tsonis, 2009). Moreover, the development of regeneration models in organisms more amenable to genetic manipulations such as this has the potential to expand our understanding of the regenerative process as a result of the availability of different technical strategies.

Learning from the Differences

In addition to the approach discussed earlier, important knowledge has been gained by comparing the differences between regenerating and nonregenerating systems. This strategy provides the opportunity to test the possibility of inducing regeneration in normally incapable tissues or animals by overcoming those differences. The case of lens regeneration in adult newts illustrates this point. In these animals, the lens regenerates through transdifferentiation of the pigmented epithelial cells at the tip of the dorsal iris (Del Rio-Tsonis and Tsonis, 2003). Upon lentectomy, these cells de-differentiate to form a lens vesicle that in turn proliferates and redifferentiates into a lens epithelium and crystalline expressing lens fibers to restore a normal structure. Interestingly, the cells of the ventral iris, although morphologically indistinguishable from their dorsal counterparts, are unable to regenerate a lens. This difference constitutes an excellent model to test potential regeneration-inducing factors, which has led for example to the discovery of the role of six3, retinoic acid, and BMP in lens regeneration (Grogg et al., 2005). When the highly conserved transcription factor six3 is overexpressed in newt ventral iris cells in the presence of retinoic acid, these cells are able to transdifferentiate and form a lens. The same is true for the inhibition of BMP signaling by treatment with chordin in the ventral iris (Grogg et al., 2005). Because six3 was found to be expressed in both the intact dorsal and ventral iris but lens removal produced a higher increase in its expression in the dorsal cells, it has been proposed that an elevation of the levels of specific factors over a particular threshold is responsible for the induction of the regenerative ability (Grogg et al., 2005), a concept that has been reinforced by proteomic analysis (Roddy et al., 2008). On the other hand, the axolotl, another salamander with otherwise remarkable regenerative abilities, is unable to regenerate its eye tissues. However, if a newt's dorsal iris is transplanted into an axolotl's eye, it is still able to regenerate a lens, indicating that the axolotl's limitation is intrinsic to its tissues, not attributable to an inhibitory environmental signal (Tsonis et al., 2004). Therefore, comparisons of eye regeneration between these salamanders could also be useful for dissecting molecular mechanisms involved in the regenerative process. In this scenario, the development of molecular biology tools specific for these animals would be greatly beneficial, and some attempts in that regard are already underway. The sequencing of axolotl expressed sequence tags (ESTs) and the development of transgenic lines constitute some technologies that will prove useful in the study of regeneration (Habermann et al., 2004; Putta et al., 2004; Sobkow et al., 2006).

Another valuable example of this comparative approach is given by the regeneration of the tail in *Xenopus* tadpoles. These animals are able to regenerate their tails upon amputation, except for a refractory period between developmental stages 45 to 47 in which regeneration does not take place. This constitutes another paradigm for testing molecular pathways involved in the induction of the regeneration process. For example, it has been shown that expression of a constitutively active form of a

BMP receptor during the refractory period was sufficient to induce the regeneration of a normal tail (Beck et al., 2003). Expression of an activated form of Msx1 had a similar effect, while activation of Notch signaling led to imperfect regeneration. Confirming the role of these pathways, inhibition of either Notch or BMP signaling during regeneration permissive stages was able to hinder the regenerative process (Beck et al., 2003). An exciting parallel with these discoveries has been found for mammalian digit tip regeneration using the fetal mouse as a model system. Han et al. (2003) showed that regeneration is defective in Msx1 mutant mice, but expression of BMP-4 is able to rescue that defect. Conversely, BMP inhibition with Noggin can inhibit regeneration in wild-type animals. Moreover, an upregulation of Msx1 expression during regeneration was also demonstrated in an in vitro assay of human fetal digit tip regeneration (Allan et al., 2006).

Further demonstration of the success of comparing regenerating and nonregenerating systems for identifying inductive signals is found in the study of newt and mouse myotubes. When cultured newt myotubes are stimulated with serum, they are able to reenter the cell cycle, progress through S phase, and arrest in G2. This capacity is attributable to the serum induced inactivation of the retinoblastoma gene product (Rb) because transfection of newt myotubes with a plasmid encoding the $p16^{INK4}$ gene, an inhibitor of a protein kinase that inactivates Rb, prevents the cells from reentering the cell cycle (Tanaka et al., 1997). On the other hand, serum stimulation has no effect on mouse myotubes unless they lack both copies of the Rb gene (Schneider et al., 1994). The involvement of this gene in both cases suggests that a serum component is able to activate a pathway in newt and not in mouse cells that leads to Rb inactivation and the subsequent progression into S phase. However, if the activation of the pathway is circumvented, the result is the same in both cases, as demonstrated by the fact that hybrid myotubes resulting from the fusion of newt and mouse cells respond to serum by the cell cycle reentry of the nuclei from both species (Velloso et al., 2001). The identity of the inducing factor remains to be elucidated, but it has been suggested to be activated by the activity of the blood-clotting factor thrombin (Tanaka et al., 1999; Brockes and Kumar, 2002; Stoick-Cooper et al., 2007). Thrombin not only activates newt myotubes in culture, but its activity is also increased in the regenerating limb blastema and even in other instances of regeneration in newts such as that of the lens (Tanaka et al., 1999; Imokawa and Brockes, 2003; Imokawa et al., 2004). In addition, after retina removal in newts, thrombin can promote cell-cycle re-entry of RPE cells in a heparin-dependent manner (Yoshikawa et al., 2012). Finally, exposure of mouse myotubes to an extract of newt regenerating limb tissue is able to induce both cell cycle reentry and cleavage of the mouse myotubes into mononucleated cells, consolidating the idea that these mammalian cells retain the intracellular signaling pathways necessary for de-differentiation (McGann et al., 2001).

These are only some examples of the insights that can be gained by comparative analysis of the regenerative mechanisms across species, pinpointing the knowledge that could be achieved by the establishment of genetic and molecular biology tools for regenerative species, and emphasizing the likelihood of applying that knowledge to the induction of regeneration in mammalian systems.

Applications to Regenerative Medicine

Even if we understand some of the signaling pathways that modulate regeneration in different species, how realistic is the expectation that we could induce (and control) extensive regeneration in humans? The answer to this question might come from a different front (Tsonis, 2007).

Regenerative medicine exists at the intersection between regenerative and stem cell biology, materials science, and bioengineering. Its goal is to replace lost or damaged cells and tissues in the human body in order to restore their normal function (Gurtner et al., 2007). Different strategies are being developed to achieve this goal, including (1) cell transplantation, (2) transplantation of cell-seeded scaffolds or in vitro constructed bioartificial tissues, and (3) induction of endogenous regeneration (Odelberg, 2002; Stocum, 2004; Baddour et al., 2012). We will discuss each of these strategies here.

Cell Transplantation

This approach involves replacing the injured tissue by transplanting aggregates of donor cells. The source of the transplant can be mature cells from a donor, embryonic or adult stem cells induced to differentiate into the appropriate cell type, or transdifferentiation of other mature cells. The importance of the knowledge gained from developmental and regenerative biology in this strategy is evident.

The transplantation of mature cells has only limited applications because these cells are generally difficult to propagate in culture, so their supply is limited. This problem could be overcome by the use of pluripotent stem cell sources such as embryonic stem cells, which have the advantage of being able to replicate indefinitely in culture and to generate many different cell types. However, there are ethical and legal issues surrounding the use of these cells for therapeutic purposes because it involves the manipulation of human embryos. In addition, if the cells are not derived from the same patient, the matter of immune rejection needs to be addressed, generally by the use of immunosuppressive therapies that can cause further complications. And finally, the protocols for inducing the appropriate differentiation of these stem cells into specific cell types need to be optimized, and the tumorigenic potential of the cells needs to be controlled. Both of these issues require a deeper understanding of developmental processes, an understanding that would benefit from the knowledge gained from organisms that use a similar approach in their regenerative strategy.

In light of these limitations, the use of adult stem cells, especially those that could be derived from the same patient, would seem to be a more welcome approach.

However, the plasticity of these cells is more restricted than that of their embryonic counterparts, which means that the number of cell types that can be generated from them is limited and that their expansion capability in culture conditions is not as extensive as that of embryonic cells. Still, their relative specialization can make it easier to obtain certain differentiated cell types, and some sources of adult stem cells, such as the bone marrow, cornea, or umbilical cord, are easily accessible.

Another source of stem cells for transplantation that would bypass ethical and immune rejection constraints could come from the de-differentiation of mature cells. Only a few years ago, transdifferentiation potential was regarded as a privilege of lower vertebrate species. However, that concept has completely changed in recent years thanks to the development of induced pluripotent stem (iPS) cells from mouse and human sources (Takahashi and Yamanaka, 2006; Okita et al., 2007; reviewed in Tsonis, 2007; Baker, 2009). In 2006, Takahashi and Yamanaka published the first account of successful reprogramming of mouse fibroblasts by retrovirus-mediated induction of a cocktail of four genes: *Oct3/4*, *Sox2*, *c-Myc*, and *Klf4*. The fact that these cells were able to acquire pluripotency and resemble embryonic stem cells generated much excitement in the scientific community, and 10 months later, the same group published an improved version of this technique in which selection of the iPS cells for Nanog, another pluripotency-maintaining gene, rendered them capable of becoming germline competent, a clear indication of their pluripotent stem cell-like state (Okita et al., 2007). Since then, numerous groups have concentrated on improving the technologies for the production and manipulation of these cells and attempting to mitigate their tendency to generate tumors. The field is now growing rapidly and moving toward the production of iPS cells without the addition of reprogramming genes by using small molecules and inductive proteins instead (Baker, 2009). In 2012, Dr. Shinya Yamanaka was awarded the Nobel Prize in Physiology or Medicine for his work on iPS cells, which demonstrated that mature cells can be reprogrammed to become pluripotent. iPS cell technology holds much promise for medical applications, but it is now necessary to carefully evaluate the current protocols and established cells and learn how to harness their potential toward the adequate and controlled production of differentiated cell types (Drews et al., 2012). In this sense, it might be possible to gain some insights from the study of animals such as newts, which have made use of similar strategies for thousands of years, remaining at the same time amazingly refractory to tumor formation (Eguchi and Watanabe, 1973; Tsonis and Eguchi, 1982). It is worth noting that some of the same pluripotency factors necessary for the generation of iPS cells, namely *Sox2*, *Klf4* and *c-myc*, are up-regulated during lens and limb regeneration in newts (Maki et al., 2009).

Finally, despite being only in its beginnings, the cell transplantation approach has already yielded some successful therapeutic possibilities in humans, and more are underway based on their promising results in animal models (Mimeault and Batra, 2006; Stocum, 2004). The most successful and commonly used stem cell therapy is bone marrow transplant, which has been around for more than 40 years, while limbal stem cell transplantation has been used for corneal reconstruction for more than a decade. Conversely, the first clinical trial for the use of embryonic stem cells in humans has recently been approved for the treatment of spinal cord injury (Wadman, 2009).

Transplantation of Cell-Seeded Scaffolds or In Vitro Constructed Bioartificial Tissues

Tissue engineering focuses on the development of biological substitutes to replace damaged tissues (Gurtner et al., 2007). This approach brings together the impressive advances made in materials science on the generation of biocompatible scaffolds and the progress in stem cell biology discussed in the previous section. Scaffolds should not only provide the appropriate three-dimensional context but also the specific adhesive properties to optimize the attachment and migration of cells, as well as the necessary factors to drive their survival and differentiation. Both natural and synthetic materials – including novel nanobiomaterials – are being used in scaffold design to try to imitate the properties of the extracellular matrix found in the native tissues, and even nanoscale surface manipulation is being incorporated to promote adequate cell adhesion and migration (Gurtner, 2007; Czarnecki et al., 2012; Ilie et al., 2012). Moreover, new biodegradable and bioabsorbable materials are being developed for scaffold design to avoid inflammatory reactions after transplantation (Koh and Atala, 2004). In addition, knowledge acquired from stem cell, regenerative, and developmental biology is crucial in the design of bioartificial organs because there needs to be a thorough understanding of stem cell survival and differentiation cues to generate the required cell types.

This type of multidisciplinary approach stands a good chance of deriving viable tissues and organs for clinical applications (Tsonis, 2007; Sanchez-Lara et al., 2012). In fact, various types of bioartifical tissues are currently used or being tested for transplantation in animals and humans (Stockum, 2004). For example, biostatic allografts of skin and bone have been used for a long time in humans to treat burns and large wounds (Moreno-Borchart, 2004; Stocum, 2004; Olender et al., 2011), myocardial restoration using embryonic stem cell–seeded artificial scaffolds has been observed in rodents (Kofidis et al., 2005), functional bioartificial renal tissue has been developed in bovines (Lanza et al., 2002), and genital tissues have been bioartificially reconstructed in rabbit models (Kreshen et al., 2002; Kwon et al., 2002; Wang et al., 2003). Moreover, in humans, auricular reconstruction is currently performed using hand-carved autologous costal cartilage grafts or polyethylene implants, but numerous innovative alternative materials are currently being developed and tested for this purpose, in order to decrease morbidity, increase compatibility and improve shape (Sun et al., 2011; Bichara et al., 2012). In addition, clinical trials are under way with promising results for the transplantation of bioengineered bone to repair craniomax-illofacial bone defects, using autologous bone marrow derived stem cells and partially demineralized bone matrix (Sun et al., 2011). Finally, bone-marrow derived stem cells seeded onto a biological scaffold have also been used for tracheal replacement in humans (Elliot et al., 2012). These are only some of the examples that illustrate the tremendous potential of the combination of materials science and stem cell biology for the purpose of treatment in humans.

Induction of Endogenous Regeneration

Finally, the knowledge accumulated on the molecular mechanisms of regeneration could be applied to the modulation of endogenous regeneration. Attempting to trigger complete regeneration upon damage in a normally nonregenerating organism might be an unrealistic expectation. However, the implantation of biodegradable acellular matrices to aid in the regenerative process together with the delivery of inducing signals could recruit and activate local stem cells or enhance the regenerative capacity of normally more restrained tissues. The lessons from regenerative models described in this chapter provide numerous examples of candidate factors, and the development of small molecule therapies shows promise for its application in the induction of regenerative pathways and in the neutralization of inhibitory signals (Stocum, 2004; Ding and Schultz, 2005; Stoick-Cooper et al., 2007).

In summary, the field of regenerative medicine is a young one, and its full potential has not yet been unleashed. But the goal of providing humans with the capacity to replace damaged tissues, once thought to be just a dream, is rapidly becoming a reality, and the classic regenerative animal models have a lot to teach us about the mechanisms to achieve that goal.

References

Adams, D.S., Masi, A., and Levin, M. (2007). H+ pump-dependent changes in membrane voltage are an early mechanism necessary and sufficient to induce Xenopus tail regeneration. *Development* 134, 1323–1335.

Agata, K., and Watanabe, K. (1999). Molecular and cellular aspects of planarian regeneration. *Semin Cell Dev Biol* 10, 377–383.

Allan, C.H., Fleckman, P., Fernandes, R.J., Hager, B., James, J., Wisecarver, Z., Satterstrom, F.K., Gutierrez, A., Norman, A., Pirrone, A., et al. (2006). Tissue response and Msx1 expression after human fetal digit tip amputation in vitro. *Wound Repair Regen* 14, 398–404.

Avaron, F., Hoffman, L., Guay, D., and Akimenko, M.A. (2006). Characterization of two new zebrafish members of the hedgehog family: atypical expression of a zebrafish indian hedgehog gene in skeletal elements of both endochondral and dermal origins. *Dev Dyn* 235, 478–489.

Baddour, J. A., Sousounis, K., and Tsonis, P. A. (2012). Organ repair and regeneration: an overview. *Birth Defects Res C Embryo Today* 96, 1–29.

Baguñà J. (1998). Planarians. In: Cellular and Molecular Basis of Regeneration. From Invertebrates to Humans. P. Ferretti and J. Geraudie (eds.). John Wiley & Sons; Chichester, NY, USA; pp. 135–165.

Baker, M. (2009). iPS cells make mice that make mice. *Nature Reports Stem Cells* published online: 6 August 2009 | doi:10.1038/stemcells.2009.106

Barbosa-Sabanero, K., Hoffmann, A., Judge, C., Lightcap, N., Tsonis, P. A., and Del Rio-Tsonis, K. (2012). Lens and retina regeneration: new perspectives from model organisms. *Biochem J* 447, 321–334.

Bayascas, J.R., Castillo, E., MunozMarmol, A.M., and Salo, E. (1997). Planarian Hox genes: Novel patterns of expression during regeneration. *Development* 124, 141–148.

Beck, C.W., Christen, B., and Slack, J.M.W. (2003). Molecular pathways needed for regeneration of spinal cord and muscle in a vertebrate. *Dev Cell* 5, 429–439.

Bely A.E., and Nyberg K.G. (2010). Evolution of animal regeneration: re-emergence of a field. *Trends Ecol Evol* 25, 161–70.

Bichara, D.A., O'Sullivan, N.A., Pomerantseva, I., Zhao, X., Sundback, C.A., Vacanti, J.P., and Randolph, M.A. (2012). The tissue-engineered auricle: past, present, and future. *Tissue Eng Part B Rev* 18, 51–61.

Bosch TC. (2007). Why polyps regenerate and we don't: towards a cellular and molecular framework for *Hydra* regeneration. *Dev Biol* 303, 421–433.

Brockes, J.P., Kumar, A., and Velloso, C.P. (2001). Regeneration as an evolutionary variable. *J Anat* 199, 3–11.

Brockes, J.R., and Kumar, A. (2002). Plasticity and reprogramming of differentiated cells in amphibian regeneration. *Nat Rev Mol Cell Biol* 3, 566–574.

Brockes, J.R., and Kumar, A. (2008). Comparative aspects of animal regeneration. *Ann Rev Cell Dev Biol* 24, 525–549.

Cai, S., Fu, X.B., and Sheng, Z.Y. (2007). Dedifferentiation: A new approach in stem cell research. *Bioscience* 57, 655–662.

Callaerts, P., Munoz-Marmol, A.M., Glardon, S., Castillo, E., Sun, H., Li, W.H., Gehring, W.J., and Salo, E. (1999). Isolation and expression of a Pax-6 gene in the regenerating and intact Planarian Dugesia(G)tigrina. *Proc Nat Acad Sci U S A* 96, 558–563.

Carlson BM. (2007). Principles of Regenerative Biology. London: Elsevier. 379 pp.

Christen, B., and Slack, J.M.W. (1997). FGF-8 is associated with anteroposterior patterning and limb regeneration in *Xenopus*. *Dev Biol* 192, 455–466.

Czarnecki, J.S., Lafdi, K., Joseph, R.M., and Tsonis, P.A. (2012). Hybrid carbon-based scaffolds for applications in soft tissue reconstruction. *Tissue Eng Part A*. 18, 946–956.

Del Rio-Tsonis, K., and Tsonis, P.A. (2003). Eye regeneration at the molecular age. *Dev Dynam* 226, 211–224.

Del Rio-Tsonis, K., Washabaugh, C.H., and Tsonis, P.A. (1995). Expression of Pax-6 during urodele eye development and lens regeneration. *Proc Nat Acad Sci U S A* 92, 5092–5096.

Deng, W., and Lin, H. (2002). miwi, a murine homolog of piwi, encodes a cytoplasmic protein essential for spermatogenesis. *Dev Cell* 2, 819–830.

Ding, S., and Schultz, P.G. (2005). Small molecules and future regenerative medicine. *Curr Topics in Med Chem* 5, 383–396.

Dinsmore, C.E. (1991). Bonnet, Charles – 18th-century science as politics. *Am Zool* 31, A139–A139.

Dinsmore, C.E. (1992). The foundations of contemporary regeneration research: historical perspectives. *Monogr Dev Biol* 23, 1–27.

Drews, K., Jozefczuk, J., Prigione, A., and Adjaye, J. (2012). Human induced pluripotent stem cells – from mechanisms to clinical applications. *J Mol Med* 90, 735–745.

Eguchi, G., and Watanabe, K. (1973). Elicitation of lens formation from ventral iris epithelium of newt by a carcinogen, N-methyl-N′-nitro-N-nitrosoguanidine. *J Embryol Exp Morphol* 30, 63–71.

Eguchi, G., Eguchi, Y., Nakamura, K., Yadav, M. C., Millan, J.L., and Tsonis, P.A. (2011). Regenerative capacity in newts is not altered by repeated regeneration and ageing. *Nat Commun* 2, 384.

Elliott, M. J., De Coppi, P., Speggiorin, S., Roebuck, D., Butler, C. R., Samuel, E., Crowley, C., McLaren, C., Fierens, A., Vondrys, D., Cochrane, L., Jephson, C., Janes, S., Beaumont, N. J., Cogan, T., Bader, A., Seifalian, A. M., Hsuan, J. J., Lowdell, M. W., and Birchall, M. A. (2012). Stem-cell-based, tissue engineered tracheal replacement in a child: a 2-year follow-up study. *Lancet* 380, 994–1000.

Endo, T., Yokoyama, H., Tamura, K., and Ide, H. (1997). Shh expression in developing and regenerating limb buds of Xenopus laevis. *Dev Dynam* 209, 227–232.

Galliot, B. (1997). Signaling molecules in regenerating hydra. *Bioessays* 19, 37–46.

Galliot B. (2012). Hydra, a fruitful model system for 270 years. *Int J Dev Biol* 56, 411–423.

Gauchat, D., Mazet, F., Berney, C., Schummer, M., Kreger, S., Pawlowski, J., and Galliot, B. (2000). Evolution of Antp-class genes and differential expression of Hydra Hox/paraHox genes in anterior patterning. *Proc Nat Acad Sci U S A* 97, 4493–4498.

Geraudie, J., and Singer, M. (1992). The fish fin regenerate. *Keys Regen* 23, 62–72 252.

Goss, R.J. (1992). The evolution of regeneration – adaptive or inherent. *J Theoret Biol* 159, 241–260.

Grogg, M.W., Call, M.K., Okamoto, M., Vergara, M.N., Del Rio-Tsonis, K., and Tsonis, P.A. (2005). BMP inhibition-driven regulation of six-3 underlies induction of newt lens regeneration. *Nature* 438, 858–862.

Gurtner, G.C., Callaghan, M.J., and Longaker, M.T. (2007). Progress and potential for regenerative medicine. *Ann Rev Med* 58, 299–312.

Habermann, B., Bebin, A.G., Herklotz, S., Volkmer, M., Eckelt, K., Pehlke, K., Epperlein, H.H., Schackert, H.K., Wiebe, G., and Tanaka, E.M. (2004). An *Ambystoma mexicanum* EST sequencing project: analysis of 17,352 expressed sequence tags from embryonic and regenerating blastema cDNA libraries. *Genome Biol* 5, R67.

Han M, Yang X, Farrington JE, Muneoka K. (2003). Digit regeneration is regulated by Msx1 and BMP4 in fetal mice. *Development* 130, 5123–5132.

Ilie, I., Ilie, R., Mocan, T., Bartos, D., and Mocan, L. (2012). Influence of nanomaterials on stem cell differentiation: designing an appropriate nanobiointerface. *Int J Nanomedicine* 7, 2211–2225.

Imokawa, Y., and Brockes, J.P. (2003). Selective activation of thrombin is a critical determinant for vertebrate lens regeneration. *Curr Biol* 13, 877–881.

Imokawa, Y., Simon, A., and Brockes, J.P. (2004). A critical role for thrombin in vertebrate lens regeneration. *Phil Trans Royal Soc Bio Sci* 359, 765–776.

Imokawa, Y., and Yoshizato, K. (1997). Expression of Sonic hedgehog gene in regenerating newt limb blastemas recapitulates that in developing limb buds. *Proc Nat Acad Sci U S A* 94, 9159–9164.

Jenkins, L.S., Duerstock, B.S., and Borgens, R.B. (1996). Reduction of the current of injury leaving the amputation inhibits limb regeneration in the red spotted newt. *Dev Biol* 178, 251–262.

Jones, M.K., Tomikawa, M., Mohajer, B., and Tarnawski, A.S. (1999). Gastrointestinal mucosal regeneration: role of growth factors. *Front Biosci* 4, D303–309.

Kaneko, Y., Matsumoto, G., and Hanyu, Y. (1999). Pax-6 expression during retinal regeneration in the adult newt. *Dev Growth Differ* 41, 723–729.

Kershen, R.T., Yoo, J.J., Moreland, R.B., Krane, R.J., and Atala, A. (2002). Reconstitution of human corpus cavernosum smooth muscle in vitro and in vivo. *Tissue Eng* 8, 515–524.

Kofidis, T., de Bruin, J.L., Hoyt, G., Ho, Y., Tanaka, M., Yamane, T., Lebl, D.R., Swijnenburg, R.J., Chang, C.P., Quertermous, T., et al. (2005). Myocardial restoration with embryonic stem cell bioartificial tissue transplantation. *J Heart Lung Transplant* 24, 737–744.

Koh, C.J., and Atala, A. (2004). Tissue engineering, stem cells, and cloning: Opportunities for regenerative medicine. *J Am Soc Nephrol* 15, 1113–1125.

Kuramochi-Miyagawa, S., Kimura, T., Ijiri, T.W., Isobe, T., Asada, N., Fujita, Y., Ikawa, M., Iwai, N., Okabe, M., Deng, W., et al. (2004). Mili, a mammalian member of piwi family gene, is essential for spermatogenesis. *Development* 131, 839–849.

Kwon, T.G., Yoo, J.J., and Atala, A. (2002). Autologous penile corpora cavernosa replacement using tissue engineering techniques. *J Urol* 168, 1754–1758.

Lanza, R.P., Chung, H.Y., Yoo, J.J., Wettstein, P.J., Blackwell, C., Borson, N., Hofmeister, E., Schuch, G., Soker, S., Moraes, C.T., et al. (2002). Generation of histocompatible tissues using nuclear transplantation. *Nat Biotechnol* 20, 689–696.

Lawrence, P.A. (2001). Morphogens: how big is the big picture? *Nat Cell Biol* 3, E151–E154.

Lepilina, A., Coon, A.N., Kikuchi, K., Holdway, J.E., Roberts, R.W., Burns, C.G., and Poss, K.D. (2006). A dynamic epicardial injury response supports progenitor cell activity during zebrafish heart regeneration. *Cell* 127, 607–619.

Levin, M. (2007). Large-scale biophysics: ion flows and regeneration. *Trends Cell Biol* 17, 261–270.

Makar'ev, E.O., Zinov'eva, R.D., and Mitashov, V.I. (2002). Expression of regulatory homeobox genes during retina regeneration in adult newts. *Biol Bull* 29, 540–544.

Maki, N., Suetsugu-Maki, R., Tarui, H., Agata, K., Del Rio-Tsonis, K., and Tsonis, P. A., (2009). Expression of stem cell pluripotency factors during regeneration in newts. *Dev Dyn* 238, 1613–1616.

McGann, C.J., Odelberg, S.J., and Keating, M.T. (2001). Mammalian myotube dedifferentiation induced by newt regeneration extract. *Proc Nat Acad Sci U S A* 98, 13699–13704.

Michalopoulos, G.K., and DeFrances, M.C. (1997). Liver regeneration. *Science* 276, 60–66.

Mimeault, M., and Batra, S.K. (2006). Concise review: Recent advances on the significance of stem cells in tissue regeneration and cancer therapies. *Stem Cells* 24, 2319–2345.

Mizuno, N., Mochii, M., Yamamoto, T.S., Takahashi, T.C., Eguchi, G., and Okada, T.S. (1999). Pax-6 and Prox 1 expression during lens regeneration from Cynops iris and Xenopus cornea: evidence for a genetic program common to embryonic lens development. *Differentiation* 65, 141–149.

Mizuno, A., Yasumuro, H., Yoshikawa, T., Inami, W., and Chiba, C. (2012). MEK-ERK signaling in adult newt retinal pigment epithelium cells is strengthened immediately after surgical induction of retinal regeneration. *Neurosci Lett* 523, 39–44.

Mochii, M., Taniguchi, Y., and Shikata, I. (2007). Tail regeneration in the Xenopus tadpole. *Dev Growth Diff* 49, 155–161.

Moreno-Borchart, A. (2004). Building organs piece by piece. *EMBO Rep* 5, 1025–1028.

Morgan, T.H. (1901). Regeneration and liability to injury. *Science* 14, 235–248.

Newmark, P.A., and Sanchez Alvarado, A. (2000). Bromodeoxyuridine specifically labels the regenerative stem cells of planarians. *Dev Biol* 220, 142–153.

Odelberg, S. (2002). Inducing cellular dedifferentiation: a potential method for enhancing endogenous regeneration in mammals. *Semin Cell Dev Biol* 13, 335–343.

Okada, T.S. (1996). A brief history of regeneration research – For admiring Professor Niazi's discovery of the effect of vitamin A on regeneration. *J Biosci* 21, 261–271.

Okita, K., Ichisaka, T., and Yamanaka, S. (2007). Generation of germline-competent induced pluripotent stem cells. *Nature* 448, 313–U311.

Olender, E., Uhrynowska-Tyszkiewicz, I., and Kaminski, A. (2011). Revitalization of biostatic tissue allografts: new perspectives in tissue transplantology. *Transplant Proc* 43, 3137–3141.

Putta, S., Smith, J.J., Walker, J.A., Rondet, M., Weisrock, D.W., Monaghan, J., Samuels, A.K., Kump, K., King, D.C., Maness, N.J., et al. (2004). From biomedicine to natural history research: EST resources for ambystomatid salamanders. *BMC Genom* 5, 54.

Reddien, P.W., Bermange, A.L., Murfitt, K.J., Jennings, J.R., and Sanchez Alvarado, A. (2005). Identification of genes needed for regeneration, stem cell function, and tissue homeostasis by systematic gene perturbation in planaria. *Dev Cell* 8, 635–649.

Reddien, P.W., Oviedo, N.J., Jennings, J.R., Jenkin, J.C., and Sanchez Alvarado, A. (2005). SMEDWI-2 is a PIWI-like protein that regulates planarian stem cells. *Science* 310, 1327–1330.

Reginelli, A.D., Wang, Y.Q., Sassoon, D., and Muneoka, K. (1995). Digit tip regeneration correlates with regions of Msx1 (Hox-7) expression in fetal and newborn mice. *Development* 121, 1065–1076.

Roddy, M., Fox, T.P., McFadden, J.P., Nakamura, K., Del Rio-Tsonis, K., and Tsonis, P.A. (2008). A comparative proteomic analysis during urodele lens regeneration. *Biochem Biophys Res Commun* 377, 275–279.

Sanchez Alvarado, A. (2000). Regeneration in the metazoans: why does it happen? *Bioessays* 22, 578–590.

Sánchez Alvarado, A., and Tsonis, P.A. (2006). Bridging the regeneration gap: genetic insights from diverse animal models. *Nat Rev Genet* 7, 873–884.

Sanchez-Lara, P.A., Zhao H., Bajpai, R., Abdelhamid, A.I., and Warburton, D. (2012). Impact of stem cells in craniofacial regenerative medicine. *Front Physiol* 3, 188, 1–9.

Schnapp, E., Kragl, M., Rubin, L., and Tanaka, E.M. (2005). Hedgehog signaling controls dorsoventral patterning, blastema cell proliferation and cartilage induction during axolotl tail regeneration. *Development* 132, 3243–3253.

Schneider, J.W., Gu, W., Zhu, L., Mahdavi, V., and Nadalginard, B. (1994). Reversal of Terminal Differentiation Mediated by P107 in Rb(-/-) Muscle-Cells. *Science* 264, 1467–1471.

Schummer, M., Scheurlen, I., Schaller, C., and Galliot, B. (1992). Hom Hox homeobox genes are present in hydra (Chlorohydra-viridissima) and are differentially expressed during regeneration. *EMBO Journal* 11, 1815–1823.

Sobkow, L., Epperlein, H.H., Herklotz, S., Straube, W.L., and Tanaka, E.M. (2006). A germline GFP transgenic axolotl and its use to track cell fate: dual origin of the fin mesenchyme during development and the fate of blood cells during regeneration. *Dev Biol* 290, 386–397.

Spence, J.R., Aycinena, J.C., and Del Rio-Tsonis, K. (2007). Fibroblast growth factor-hedgehog interdependence during retina regeneration. *Dev Dyn* 236, 1161–1174.

Spence, J.R., Madhavan, M., Aycinena, J.C., and Del Rio-Tsonis, K. (2007). Retina regeneration in the chick embryo is not induced by spontaneous Mitf downregulation but requires FGF/FGFR/MEK/Erk dependent upregulation of Pax6. *Mol Vis* 13, 57–65.

Spence, J.R., Madhavan, M., Ewing, J.D., Jones, D.K., Lehman, B.M., and Del Rio-Tsonis, K. (2004). The hedgehog pathway is a modulator of retina regeneration. *Development* 131, 4607–4621.

Stocum, D.L. (2004). Tissue restoration through regenerative biology and medicine. *Adv in Anat, Embryol and Cell Biol* 176:1–104.

Stoick-Cooper, C.L., Moon, R.T., and Weidinger, G. (2007). Advances in signaling in vertebrate regeneration as a prelude to regenerative medicine. *Genes Dev* 21, 1292–1315.

Sun, H., Liu, W., Zhou, G., Zhang, W., Cui, L., and Cao, Y. (2011) Tissue engineering of cartilage, tendon and bone. *Front Med* 5, 61–69.

Takahashi, K., and Yamanaka, S. (2006). Induction of pluripotent stem cells from mouse embryonic and adult fibroblast cultures by defined factors. *Cell* 126, 663–676.

Tanaka, E.M., Drechsel, D.N., and Brockes, J.P. (1999). Thrombin regulates S-phase re-entry by cultured newt myotubes. *Curr Biol* 9, 792–799.

Tanaka, E.M., Gann, A.A.F., Gates, P.B., and Brockes, J.P. (1997). Newt myotubes reenter the cell cycle by phosphorylation of the retinoblastoma protein. *J Cell Biol* 136, 155–165.

Torok, M.A., Gardiner, D.M., Izpisua-Belmonte, J.C., and Bryant, S.V. (1999). Sonic hedgehog (shh) expression in developing and regenerating axolotl limbs. *J Exp Zool* 284, 197–206.

Tsonis, P.A. (2000). Regeneration in vertebrates. *Dev Biol* 221, 273–284.

Tsonis, P.A. (2007). Bridging knowledge gaps on the long road to regeneration: Classical models meet stem cell manipulation and bioengineering. *Mol Intervent* 7, 249–250.

Tsonis, P.A., and Eguchi, G. (1982). Abnormal limb regeneration without tumor production in adult newts directed by carcinogens, 20-methylcholanthrene and benzo (alpha) pyrene. *Dev Growth Diff* 24, 183–190.

Tsonis, P.A., Madhavan, M., Tancous, E.E., and Del Rio-Tsonis, K. (2004). A newt's eye view of lens regeneration. *Int J Dev Biol* 48, 975–980.

Tsonis, P.A., Sargent, M.T., DelRioTsonis, K., and Jung, J.C. (1996). 9-cis retinoic acid antagonizes the stimulatory effect of 1,25 dihydroxyvitamin D-3 on chondrogenesis of chick limb bud mesenchymal cells: Interactions of their receptors. *Int J Dev Biol* 40, 1053–1059.

Tsonis, P.A., Vergara, M.N., Spence, J.R., Madhavan, M., Kramer, E.L., Call, M.K., Santiago, W.G., Vallance, J.E., Robbins, D.J., and Del Rio-Tsonis, K. (2004). A novel role of the hedgehog pathway in lens regeneration. *Dev Biol* 267, 450–461.

Tsonis P.A. and Fox T.P. (2009). Regeneration according to Spallanzani. *Dev Dyn* 238, 2357–2363.

Velloso, C.P., Simon, A., and Brockes, J.P. (2001). Mammalian postmitotic nuclei reenter the cell cycle after serum stimulation in newt/mouse hybrid myotubes. *Curr Biol* 11, 855–858.

Vergara, M.N., Arsenijevic, Y., and Del Rio-Tsonis, K. (2005). CNS regeneration: a morphogen's tale. *J Neurobiol* 64, 491–507.

Vergara, M.N., and Del Rio-Tsonis, K. (2009). Retinal regeneration in the *Xenopus laevis* tadpole: a new model system. *Mol Vision* 15, 1000–1013.

Wadman, M. (2009). Stem cells ready for prime time. *Nature* 457, 516–516.

Wang, T., Koh, C.J., Yoo, J.J. et al. (2003). Creation of an engineered uterus for surgical reconstruction [abstr]. Presented at the Proceedings of the American Academy of Pediatrics, Section on Urology, New Orleans.

Yokoyama H. (2008). Initiation of limb regeneration: the critical steps for regenerative capacity. *Dev Growth Differ* 50, 13–22.

Yoshikawa, T., Mizuno, A., Yasumuro, H., Inami, W., Vergara, M. N., Del Rio-Tsonis, K., and Chiba, C. (2012). MEK-ERK and heparin-susceptible signaling pathways are involved in cell-cycle entry of the wound edge retinal pigment epithelium cells in the adult newt. *Pigment Cell Melanoma Res* 25, 66–82.

Index